ALTERNATIVE TREATMENT *for* CANCER

ANNALS OF TRADITIONAL CHINESE MEDICINE

Series Editors: Ping-Chung Leung
(The Chinese University of Hong Kong, Hong Kong)
Charlie Changli Xue
(RMIT University, Australia)

Published

Volume 1 Chinese Medicine — Modern Practice
Edited by Ping-Chung Leung & Charlie Changli Xue
ISBN: 978-981-256-018-6
Publication date: February 2005 252 pp.

Volume 2 Current Review of Chinese Medicine: Quality Control of Herbs and Herbal Material
Edited by Ping-Chung Leung, Harry Fong & Charlie Changli Xue
ISBN: 978-981-256-707-9
Publication date: May 2006 308 pp.

Annals of Traditional Chinese Medicine – Vol. 3

ALTERNATIVE TREATMENT *for* CANCER

Editors

Ping-Chung Leung
The Chinese University of Hong Kong

Harry Fong
University of Illinois at Chicago, USA

World Scientific

NEW JERSEY • LONDON • SINGAPORE • BEIJING • SHANGHAI • HONG KONG • TAIPEI • CHENNAI

Published by

World Scientific Publishing Co. Pte. Ltd.
5 Toh Tuck Link, Singapore 596224
USA office: 27 Warren Street, Suite 401-402, Hackensack, NJ 07601
UK office: 57 Shelton Street, Covent Garden, London WC2H 9HE

British Library Cataloguing-in-Publication Data
A catalogue record for this book is available from the British Library.

Annals of Traditional Chinese Medicine — Vol. 3
ALTERNATIVE TREATMENT FOR CANCER

ISBN-13 978-981-270-929-5
ISBN-10 981-270-929-0

Printed by FuIsland Offset Printing (S) Pte Ltd, Singapore

Contents

Contributors		xi
Preface to Series		xvii
Preface to Volume 3		xix
Chapter 1	The Scientific Basis of Chinese Medicine and Cancer Care: A Western Medicine Perspective *Stephen M. Sagar & Raimond Wong*	1
Chapter 2	Recent Status and Outlook of Traditional Chinese Medicine in Cancer Treatment *Dai-Han Zhou*	55
Chapter 3	Chinese Medicine and Cancer Treatment in Hong Kong: A General Review *Ping-Chung Leung, Vincent Ooi, Eliza L.-Y. Wong, Wai-Chun Au, Chun-Kwok Wong, Wai-Kei Lam, Sing-Fai Leung & Tony S.-K. Mok*	65
Chapter 4	Advancements of Ayurveda in Cancer Management with Special Focus on Hepatocellular Carcinoma *Premalatha Balachandran*	77
Chapter 5	Complementary Approaches to Cancer in Italy *Ralph W. Moss*	107

Chapter 6	Kampo Treatment for Cancer *Kenji Watanabe*	117
Chapter 7	Risk Management of Complementary Alternative Medicines in Cancer *Ursula Werneke*	129
Chapter 8	Complementary Therapies for Cancer Patients *Barrie R. Cassileth, Jyothirmai Gubili & K. Simon Yeung*	163
Chapter 9	Positive Findings about Herbs and Natural Products Action on Cancer *Muriel J. Montbriand*	179
Chapter 10	Mechanistic Studies on Combination of Phytochemicals and Synthetic Drugs as Anti-Cancer Agents *Shanmugam HemaIswarya & Mukesh Doble*	233
Chapter 11	Ethnopharmacology Approaches for Botanical Immunomodulators and Chemoprotectants in Cancer Therapy *Patwardhan Bhushan & Gautam Manish*	255
Chapter 12	Bioactive Polysaccharides from TCM Herbs as Anti-Cancer Adjuvants *Raymond Chang*	285
Chapter 13	Clinical Evaluation of Herbal Formula Decoction in Treating Non-Small Cell Lung Cancer by Various Rating Scales *Jie You & Zhi-Ming Shi*	301
Chapter 14	New Approach for Evaluating the Anti-Breast Cancer Activity of Traditional Chinese Medicine *John M. Pezzuto, Richard C. Moon, Charles K.-H. Chang & Ching-Jer Chang*	321

Chapter 15 Functional Magnetic Resonance Imaging Studies of Acupuncture 347
Gary Deng & Barrie Cassileth

Index 359

Contributors

Wai-Chun Au
Centre for Clinical Trials on Chinese Medicine
The Institute of Chinese Medicine
School of Public Health
The Chinese University of Hong Kong
Shatin, New Territories, Hong Kong, SAR China

Premalatha Balachandran
National Center for Natural Products Research
Research Institute of Pharmaceutical Sciences, School of Pharmacy
University of Mississippi
University, MS 38677, USA

Patwardhan Bhushan
Interdisciplinary School of Health Sciences
University of Pune
Pune 411 007, India

Barrie R. Cassileth
Integrative Medicine Service
Memorial Sloan-Kettering Cancer Center
New York, NY 10021, USA

Charles K.-H. Chang
Mintong Pharmaceutical Company, Taichung, Taiwan

Ching-Jer Chang
Department of Medicinal Chemistry and Molecular Pharmacology
School of Pharmacy and Pharmaceutical Sciences
Purdue University
West Lafayette, IN 47907-2091, USA

Raymond Chang
Institute of East-West Medicine
New York, NY 10016, USA

Gary Deng
Integrative Medicine Service
Memorial Sloan-Kettering Cancer Center
New York, NY 10021, USA

Mukesh Doble
Department of Biotechnology
Indian Institute of Technology Madras
Chennai-600036, India

Jyothirmai Gubili
Integrative Medicine Service
Memorial Sloan-Kettering Cancer Center
New York, NY 10021, USA

Shanmugam HemaIswarya
Department of Biotechnology
Indian Institute of Technology Madras
Chennai-600036, India

Wai-Kei Lam
Department of Chemical Pathology
Faculty of Medicine
Prince of Wales Hospital
The Chinese University of Hong Kong
Shatin, New Territories, Hong Kong, SAR China

Ping-Chung Leung
Centre for Clinical Trials on Chinese Medicine
The Institute of Chinese Medicine
School of Public Health
The Chinese University of Hong Kong
Shatin, New Territories, Hong Kong, SAR China

Sing-Fai Leung
Department of Clinical Oncology
Faculty of Medicine
Prince of Wales Hospital
The Chinese University of Hong Kong
Shatin, New Territories, Hong Kong, SAR China

Gautam Manish
Interdisciplinary School of Health Sciences
University of Pune
Pune 411 007, India

Tony S.-K. Mok
Department of Clinical Oncology
Faculty of Medicine
Prince of Wales Hospital
The Chinese University of Hong Kong
Shatin, New Territories, Hong Kong, SAR China

Muriel J. Montbriand
Applied Research/Psychiatry
College of Medicine
University of Saskatchewan
Royal University Hospital
Saskatoon, SK, Canada S7N 0W8

Richard C. Moon
Department of Medicinal Chemistry and Molecular Pharmacology
School of Pharmacy and Pharmaceutical Sciences
Purdue University
West Lafayette, IN 47907-2091, USA

Ralph W. Moss
Cancer Communications, Inc.
PO Box 1076
Lemont, PA 16851, USA

Vincent Ooi
Department of Biology
Faculty of Science
The Chinese University of Hong Kong
Shatin, New Territories, Hong Kong, SAR China

John M. Pezzuto
Department of Medicinal Chemistry and Molecular Pharmacology
School of Pharmacy and Pharmaceutical Sciences
Purdue University
West Lafayette, IN 47907-2091, USA
Department of Pharmaceutical Sciences, College of Pharmacy
University of Hawaii at Hilo
Hilo, HI 96720, USA

Stephen M. Sagar
Departments of Oncology and Medicine
McMaster University
Juravinski Cancer Centre
Hamilton, ON, Canada L8V 5C2

Zhi-Ming Shi
Tumor Department
Clinical Oncology Centre
Longhua Hospital Affiliated to
Shanghai University of Traditional Chinese Medicine
Shanghai 200036, P. R. China

Kenji Watanabe
Department of Kampo Medicine
Keio University School of Medicine
Tokyo 160-8582, Japan

Ursula Werneke
Department of Psychiatry
Homerton University Hospital
London E9 6SR, UK

Chun-Kwok Wong
Department of Chemical Pathology
Faculty of Medicine
Prince of Wales Hospital
The Chinese University of Hong Kong
Shatin, New Territories, Hong Kong, SAR China

Eliza L.-Y. Wong
Department of Community and Family Medicine
School of Public Health
Faculty of Medicine
Prince of Wales Hospital
The Chinese University of Hong Kong
Shatin, New Territories, Hong Kong, SAR China

Raimond Wong
Departments of Oncology and Medicine
McMaster University
Juravinski Cancer Centre
Hamilton, ON, Canada L8V 5C2

K. Simon Yeung
Integrative Medicine Service
Memorial Sloan-Kettering Cancer Center
New York, NY 10021, USA

Jie You
Tumor Department
Clinical Oncology Centre
Longhua Hospital Affiliated to
Shanghai University of Traditional Chinese Medicine
Shanghai 200036, P. R. China

Dai-Han Zhou
Cancer Centre, No. 1 Affiliated Hospital
Chinese Medicine University
Guangzhou 510405, P. R. China

Preface to Series

Does Traditional Chinese Medicine Work?

History should be acknowledged and respected. Despite this, the historical value of Chinese medicine in China and some parts of Asia should not be used as the only important evidence of efficacy.

While clinical science has followed closely the principles of deductive research in science and developed its methodology of wide acceptance, there is a natural demand from both users and service providers that the same methodology be applied to the traditional art of healing. There should be only one scale for the measurement of efficacy. Thus, evidence-based medicine, which apparently is the only acceptable form of treatment, would also claim its sovereignty in Chinese medicine.

In spite of influential proponents and diligent practitioners, efforts relating to the application of evidence-based medicine methodology to Chinese medicine research have been slow and unimpressive. This should not come as a surprise. Evidence-based medicine requires the knowledge of the exact chemistry of the drug used, the exact physical or chemical activities involved and above all, the biological responses in the recipient. All these are not known. Working back from the black box of old historical records of efficacy requires huge resources and time, if at all possible. Insistence on this approach would result in either unending frustrations or utter desperation.

Parallel with the modern attempts, respectable Chinese medicine practitioners have unendingly and relentlessly cried out their objection to the evidence-based approach. They insisted that all the evidences were already there from the Classical Records. Forcing the classical applications through a rigid modern framework of scrutiny is artificially coating Chinese medicine with a scientific clothing that does not fit.

Thus, the modern proponents are facing an impasse when they rely totally on modern scientific concepts. The traditional converts are persisting to push their pilgrims of defense. Where do we stand so as to achieve the best results of harmonisation?

There must be a compromise somewhere. Classic evidences can be transformed into a universal language to be fairly evaluated and to be decided whether suitable for further research, using the deductive methodology or an innovative one after intelligent modifications.

There is a need for a platform on which a direction can be developed in the attempt to modernise the traditional art and science of healing, while remaining free and objective to utilise the decaying wisdom without prejudice.

With the growing demand for complementary/alternative medicine from the global public and a parallel interest from the service providers, there is an urgent need for the provision of valuable information in this area.

The Annals of Chinese Medicine is a timely serial publication responding to this need. It will be providing authoritative and current information about Chinese medicine in the areas of clinical trials, biological activities of herbs, education, research and quality control requirements. Contributors are invited to send in their reports and reviews to ensure quality and value. Clinicians and scientists who are willing to submit their valuable observations, resulting from their painstaking researches are welcome to send in their manuscripts. *The Annals of Chinese Medicine* has the objective of providing a lasting platform for all who concentrate their efforts on the modernization of Chinese medicine.

Professor Ping-Chung Leung
Institute of Chinese Medicine
The Chinese University of Hong Kong

Preface to Volume 3

The third volume of the *Annals of Traditional Chinese Medicine* carries the theme of Cancer Treatment. Since the commencement of this book series, the Editorial Board has emphasized its main objective, that is to help modernize Chinese medicine, thus providing a convenient platform for all scientists, including those who belong to the traditional camp as well as members of the modern scientific community who insist on strict deductive approaches.

Cancer is obviously one of the most common areas where demand for alternative treatment is overwhelming. A significant portion of the American and European populations regularly consumes health supplements to either prevent cancer or as adjuvant therapy during cancer treatment. Health surveys conducted in Hong Kong (a city of predominantly Chinese people) have shown that over 90% of cancer patients consume products of Chinese medicine, either prescribed by Chinese medicine practitioners or purchased over-the-counter. Choosing Cancer as the theme of our third volume is therefore appropriate. There is no intention of guiding the reader on the choice of therapy, nor is there any suggestion of preferences of the available options of treatment (although a few solid examples are given). Instead we want to introduce the justification and logic of using Chinese medicine as an adjunct, discuss about the basic principles and the options that are available, expose the regional and cultural varieties, and some problems related to their use, describe some natural products of particular interests and lastly, give examples of specific cancers being treated with herbal therapy.

Using modern scientific concepts to understand and explain traditional or alternative medicine is logical and unavoidable. Indeed, the *Annals* has already adopted this principle. Nevertheless, we welcome distinguished scholars of the very traditional stream to explain their views, particularly at this time, in the popular field of cancer.

Professor Dai-Han Zhou is a learned scholar in Chinese medicine who has written extensively on the principles and practice of Chinese medicine for cancer patients. Readers will find his articles quite out-of-the-norm as he stresses on holistic care and the importance of individualized therapy. On the other hand, Prof. Zhou tries to equate herbalists' observations as evidence-based medicine, and assumes that some herbs work via specific channels resembling those being targeted by new therapies like Iressa, Tarceva and Avastin. Professor Zhou quoted one clinical trial using a proprietor herbal medicine. In that situation, he accepts generalization and ignores individualization. The article is really interesting because it exposes the complexity of thoughts of the modern day Chinese medicine expert. While the discrepancies observed may be controversial, Prof. Zhou's strong criticisms against over-treatment in modern medicine and his call for higher rates of survival among cancer patients should be established as good advice for all.

Professor Zhou's orthodox account is well balanced with Professor Stephen Sagar's Western medicine perspectives on the scientific basis of cancer care in Chinese medicine.

This volume attempts to give very rich accounts of the varieties of cancer treatment available, as well as the cultural differences in China, Hong Kong, Japan, India, Italy, the United Kingdom and the United States. There are altogether seven chapters sharing this load.

Since herbal medicine can be the main basis for the maintenance of survival in spite of the persistence of cancer or cancer metastases, natural products and phytochemistry that contribute toward survival via various channels should be explored. This volume provides a number of high quality articles (by authors from Canada, India and the US) on the subject. Lastly, there are some real examples of integrated treatment for specific cancers that will be of interest to readers. Two good examples from China are chosen.

With the growing demand for complementary and alternative medicine from the global public and a parallel interest from the service providers, we believe that this volume will provide valuable information in the area of cancer for all.

Chapter 1

The Scientific Basis of Chinese Medicine and Cancer Care: A Western Medicine Perspective

Stephen M. Sagar & Raimond Wong

Abstract

Traditional Chinese medicine (TCM) may be integrated with conventional Western medicine to enhance the care of patients with cancer. Recent evidence confirms a scientific basis for the use of acupuncture, herbs, diet and energy therapies. We suggest a holistic care plan based on the concepts of biological response modification, enhancement of psycho-immunological function, better symptom control, and improvement of psycho-spiritual well-being. There is enough preliminary evidence to encourage good quality clinical trials to evaluate the efficacy of integrating TCM into Western cancer care.

Keywords: Traditional Chinese Medicine (TCM); Western Medicine; Cancer Treatment.

1.1 Introduction

Recent evidence suggests that many traditional Chinese medical therapies can be effective for the supportive care of cancer patients. This is a review of the published literature (indexed in Medline) and our own practical experience. It provides various levels of evidence that support further research into a developing model of integrative care. Most published studies are at evidence level III, in other words trials without randomization, single group pre-post, cohort, time series, or matched case-controlled studies. Levels I and II evidence from well designed randomized controlled trials of appropriate size is emphasized in the text of this review. In view of the paucity of quality data from levels I and II evidence, meta-analysis of the data is usually not possible. Well-designed randomized controlled trials are encouraged in view of the promising initial observations. It is important not to discount TCM as a system simply because an individual study is negative. The same applies to Western biomedical medicine. A negative drug study does not negate the whole of biomedicine. The challenge for TCM is to develop repeatable and provable outcomes, standardization, and quality assurance. The scientific bases of herbs and acupuncture are rapidly being established, but well designed, pragmatic, controlled clinical studies are lacking in most domains.

Traditional Chinese medicine (TCM) may be practiced alongside conventional Western medicine to enhance patient care. The philosophy of TCM proposes novel hypotheses that will support the development of a science-based holistic medicine.

1.2 Cancer as a Systemic Disease

In Western medicine, cancer is conventionally viewed from the somatic point of view as a clone of cells which has outgrown its environmental constraints and control mechanisms. These cells are abnormal and are considered to be foreign to the body. The main philosophy of cancer treatment is direct annihilation of the cancer cells using aggressive and destructive therapies. Chinese medicine emphasizes the importance of the body-mind communication network. The science of psychoneuro-immunology (PNI) has demonstrated a potential physiological basis for cancer cell progression through the effects of emotions on cellular immunity and other mechanisms.

In TCM, the development of cancer is viewed as a part of the presenting features of a syndrome representing an imbalance of the whole body-mind network (Macek, 1984). In other words, cancer is a systemic disease from the start, and the terrain is considered to be as important as the tumor itself (Schipper *et al.*, 1995). It is believed that if one can strengthen and rebalance the body-mind network, the normal pattern will be restored and this will help to resolve the cancer. This concept is currently being incorporated into a more holistic science, where the whole picture is as important as the parts. To quote Hanahan and Weinberg

(2000), "The metaphors used to conceptualize cancer cell function will also shift dramatically. For decades now, we have been able to predict with precision the behavior of an electronic integrated circuit in terms of its constituent parts — its interconnecting components, processing, and emitting signals. Having fully charted the wiring of every cellular signaling pathway, it will be possible to lay out the complete 'integrated' circuit. We will then be able to apply the tools of mathematical modeling to cancer cells. With holistic clarity of mechanism, cancer prognosis and treatment will become a rational science." Recent evidence suggests that bone marrow stem cells may play a significant role in the perpetuation of some cancers, including the production of pro-angiogenic peptides. Thus Western science is now exploring the possibility that both hematological and solid cancer may sometimes be a systemic disease from the outset (Rafii and Lyden, 2003; Kerbel and Kamen, 2004; Houghton *et al.*, 2004).

1.3 The Body-Mind Network

TCM recognizes that the human being functions as a body-mind network (Ikemi and Ikemi, 1986). The philosophy of TCM analyzes the *process* of body-mind communication, rather than a "snap shot" of structural, material entities such as molecules. If Western medicine is viewed as the hardware of a computer, then TCM could represent the software. It recognizes a correspondence between patterns of information that are independent of the carrier of the information. For example, the pattern of information may be similar regardless of whether it is mediated by pulses of hormones and neuropeptides, or the electrophysiological frequency pattern of the heart (Watkins, 1995; Dardik, 1996; Pennisi, 1997; Pert *et al.*, 1998; Song *et al.*, 1998). Acupuncture stimulation of specific points on the body releases neuropeptides (such as somatostatin and vasoactive intestinal peptide) within the central nervous system (Zhang *et al.*, 1997 and 1999). The body-mind information system may be partly regulated by the relative contributions of the sympathetic and parasympathetic components of the autonomic nervous system. This corresponds to the traditional Chinese concept of a balance between yin and yang, which represents a pattern of information, rather than concrete material entities. Analysis of the pulse, using the classical Chinese technique, may indicate the relative imbalance.

This has been demonstrated indirectly by spectral analysis of the electrocardiogram, using appropriate computer software. Acupuncture has been shown to rebalance the relative contributions of the sympathetic and parasympathetic nervous systems (Haker *et al.*, 2000). The patterns of information transfer may interact to entrain and reinforce information flow in a complex dynamical system (Lee and Wei, 1983; McCraty *et al.*, 1995; Rubik, 1995). The system is an autopoietic process. In other words, it can recreate itself and evolve through learning, so that the body can adapt to changing circumstances.

When the person is healthy, communication between systems flows freely through a complex, non-linear heterarchical and hierarchical process of information transfer, via physiological interactions. Metaphorically, mind-body communication is represented by an informatics system of energy-in-motion, in other words, "e-motion." Cancer may be associated with a disturbance in information flow, manifest by an over-plastic system that loses process structure and becomes irreversibly chaotic (Coffey, 1998; Cuzick *et al.*, 1998). Experiments in rats show that chronic restraint stress promotes lymphocyte apoptosis through modulating CD95 gene expression via a pathway that involves opioid receptors (Yin *et al.*, 2000). In other words, stress can influence both the function and structure of the nervous system that, in turn, may modulate lymphocyte gene expression, thereby influencing immunity and resistance to cancer (Yin *et al.*, 2000). Intervention with a technique, such as acupuncture, may restore the imbalance in information flow, for example through the autonomic nervous system by balancing the sympathetic and parasympathetic components (Thomas *et al.*, 1992; Chao *et al.*, 1999). The same model may help us understand how the compassionate intentionality of a healer can restore health through entrainment and normalization of the imbalanced system (Watkins, 1996). In order to understand these processes, we will need to consider systems outside of our current reductionist pharmacological model. These may include electromagnetic and non-local effects between molecules, and the analysis of information flow between cells by novel mechanisms, such as quantum mechanics (Jovanovic-Ignjatic and Rakovic, 1999). In order to understand the concurrent, synergistic contributions of multiple systems, it is necessary to develop computerized algorithmic modeling, such as power spectral analysis (Haker *et al.*, 2000), neural networks (Riess and Abbas, 2000), and fuzzy logic (Kosko and Isaka, 1993).

The beauty of this body-mind network model is that it can combine constitutional personality factors (such as emotions and feelings) with bodily symptoms, into a single diagnostic and treatment paradigm. This is represented in TCM terms by patterns of disharmonies in the main organ systems, as well as abnormalities of *qi* (energy flow), essence (energy reserves), blood, heat and moisture. It is interesting that there is correspondence with the TCM model of cancer predisposition being associated with rising *qi* (sheng qi) or Liver fire (representing anger), and the scientific evidence that repressed anger both suppresses the immune system and may increase the risk of breast cancer in the so-called Type C personality (Amkraut and Solomon, 1972; Temoshok, 1985; Temoshok and Dreher, 1992).

1.4 Pharmacology of Chinese Herbs

In TCM, herbs are used in combinations that enhance their benefits while reducing their side effects (Rosenberg, 1997). In effect, multiple low dose pharmacological agents are being administered synergistically. Western medicine usually focuses on maximally tolerated doses of single agents. Although chemotherapy drugs are usually combined, the reason is to minimize drug resistance and the consequence can be to further increase drug toxicity. According to TCM practitioners, combinations of herbs can reduce the side effects of anti-cancer drugs, but further research is indicated to determine their pharmaco-kinetic interactions with drugs and any potential adverse effects.

A scientific approach to introducing Chinese herbs into Western practice involves a rigorous and systematic approach to phytochemical profiling, quality control, preclinical evaluation, safety evaluation, and Phases I to III clinical trials (Fig. 1.1). More data is required to establish optimal combinations of herbs that produce synergistic activity. Traditionally, Chinese herbs have been used as complex mixtures. One study evaluated the DNA microarray data for 12,600 genes to examine the anti-proliferative activity of the single herb *Coptidis rhizoma* and eight constituent molecules against eight human pancreatic cancer cell lines (Hara, 2005). They identified 27 genes showing a strong correlation with the 50% inhibitory dose (ID50) of *C. rhizoma* after 72-h exposure. Hierarchical cluster

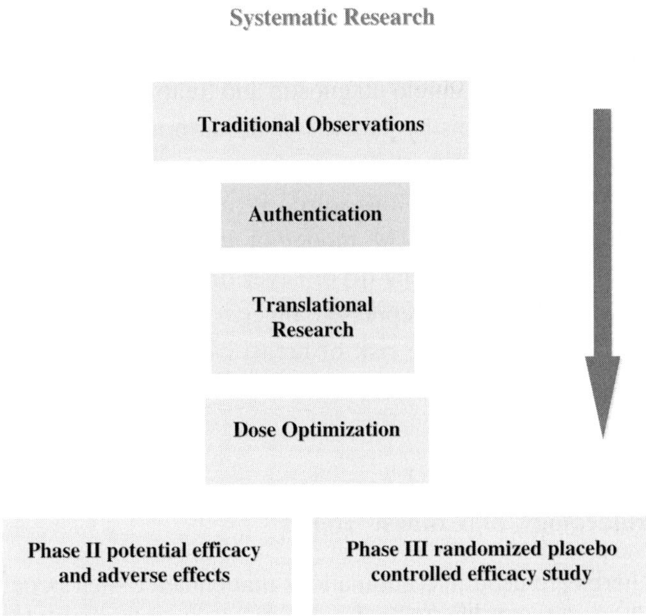

Figure 1.1. Scientific approach to introducing Chinese herbs into Western practice.

analysis with correlation coefficients between expression levels of these 27 *C. rhizoma-related genes* and the ID50 of each constituent molecule classified these test molecules into two clusters, one consisting of *C. rhizoma* and *berberine* and the other consisting of the remaining seven molecules. Their results suggest that one specific phytochemical, *berberine*, can account for the majority of the anti-proliferative activity of *C. rhizoma* and that DNA microarray analyses can be used to improve our understanding of the actions of an intact herb. In contrast, there appears to be merit in using combinations of herbs and their derivatives. For example, PHY106 (*Radix scutellariae*, *Paeonia lactiflora pall*, *Fructus*, *ziziphi*, *Radix glycyrrizae*) is an authenticated combination of herbs that may increase the efficacy and reduce the adverse effects of the cytotoxic drug, Capecitabine, which is used in treating colorectal cancer (Farrell, 2003). The biotech company, Phytoceutica Inc.® (Newhaven, CT, USA) has systematically profiled the phytochemical content of each herb and tested various combinations at the preclinical stage to optimize the complex mixture. Quality has been assured by establishing profiles using chemical chromatography and spectroscopy, along with biologic, proteomic and genomic profiling. Through these techniques, they have developed a Phytomics Similarity Index.® Interestingly, their modern technological approach confirms traditional Chinese medical theory of optimizing efficacy through a hierarchy of herb combinations. The combination enhances anti-tumor activity, reduces toxicity, and enhances the pharmacokinetics of the chief herb (the Emperor herb). The mechanisms include inhibiting drug resistance proteins that may decrease absorption, inhibiting cytochrome p450 enzymes that metabolize phytochemicals, inhibiting microfloral beta-glucuronidase, chemical stabilization, and modification of solubility. Initial clinical trials demonstrate a reduction of gastrointestinal toxicity and enhancement of the tumoricidal effect of the chemotherapy. Many preclinical studies are now demonstrating that specific combinations of Chinese herbs can be synergistic with cytotoxic chemotherapy through pharmacodynamic, as well as pharmacokinetic, interactions. For example, *Phellinus linteus* is a mushroom, which mainly consists of polysaccharides. It sensitizes apoptosis induced by doxorubicin in an *in vitro* prostate cancer cell line (Collins, 2006). *P. linteus* or doxorubicin, at relatively low doses, do not independently induce apoptosis in the cells. However, combination treatment with both low doses of *P. linteus* and doxorubicin result in a synergistic effect on the induction of apoptosis. *P. linteus* has a synergistic effect with doxorubicin to activate caspases in prostate cancer LNCaP cells. Sensitization can be obtained at subtoxic concentrations of doxorubicin. *P. linteus* is an apoptotic synergiser for conventional chemotherapeutics such as doxorubicin, which can keep normal, surrounding cells unharmed.

Gene expression profiling coupled with promoter assays can evaluate the effect of a herbal mixture on cancer. Such approaches may be used for the standardization of herbal extract activity. An example is the comparison of the gene profile of PC-SPES with that of PC-CARE, a product with a similar herbal composition. Prior studies have shown that PC-SPES contains estrogenic organic compounds, and such compounds are known to affect prostate cancer. An important question is whether these are the primary drivers of the gene profile. The data suggest that gene expression profiles of LNCaP human prostate cancer cells in response to PC-SPES are different from those found when diethylstilbestrol (DES), a synthetic estrogen, is used, suggesting that the estrogenic moieties within PC-SPES do not drive this expression signature (Bigler *et al.*, 2003). In contrast, the expression profile of PC-CARE is almost identical to that of DES, highlighting that mixtures containing similar herbal compositions do not necessarily result in similar biological activities. To validate the expression profiling data, the investigators evaluated the protein expression and promoter activity of prostate-specific antigen (PSA), a gene induced by PC-SPES but repressed by DES. In order to gain a mechanistic understanding of how PC-SPES and DES affect PSA expression differently, LNCaP cells were transiently transfected with wild-type and mutagenized PSA promoter, ARE concatemers and appropriate controls. The evidence suggests that the androgen response elements (ARE) II and III within the promoter region are responsible for the suppressive effects of DES and stimulatory effects of PC-SPES. The effects on PSA transcription are specific to ARE in the case of DES, while PC-SPES affects this promoter non-specifically. The expression profiling coupled with mechanistic target validation yields valuable clues as to the mode of action of complex botanical mixtures and provides a new way to compare objectively mixtures with similar components either for effect or quality assurance prior to their use in clinical trials. In the case of PC-SPES, the effectiveness of the complex mixture of herbs has been shown in a randomized controlled clinical trial to be more effective than DES alone (Oh, 2004).

Current technology is demonstrating the multi-dimensional activities of Chinese herbs as anti-cancer agents. Many are potent antioxidants that can induce apoptosis and others are anti-angiogenic agents (Cai, 2004; Yance, 2006). Many of the herbs that are traditionally considered effective against cancer cells are now being shown to have subtle effects on genetic expression and may play a key synergistic role in anti-cancer treatment through synergistic activity with cytotoxic agents and maintenance regimens for prevention of recurrence (Yonghe, 2004). Future research should maximize the use of technology to validate scientific mechanisms for quality assurance, safety, optimization and clinical effectiveness within the modern cancer treatment environment. Rigorous adherence to the development of research protocols and standards of reporting are necessary, as stated by a recent publication of the CONSORT group, which establishes the standards for clinical trials (Gagnier, 2006). Further development of Chinese herbal medicine for administration in Western cancer clinics will require both international collaboration and an improved working relationship between national governments, industries and universities.

1.5 Physiology of Acupuncture

Acupuncture is a technique that allows us to modulate communication within the body-mind network through concurrent changes in multiple signaling pathways.

Most evidence suggests that acupuncture modulates neurotransmitters, cytokines and neuropeptides through electrophysiological changes in the nervous system (Bucinskaite *et al.*, 1996; Dawidson *et al.*, 1997). Interaction with the brain stem, hypothalamus, limbic system and autonomic nervous system occurs through either stimulating or suppressing the activity of afferent peripheral nerves (Kerr *et al.*, 1978; Kumar *et al.*, 1994; Alavi *et al.*, 1997; Cho *et al.*, 1998; Wu *et al.*, 1999; Zonenshayn *et al.*, 2000). Acupuncture may also modify the somatic electromagnetic field (Jessel-Kenyon *et al.*, 1992). Recent research suggests that the initial transduction of the acupuncture needle is through myofascial tissue planes. The network of acupuncture points and meridians can be viewed as a representation of the network formed by interstitial connective tissue. Langevin *et al.* (2002) mapped acupuncture points in serial gross anatomical sections through the human arm. They found an 80% correspondence between the sites of acupuncture points and the location of intermuscular or intramuscular connective tissue planes in postmortem tissue sections. The surface points appear to connect to a web of vessels that cover internal organs. This is demonstrated by special DNA staining (Shin *et al.*, 2005). The de qi or "needle grasp" may be due to mechanical coupling between the needle and connective tissue with winding of tissue around the needle during needle rotation. Needle manipulation could transmit a mechanical signal to connective tissue cells via mechanotransduction (Langevin *et al.*, 2001). This may be converted into an electrophysiological response through a change in electrical impedance that spreads through the connective tissue planes, interacts with cellular genomic expression, and releases local cytokines and other messenger molecules that may initiate neurological transmission (Ahn *et al.*, 2005).

In view of the power of the placebo effect, a sham acupuncture control arm is required as a standard for randomized controlled trials of acupuncture. Sham needles have been validated to a limited extent. The results may depend on whether the subject has past experience of acupuncture. These devices, withdraw a blunt needle back into the sheath during application. This is a more valid sham technique than using superficial penetration of the skin or randomly assigning points away from known meridians. Evaluation of the widely used Streitberger sham needle concluded that most patients were unable to discriminate between the needles by penetration; however, nearly 40% were able to detect a difference in treatment type between needles. No major differences in outcome between real and placebo needling could be found. The fact that nearly 40% of subjects did not find that the two interventions were similar, however, raises some concerns with regard to the wholesale adoption of this instrument as a standard acupuncture placebo. The authors conclude that further work on inter-tester reliability and standardization of technique is highly recommended before we can be confident about using this needle in further studies (White *et al.*, 2003).

1.6 Roles of TCM in Cancer Supportive Care

The goals of cancer treatment should be to increase patients' survival, when possible, and to improve their quality of life. TCM is able to support patients being treated with conventional Western medicine (surgery, radiotherapy and chemotherapy) through four major approaches:

(1) modification of biological response to improve therapeutic gain;
(2) improved psycho-neuro-immunological response;
(3) enhancement of symptom control;
(4) psychospiritual integration.

Very often, TCM therapy works through more than one approach synergistically.

(1) Biological Response Modification

[I] Adjunctive Cancer Treatment

(a) Modification of Tumor Physiology

(i) *Herbs*

There is increasing evidence that suggests TCM can favorably modify the tumor response to conventional Western cancer treatment. There is a correspondence between the TCM theory of cancer and recent medical research findings.

TCM herbs have been extensively investigated in the laboratory and are known to have multiple pharmacological effects (Wang *et al.*, 1992; Tode *et al.*, 1993; Lao *et al.*, 1994; Boik, 1996 and 1997; Kang *et al.*, 2000). It is often important to specify the botanical parts from which the herbal agent is prepared, since the active pharmacological agents depend on their source. Radix (Rx) denotes the root, Cortex (Cx) denotes the bark or rind, and Rhizome (Rh) denotes the rhizome. There are plenty of examples of anti-cancer multiplicity. *Rx Ginseng* has anti-tumor activity, inhibits platelet aggregation, and inhibits chemotherapy-induced immunosuppression. *Glycyrrhizic* acid has anti-tumor activity, is anti-inflammatory through increasing serum cortisol, and also increases natural killer (NK) cell activity against cancer cells. *Rx Astragali membranaceus* is a powerful stimulator of the immune system, has anti-tumor activity and inhibits platelet aggregation. *Rx Angelica sinensis* stimulates the immune system, has anti-tumor activity, inhibits platelet aggregation, and inhibits vascular permeability. *Rh Atractylodis macrocephala* has anti-tumor activity, and is an anti-thrombotic and fibrinolytic agent. *Ginkgo biloba* has multiple effects including inhibition of platelet activation factor (PAF), stimulation of the immune system, fibrinolyis and anti-thrombosis, scavenging of free radicals, and dilation of blood vessels to increase perfusion. The effects on the hemostatic coagulation system are interesting as we learn more about the interactive roles of the bone marrow, hemopoietic system, and angiogenesis in the progression of cancer (Yance and Sagar, 2006).

Extracts of multiple Chinese herbs traditionally used for anti-cancer therapy (*Anemarrhena asphodeloides*, *Atremisia argyi*, *Commiphora myrrha*, *Duchesnea indica*, *Gleditsia sinensis*, *Ligustrum lucidum*, *Rheum palmatum*, *Rubia cordifolia*, *Salvia chinensis*, *Scutellaria barbata*, *Uncaria rhychophylla*, *Vaccaria segetalis*) demonstrate growth inhibitory activity against various cancer cell lines, but limited inhibitory activity against normal cell proliferation (Shoemaker *et al.*, 2005). Occasionally herbs alone are associated with tumor regression. For example, a 51-year-old lady with pathological proven squamous cell carcinoma of the lung attained complete regression with sole treatment using a combination of herbs (*Herba Hedyotis diffusae*, *Radix ophiopogonis*, *Herba taraxaci*, *Radix notoginseng*, *Pseudobulbus cremastrae seu pleiones*, *Radix panacis quinquefolii*, *Herba houttuyniae*, *Bulbus Fritillariae thunbergii*, *Rhizoma Pinelliae preparata*) (Liang *et al.*, 2004).

These herbs contain a variety of chemicals that may act synergistically to inhibit tumor cell division, increase tumor cell death (apoptosis), increase the proportion of immune cells within the tumor, and increase blood flow through the tumor. This is associated with a change in the balance of cytokines (communicating peptides released by the immune cells) that may improve the *therapeutic gain*. This means that they reduce the proliferation of tumor cells, increase tumor cell death, whilst minimizing many side effects for normal tissues. Recent meta-analyses confirm the utility for Chinese herbs to both enhance the control of particular cancers (particularly viral-induced cancers such as hepatocellular carcinoma and nasopharyngeal cancers) and reduce side effects of chemotherapy (Taixang *et al.*, 2005; Shu *et al.*, 2005). This synergy appears to be secondary to inducing apoptosis, anti-angiogenesis, antagonism of the viral genome, and induction of an immune response. In addition, some herbs can reverse multidrug resistance (Zhou and Liu, 2005). Examples of some studies that illustrate these principles are discussed elsewhere in this chapter.

In TCM, the malignant tumor is viewed as being associated with stagnation of *qi* (energy) and blood. *Qi* may be viewed as a model for intra- and intercellular information and potential energy transfer. This would correlate with the known abnormalities of signal transduction, cell contact, and electrophysiology of cancer cells (Coffey, 1998; Cuzick *et al.*, 1998; Kang *et al.*, 2000). It has been shown that there is increased fluid content and a stagnant blood supply in malignant tumors (Baxter and Jain, 1989; Boucher and Jain, 1992; Sagar *et al.*, 1993; Milosevic *et al.*, 1998). The microcirculation within a tumor is very abnormal, and there are regions within the tumor where the blood flow is sluggish. In TCM, stagnation of blood is classically associated with tumors. The impaired blood circulation leads to areas of poor oxygenation in the tumor. Cancer cells that survive in a low oxygen tension environment are also found to be more resistant to radiotherapy and some types of chemotherapy (Brizel *et al.*, 1997; Fyles *et al.*, 1998).

In TCM, destagnation or detoxification herbs are used to move the blood and *qi* within the malignant tumor. Interestingly, the use of anti-coagulants, such as heparin and coumadin (warfarin), as an adjunctive treatment to chemotherapy, has been shown to prevent the development of blood-borne metastases in animal laboratory studies, and to improve the survival of cancer patients in clinical studies (Lebeau *et al.*, 1994; Hejna *et al.*, 1999). Many of these herbs are proving to be anti-angiogenic agents (Yance and Sagar, 2006).

The possible usefulness of *destagnation herbs* was demonstrated in a randomized controlled clinical trial evaluating the combined modality treatment of Chinese herbal destagnation formula and radiotherapy in patients with nasopharyngeal carcinoma (Xu *et al.*, 1989). In this trial, 90 patients received combined herbal and radiation treatment compared to 98 patients who were randomized to receive radiation treatment alone. The ingredients of the herbal formula included *Rx Astragali membranaceus*, *Rx Paeoniae rubrae*, *Rx Ligustici Chuan xiong*, *Rx Angelicae sinensis*, *Semen persica*, *Flos Carthami tinctorii*, *Rx et Caulis Jixueteng*, *Rx Puerariae*, *Pericarpium citri reticulatae*, and *Rx Codonopsitis pilosulae*. The combined treatment group showed a statistically significant increase in local tumor control and overall five-year survival as compared with the group treated with radiation alone (p-value < 0.05). The rate of local recurrence in the intervention group was halved from 29% in those receiving radiation alone, to 14% in the group receiving destagnation herbs as well. The five-year disease free survival was increased from 37% in the control group to 53% in the group receiving destagnation herbs. It is postulated that this herbal destagnation formula may have improved tumor microcirculation and increased tumor blood flow leading to an improvement in the oxygen tension inside the tumor. The oxygen tension increases the radiosensitivity of the tumor. In other words, the destagnation formula has acted as a radiation sensitizer.

In animal experiments, *Gingko biloba* has also been shown to increase perfusion and radiosensitivity (Kleijnen and Knipschild, 1992; Sung *et al.*,

1996). Chinese herbs, such as *Salviae miltiorrhizae*, which inhibit tumor edema caused by free radicals may also increase tumor perfusion, oxygenation and response to radiotherapy (Sagar *et al.*, 1995; Peigen *et al.*, 1996). Other herbs may directly sensitize neoplastic cells to radiotherapy (Huali *et al.*, 1994). Some herbs may protect normal tissues from radiotherapy. For example, *Panax ginseng* and *Panax quinquefolium* water extract (especially Rh2 ginsenoside) may radioprotect through mechanisms involving antioxidative and immunomodulating properties (Lee *et al.*, 2005).

More clinical trials need to be done to further evaluate this promising role of herbs in potentially improving the therapeutic gain. Novel non-invasive techniques such as functional MRI and positron emission tomography may be useful (Sagar *et al.*, 1993).

(ii) *Acupuncture*

The interaction of acupuncture with appropriate acupoints modulates blood flow (Thomas *et al.*, 1992; Chao *et al.*, 1999; Zhou *et al.*, 1995; Stener-Victorin *et al.*, 1996). This may be through a local effect via release of cytokines, or through neurological reflexes that adjust the balance between the sympathetic and parasympathetic nervous system. Its effect on tumor physiology and response to therapy remains to be investigated. However, we do know that electric pulses to the tumor can increase the response to chemotherapy. A Phase II study of electrochemotherapy using cisplatin in patients with skin nodules from malignant melanoma demonstrated a significantly increased control rate compared to cisplatin alone (Sersa *et al.*, 2000). However, the effect of acupuncture may be more diverse through the promotion of local cytokines at physiological levels.

(b) Enhancement of Immunity

(i) *Herbs*

Another strategy that TCM uses in cancer therapy is to strengthen the whole body-mind system by enhancing and harmonizing the energy balance between all the organs. This may be viewed as correcting an imbalance in the body-mind communication network and is reflected by an enhancement in immunity. This is called *Fu Zheng* treatment and is mediated by the specific group of TCM herbs called *Fu Zheng* herbs

(Ning *et al.*, 1988; Ling *et al.*, 1989; Chen, 1990; Yu *et al.*, 1990; Hou *et al.*, 1991; Rao *et al.*, 1991; Li, 1992; Yu *et al.*, 1993; Cao *et al.*, 1994; Cheng, 1994; Horie *et al.*, 1994; Lin *et al.*, 1995). There is some limited evidence that improvement of the immunological function of cancer patients is associated with an improvement in their survival. In China, *Fu Zheng* herbs have been reported to increase survival when combined with radiotherapy for patients with nasopharyngeal cancer, and when combined with chemotherapy for patients with stomach and liver cancer (Macek, 1984; Wang, 1990).

Fu Zheng herbs, including *Rx Ginseng*, *Ganoderma*, *Rx Astragali membranaceus*, *Rx Angelicae sinensis*, *Cordyceps sinensis* and *Fructus Lycii*, have been shown to enhance the body's defense mechanisms. Clinical studies, including two randomized trials, have found that the NK cell and OKT4 (immune-enhancing lymphocyte) cell counts were increased with the use of *Fu Zheng* herbs (Ning *et al.*, 1988; Ling *et al.*, 1989; Chen, 1990; Yu *et al.*, 1990; Hou *et al.*, 1991; Rao *et al.*, 1991; Li, 1992; Yu *et al.*, 1993; Cao *et al.*, 1994; Cheng, 1994; Horie *et al.*, 1994; Lin *et al.*, 1995). These immunocytes are known to attack cancer cells. In a study of gastric cancer patients, increased survival was found in the combined treatment group receiving both *Fu Zheng* herbs and chemotherapy versus the chemotherapy alone group. Many of these herbs are associated with an increase in cytokines, such as interferon and interleukin (Kawakita *et al.*, 1990; Jin *et al.*, 1994; Feng *et al.*, 1995). Chinese studies also suggest that healing of normal tissues may be enhanced. Anti-inflammatory constituents may diminish radiation-induced ulcers and chemotherapy-induced stomatitis (Zhu and Zhang, 1993; Zhu, 1994). However, these studies still need to be verified in the West, using acceptable standards and quality assurance.

Recently, the concept of immune enhancement has gained new ground with the discovery that both the cytotoxic therapies and the cancer suppress immunity, and that low immune levels may increase the probability of relapse. In addition, an intact innate immune system is necessary for the activity of new cancer vaccines. The interaction of host immunity with the natural history of cancer is suggested by Burnet's immune surveillance theory; the fact that immunodeficiency diseases are associated with an increased risk of cancer; and the fact that immune-enhancing therapies in malignant melanoma and renal cell carcinoma have produced anti-tumor responses. There is evidence that the healthy immune system is necessary for the control of malignant disease and that immune suppression associated with cancer contributes to its progression. Natural immune mediators are implicated in resistance against tumor development (Whiteside, 2006). Adaptive immunity is often suppressed in tumor-bearing hosts, and specially designed agents are required to boost this defense (Berkzy *et al.*, 1998). Hormonal manipulation of the host can result in the elevation of immune defenses against cancer. Such manipulation strengthens both the adaptive and natural immune defenses of the host, both of which play significant roles. Cytokines and hormones boost natural defense mechanisms during febrile reactions, which are now known as the acute phase response. Hormonal stimulation of immune mechanisms coupled with the other immunostimulants may be employed to good advantage for the combination immunotherapy of cancer. Many Chinese herbs contain glycoproteins and polysaccharides that can modulate metastatic potential and the innate immune system. Metastasis of malignant tumors may be a specific receptor-mediated process in which organ-specific lectins play a role in the adhesion of disseminated tumor cells. Glycoprotein-mediated membrane identity is part of the HLA antigen histocompatibility system. The abnormal carbohydrate group on the tumor cell could have formed during malignant transformation. The metastatic tumor cell, with its membrane-associated glycoprotein (often identical with the tumor marker) is recognized by the organ specific lectins as belonging to the organ, and is thereby captured. *In vitro* experiments show that galactoglycoconjugates can inhibit the adhesion of tumor cells to hepatocytes (Beuth, 1988). Immune suppression in cancer contributes to progression and relapse (Kebudi *et al.*, 1995; Vucković-Deki *et al.*, 1992; Maier *et al.*, 1995; Miyazaki *et al.*, 1995; Baniyash, 2006; Whiteside, 2006; Sasada *et al.*, 2003; Wichmann *et al.*, 2003; Bang *et al.*, 2006; Koukourakis *et al.*, 2003). There are currently multiple strategies to identify candidate tumor antigens, and we now understand more about activation and regulation of immunity against cancer. Vaccines can target tumor-specific antigens, but adjuvants are required to boost the innate immune response, especially in patients who already have depressed immunity from tumor-derived signaling molecules and the effects of cytotoxic therapies (Stevenson, 2005; Minev, 2002; Hoffmann *et al.*, 2004). Phytochemicals, such as specific polysaccharides, have been shown to boost the innate immune system, especially through interaction with Toll-like receptors (TLRs) in mucosa associated lymphoid tissue (MALT) (Tsan, 2006; Sen *et al.*, 2005; Rezaie, 2006). TLRs evolved to interact with polysaccharides found in the walls of bacteria and are an essential part of developing and maintaining a competent immune system (Heine and Almer, 2005). Polysaccharide extracts and complexes from Chinese medicinal herbs and mushrooms may have a potential role for enhancing innate immunity. There is some evidence from clinical trials that they can improve survival (Chang, 2002). The polysaccharide complexes and extracts include constituents of *Coriolus versicolor* (extract is Krestin, PSK or PSP) (Zeng *et al.*, 2005; Ito *et al.*, 2004; Ohwada *et al.*, 2004; Koda *et al.*, 2003; Tsang *et al.*, 2003; Kanazawa *et al.*, 2004; Wong *et al.*, 2004 and 2005; Munemoto *et al.*, 2002; Hayakawa *et al.*, 1997; Ogoshi *et al.*, 1995; Mitomi *et al.*, 1992; Nakazato *et al.*, 1994), *Ganoderma lucidum* (Shao *et al.*, 2004a; Lin, 2005; Kuo *et al.*, 2006; Gao *et al.*, 2003; Kodama *et al.*, 2005a), *Grifola frondosa* (maitake MD-fraction) (Kodama *et al.*, 2002, 2003, 2005a and b; Atsuyuki *et al.*, 2002), *Astragalus membranaceus* (Shao *et al.*, 2004b), *Panax ginseng* (Shin *et al.*, 2002 and 2004; Han *et al.*, 2005; Lim *et al.*, 2004), and various other medicinal mushrooms (Ooi and Liu, 2000; Zaidman *et al.*, 2005; Lindquist *et al.*, 2005). Molecular mechanisms for the immunobiological functions may be through various receptors on macrophages, monocytes and NK cells, which activate NF-kB and anti-tumor cytokine secretion. Interactions may include complement receptor type 3, CD14, mannose, and beta-glucan receptors. There is evidence of interaction with TLRs, especially TLR4, with polysaccharides derived from *Astragalus membranaceus*, *Acanthopanax senticosus/koreanum*, *Ganoderma lucidum* and *Platyloden grandiflorum* (Han *et al.*, 2003; Schepetkin and Quinn, 2006; Ahn *et al.*, 2006). Immuno-suppression in cancer patients can reduce the efficacy of anti-cancer vaccines and increase complications from opportunistic infections. Polysaccharides (mainly beta-D-glucans alone or linked to proteins) from the cell walls of various traditional Chinese medicinal mushrooms and plants show anti-tumor and anti-infection activities through activation of monocytes, macrophages and NK cells. A future research strategy should authenticate the source of these polysaccharide extracts and screen them for interaction with TLRs in the gastrointestinal tract of animals. Oral agents that boost cell-mediated immunity through the MALT may be subsequently evaluated in human Phase I studies for dose-response (cytokine and immune cell assays) and safety. Optimized, authenticated polysaccharides may play a role in enhancing the potency of anti-cancer vaccines and other therapeutic modalities. These non-cytokine molecules appear to signal primarily through the TLRs, which are expressed by dendritic cells. In the MALT, these agonists can induce a host of proinflammatory cytokines such as tumor necrosis factor-alpha, IL-12, and IL-6, as well as CD4+ and CD8+ T cells. Combining radiation therapy and TLR agonists may reduce the amount of radiation therapy required to eradicate tumors, thus acting as an "immunosensitizer" (Koski and Czerniecki, 2005; DeMaria *et al.*, 2005). Further evidence of the potential usefulness of polysaccharides in stimulating an enhanced immune response comes from a study of orally administered betaglucans (from maitake mushroom) that demonstrates an enhancement of anti-tumor effects of monoclonal antibodies (Cheung *et al.*, 2002). Ganopoly (a *Ganoderma lucidum* polysaccharide extract) modulated immune function in advanced-stage cancer patients. Treatment for 12 weeks resulted in a significant increase in the mean plasma concentrations of Il-2, Il-6, and IFN- gamma, whereas Il-1 and TNF-alpha were decreased. NK activity was increased, but there was no significant change in the levels of CD4+, CD8+ or the CD4+/CD8+ ratio (Gao *et al.*, 2003). Lymphoproliferative neoplasms, such as lymphomas and leukemias, may be particularly sensitive to changes in cytokine balance. The Memorial Sloan-Kettering Cancer Center (New York, NY, USA) has commenced an NCI-sponsored Phase I study of beta-glucan and rituximab in pediatric patients with relapsed or progressive CD-20 positive lymphoma or leukemia (Clinical Trials Government, 2006).

Evidence indicates that the healthy immune system is necessary for control of malignant disease and that immune suppression associated with cancer contributes to its progression. Tumors have developed strategies to successfully evade the host immune system, and various molecular and cellular mechanisms responsible for tumor evasion have been identified. Some of these mechanisms target immune anti-tumor effector cells. Dysfunction and apoptosis of these cells in the tumor-bearing host creates an immune imbalance that cannot be corrected by immunotherapies aimed only at activation of anti-tumor immune responses. Reversal of existing immune dysfunction and normalization of lymphocyte homeostasis in patients with cancer needs to be a part of future cancer immunotherapy (Whiteside, 2006). Therapeutic strategies are being designed to correct the immune imbalance, deliver adequate *in vivo* stimulation, transfer effector T cells capable of *in vivo* expansion and provide protection for the immune effector cells re-populating the host. Survival of these cells and long-term memory development in patients with malignancy are necessary for improving clinical benefits of cancer immunotherapies. Polysaccharides derived from Chinese herbs and mushrooms are emerging agents that seem to enhance cytotoxic drugs, radiotherapy, surgery, and the newer targeted therapies and vaccines (Chang, 2002; Chan, 2005a and b; McCulloch, 2006).

(ii) *Acupuncture*

Multiple animal and clinical studies have also suggested that acupuncture has a positive immune-modulating effect in cancer patients (Bianchi *et al.*, 1991; Yuan and Zhou, 1993; Wu *et al.*, 1994 and 1996a; Yang *et al.*, 1994; Liu *et al.*, 1995; Wu, 1995; Sato *et al.*, 1996; Petti *et al.*, 1998; Zhou *et al.*, 1999a). In these studies, acupuncture has been shown to increase T-lymphocyte proliferation, increase NK cell activities, activate the complement system and heat-stable mitogenic humoral factor, and increase OKT4 cell counts. Inhibition of the growth of transplanted mammary cancer has also been shown in mice with the use of acupuncture. The main acupoints that were used in these studies were those that support blood formation and Spleen function. These points include LI 4, LI 11, St 36, Sp 6, Sp10, P6, UB 20, GB39 and GV14. An increased level of all components (red blood cells, white blood cells and platelets) was found.

(c) *Hormonal effects*

Some Chinese herbs inhibit hormone-responsive tumor cells. PC-SPES is a combination of herbs with partial estrogenic activity associated with activity against prostate cancer. One study correlated laboratory activity with clinical response (DiPaola *et al.*, 1998). On the basis of these findings, a National Cancer Institute (NCI) randomized controlled trial was initiated. Unfortunately, the clinical trial was terminated when a batch of PC-SPES was contaminated with the hormone stilboestrol and other pharmacological agents. It is not certain whether there was deliberate adulteration or accidental contamination (Guns, 2002).

Acupuncture may stimulate steroid levels and other hormones, such as melatonin, somatostatin, and vasoactive intestinal peptide, which could potentially have anti-tumor effects (Massion *et al.*, 1995; Zhang *et al.*, 1997 and 1999). Exposure of the popliteal fossa (over the Bladder meridian) to bright light modulates the circadian release of melatonin from the pineal gland (Campbell and Murphy, 1998).

[II] Cancer Prevention

TCM also emphasizes appropriate nutrition according to specific constitutional and disease patterns. Green tea (*Camellia sinensis*) and *Panax Ginseng* are two dietary supplements which have been extensively investigated in both the laboratory and in epidemiological studies. Both reduce the risk of cancer induction, and they both may prevent cancer recurrence (Yang and Wang, 1993; Kaegi, 1998; Yun and Choi, 1998).

Green tea (*Camellia sinensis*) contains isoflavones and a powerful antioxidant called epigallocatechin (EGC) (McKenna *et al.*, 2000). The latter may potentiate the destruction of cancer cells through the process of apoptosis (natural programmed cell death) and by inhibiting angiogenesis (new blood vessel formation that enhances tumor growth and metastasis) (Cao and Cao, 1999; Fujiki *et al.*, 1999). *Panax Ginseng* may induce the differentiation of neoplastic cells into normal tissue (Lee *et al.*, 1996). Both EGC and Ginseng appear to restore normal intercellular communication through the gap junctions (Kang *et al.*, 2000). Both dietary supplements seem to work through novel mechanisms of signaling and communication through the body-mind network.

The soy bean contains genistein, which is an isoflavone with multiple anti-cancer effects demonstrated in the laboratory (Boik, 1996). These include the induction of tumor cell death through the process of apoptosis, inhibition of cancer cell proliferation through decreasing the availability of sex hormones, inhibition of angiogenesis, inhibition of tyrosine kinase (involved in intracellular signaling from the membrane to the nucleus), and inhibition of platelet aggregation (Kim *et al.*, 1998; Li *et al.*, 1999a and b). Some epidemiological studies suggest that populations with a high soy or tofu content in their diet may have a reduced risk of breast cancer (Wu *et al.*, 1996b; Witte *et al.*, 1997; Lu *et al.*, 2000), whereas other studies cannot confirm this link (Key *et al.*, 1999). The phytoestrogens contained within soy may reduce the symptoms of hot flashes associated with chemotherapy-induced menopause (Scambia *et al.*, 2000), although not all studies support this (Quella *et al.*, 2000). The isoflavones and phytoestrogens in soy also appear to reduce the incidence of prostate cancer, and may play a role in prevention and as an adjunctive therapy to reduce the risk of recurrence (Jacobsen *et al.*, 1998; Kamat and Lamm, 1999; Moyad, 1999; Stephens, 1999; Adlercreutz *et al.*, 2000). Cell culture and animal xenograft studies show that treatment with soy is associated with inhibition of prostate specific antigen, deactivation of NF-kappa B (a nuclear transcription factor), induction of apoptosis (programmed cell death), and inhibition of angiogenesis (Aronson *et al.*, 1999; Davis *et al.*, 1999 and 2000; Zhou *et al.*, 1999b).

TCM herb combinations may reduce the risk of lung cancer in ex-smokers. An NCI sponsored study through the British Columbia Cancer Agency, led by Dr. Stephen Lam, is recruiting participants aged 45–74 years, who are ex-smokers, to evaluate the efficacy of a herbal combination called Anti-Cancer Preventive Health Agent (ACAPHA) (personal communication). This contains *Sophora tonkinensis*, *Polygonum bistorta*, *Prunella vulgaris*, *Sonchus brachyotus*, *Dictamnus dasycarpus*, and *Dioscorea bulbifera*. In Chinese studies, ACAPHA reduced the risk of esophageal cancer by 50%, through reversing severe esophageal dysplasia. In addition, a pilot study of 20 former heavy smokers with bronchial dysplasia treated with ACAPHA showed that, after 6 months, 50% had complete regression of dysplasia, compared to only 13% in the placebo group. *Panax quinquefolium* (American ginseng) appears to reduce death and increases quality of life in survivors of breast cancer, suggesting that some botanicals may prevent recurrence (Cui *et al.*, 2005).

(2) Psychoneuroimmunology (PNI)

Psychoneuroimmunology (PNI) is a scientific discipline that has produced evidence for a dynamic mutual interaction between the mind, nervous system, endocrine system, and immunity. The interaction of emotions and immunocytes through molecules, such as neuropeptides, is now well recognized. In fact, the immune system can be viewed as a complex evolutionary communication system within the body-mind network (Page and Ben-Eliyahu, 1997; Jessop, 1998; Nutt, 1998; Pert *et al.*, 1998; Rabin, 1999). TCM recognizes this complex interaction between personality, mood states, and susceptibility to illness through malfunction of the body-mind network.

There is accumulating evidence that psychological function is linked with outcomes in cancer patients (Shekelle *et al.*, 1981; Levy and Wise, 1987; Ramirez *et al.*, 1989; Orsi *et al.*, 1996; Anderson *et al.*, 1998; Watson *et al.*, 1999). There is evidence to suggest a link between mood disorders and function of the immune system. Indeed, the experience of pain and suffering is intimately connected to immunity. A mood disorder such as helplessness and hopelessness may lead to a depressed immune system. Treatment of depression and feelings of hopelessness may not only increase quality of life, but may also increase survival (Spiegel *et al.*, 1989; Fawzy *et al.*, 1995; Fawzy, 1999). In a cancer practice, 50% of patients suffer from clinically recognized depression. In 15% of these patients, the degree of depression is severe. Therefore treatment of depression is an important intervention in the management of the body-mind network of cancer patients.

Conventionally, clinical depression is treated with oral medication, such as amitriptyline or the newer serotonin reuptake inhibitor drugs. Studies indicate that acupuncture treatment may be an equally effective alternative treatment modality to drugs in patients suffering from mild depression. In one study, the profile of side effect associated with acupuncture treatment was shown to be better than amitriptyline (Han, 1986). In a single-blind placebo-controlled study of the antidepressant, mianserin, supplementary acupuncture improved the course of depression more than pharmacological treatment with the drug alone (Roschke *et al.*, 2000). Since pharmaceutical antidepressants are not usually effective until two weeks after starting therapy, their combination with acupuncture may enable more rapid results with less side effects.

(3) Symptom Control

Cancer patients experience multiple symptoms related either to the cancer itself or late treatment side effects. Even if a patient's cancer were clinically "cured", the person may still be suffering from late treatment side effects. For example, radiation may cause xerostomia, trismus and skin ulceration. These side effects have an adverse effect on quality of life, and are often not effectively managed by conventional Western medicine.

Chinese medicine plays a useful role in symptom supportive care for cancer patients. Symptoms that can be effectively managed include general constitutional symptoms, such as fatigue and depression, pain, and specific symptoms such as gastrointestinal side effects and myelosuppression.

Cancer patients receiving chemotherapy usually develop myelosuppression (with risk of infection and bleeding) and gastrointestinal side effects (nausea, vomiting and diarrhea). They easily become fatigued and develop a reduced appetite. In TCM terms, the chemotherapeutic agents are causing Spleen and Kidney deficiency leading to a general decrease in *qi* and blood. Radiotherapy and chemotherapy act as "heat toxins" that damage the *yin* and *qi*. "Heart fire" is expressed as stomatitis; "deficient Spleen *qi*" is manifest as diarrhoea. Chemotherapy drugs "disturb Spleen and Stomach *qi*", expressed physically as damage to the lining of the stomach and intestines (Rosenberg, 1997). These physical expressions are only part of the disturbance in the body-mind network and will inevitably be accompanied by emotional disorders (such as depression, anxiety, insomnia), and constitutional change (such as fatigue or hyper-excitability and poor concentration). After an evaluation and diagnosis of the disturbance in the body-mind network, appropriate combinations of herbs, acupuncture, nutrition, and Qigong may be utilized.

(i) *Herbs*

Spleen and Stomach *qi* are supported by appropriate formulas containing *Rx Ginseng*, *Poria*, and *Rh atractylodis macrocephala* (Rosenberg, 1997). Depleted *yin* leads to dry and sore mouth, thirst, constipation and scanty dark urine. The harmonious relationship between Kidney and Heart is disturbed, leading to insomnia, restlessness, disorientation, palpitations and low back pain. This combination of symptoms is traditionally alleviated with combinations of *Rh Anemarrhenae*, *Cx Phellodendron*, and *Rx Rehmanniae*. The weakening of *qi* is associated with depressed immunity and susceptibility to infection and cancer progression. Medicinal mushrooms, such as *Ganoderma*, *Cordyceps sinensis*, and *Shitaki* strengthen the *qi*, which is associated with an improved immune profile and anti-tumor activity. Another herb with potent immune-stimulating properties is *Rx astragali membranaceus*.

At least five randomized controlled trials have shown that Chinese herbal treatment can decrease the degree of myelosuppression, reduce gastrointestinal side effects and increase the patient's appetite (Ning *et al.*, 1988; Ling *et al.*, 1989; Chen, 1990; Yu *et al.*, 1990; Wang, 1990; Hou *et al.*, 1991; Rao *et al.*, 1991; Li, 1992; Yu *et al.*, 1993; Cao *et al.*, 1994; Cheng, 1994; Horie *et al.*, 1994; Lin *et al.*, 1995). Importantly, it can also increase the probability of patients completing the scheduled chemotherapy. One randomized trial recruited 669 patients with late-stage gastric cancer (Yu *et al.*, 1993). One group of patients was treated with herbs that support the Spleen and Kidney function (*Jian Pi Yi Shen prescription*) twice daily for four to six weeks with concurrent chemotherapy, while another group was treated with the same type of chemotherapy alone. The combined treatment group showed significantly higher leukocyte and platelet counts with less general and gastrointestinal side effects. The percentage of patients completing the scheduled chemotherapy was 95% in the combined treatment group versus 74% in the chemotherapy alone group (p-value < 0.01). Unfortunately, the quality and verification of the data from these studies, which were reported from China, are not at a high enough standard that a definitive meta-analysis can be done at this stage.

In TCM, systemic Chinese herbal treatments and topical herbal applications appear to be effective in treating cancer-related pain. In one study, the effectiveness in pain control was shown to be over 90% (Yang *et al.*, 1995).

Ginger root has been shown in many clinical studies to have anti-emetic activity (Mowrey and Clayson, 1982; Grontved and Hentzer, 1986; Grontved *et al.*, 1988; Bone *et al.*, 1990; Fischer-Rasmussen *et al.*, 1991). It appears to particularly help nausea that may be intransigent to standard anti-emetics. Ginger syrup is shown to be effective in a randomized controlled trial (Keating and Chez, 2002). Caution should be used with patients on anticoagulants and those with low platelet levels, since it does have anticoagulant effects at higher doses.

Vitexina (*Vigna radiata*) is a flavonoid herb with radio-protective effects that may be useful for reducing some side effects of radiotherapy.

It treats the heat or yin-deficiency side effects of anti-cancer treatment, such as fatigue, restlessness, insomnia and constipation. This empty heat syndrome is characterized through tongue diagnosis, which reveals a red, denuded and cracked tongue. Since the tongue is the most densely innervated organ in the body, it may reflect the imbalance between yin and yang, via the autonomic nervous system, which in turn may influence blood flow and epithelial cell turnover through the local release of neuropeptides and cytokines. A randomized controlled trial of breast cancer patients receiving radiotherapy showed that Vitexina prevented the empty heat syndrome, reduced weight loss, and protected against a reduction in peripheral lymphocytes and platelets (Tran, 2002).

The role of Chinese herbs, together with conventional Western pharmaceuticals, for symptom control is currently unclear. Laboratory data suggests that they can be effective modifiers of biochemical pathways, immunostimulants, and signal transduction modulators. Potential detrimental interactions and idiosyncratic toxicity are possible. Future studies need to be done using more rigorous methodology and quality assurance. The use of appropriate modeling and suitable evaluative methodologies should enable the integration of Chinese herbology into an emerging model of holistic Western medicine.

(ii) *Acupuncture*

Acupuncture treatment at acupoint P6 has been shown to increase the anti-emetic effect of drugs for peri-operative and chemotherapy-induced nausea and vomiting (Dundee *et al.*, 1986 and 1989). Innovative randomized single blind controlled trials have since confirmed these results (Al-Sadi *et al.*, 1997; Schlager *et al.*, 1998; Lee and Done, 1999) and led to the NIH (US) consensus statement that, "acupuncture is a proven effective treatment modality for nausea and vomiting" (NIH Consensus Development Panel on Acupuncture, 1998). A three-arm randomized controlled trial of conventional modern anti-emetics (such as the 5-HT_3 antagonists), versus electro-acupuncture, versus the combination of anti-emetic drugs plus acupuncture, clearly demonstrated that the combination arm was the most effective for preventing nausea and vomiting (Shen *et al.*, 2000). Stimulation of P6 may be done more conveniently with a small transcutaneous nerve stimulation (TENS) device, such as the

Reliefband^{TM}. A recent randomized controlled trial could not confirm its efficacy in the control of chemotherapy-induced nausea in women with breast cancer (Roscoe *et al.*, 2005). This may have been due to tolerance or because these patients were already maximally controlled by pharmaceutical anti-emetics, and therefore provided no advantage over medication alone. A meta-analysis of acupuncture-point stimulation for chemotherapy-induced nausea or vomiting shows a benefit over and above drug therapy (Ezzo *et al.*, 2005). However, not all the studies used optimal drug therapy, and this may need to be optimized before using acupuncture for refractory cases. Self-administered acupressure appears to have a protective effect for acute nausea.

Pain is a common symptom of cancer. Causes of pain can be disease- or treatment-related. Acupuncture has been shown to be effective in managing pain and other symptoms in cancer patients (Thompson and Filshie, 1998). In a retrospective study from the Royal Marsden Hospital (London, UK), 183 cancer patients with malignant pain, iatrogenic pain and radiation-induced chronic ulcers were treated with acupuncture (Filshie, 1984; Filshie and Redman, 1985). There was an improvement in 82% of the patients, but effectiveness only lasted for more than three days in half of the patients. Iatrogenic pain (for example, pain due to radiation fibrosis or skin ulceration) and pain due to secondary muscle spasm responded better than malignant pain. Furthermore, increased blood flow with improved healing of skin ulcers was demonstrated after treatment with acupuncture. A randomized controlled trial using ear acupuncture showed a profound effect on cancer pain (Alimi *et al.*, 2003). We also have similar experience with the high but short lasting effectiveness of acupuncture treatment in malignant pain. We suggest that acupuncture is a useful treatment modality that may best be combined with other treatments to improve pain control, resulting in reduced doses of pharmaceutical analgesics. This has the benefit of reducing the incidence and degree of drug-induced side effects. A systematic review could not demonstrate the effectiveness of acupuncture as an adjunctive analgesic method for cancer patients (Lee, 2005). However, there was only the one randomized controlled trial (Alimi *et al.*, 2003), and all the other studies were generally of poor scientific quality (Lee *et al.*, 2005). The intensity of stimulation, especially electrostimulation, may be important (Barlas, 2006).

Some patients may not be able to access an acupuncturist because of geographic restrictions or poor performance status. In addition, some patients may not tolerate needle insertions. For these patients, a transcutaneous nerve stimulator (TENS) has the advantage of easy administration by patients or staff with minimal basic training. Recently acupuncture-like TENS (AL-TENS) devices have been developed to mimic the treatment of acupuncture using low-frequency (e.g. 4 Hz), high-intensity stimulation (Pomeranz and Niznik, 1987). The goal is to recruit the high threshold type III afferent nerve fibers that are potent releasers of endorphins. Recent meta-analyses (including a Cochrane Database systematic review) have shown that AL-TENS is more effective than placebo, and improves function more than standard TENS, when treating chronic pain (Patel *et al.*, 1989; Gadsby and Flowerdew, 1997; Ernst and White, 1998; Ghoname *et al.*, 1999). AL-TENS devices are very simple machines that patients can learn to operate in less than an hour's training. An acupoint prescription may then be given to the patient who can administer the appropriate treatments with AL-TENS at home. The Codetron™ is a sophisticated AL-TENS device that has the advantage of reducing tolerance to its analgesic effect, by electronically rotating through a series of random electrical stimulation patterns and acupoint locations.

Other symptoms that may be helped by acupuncture include constipation, trismus (post-radiotherapy contracture of the masseter muscle) (Ernst and White, 1999), radiotherapy-associated proctitis (Zhang, 1987), hiccups (Yan, 1988), persistent yawning (Wong and Sagar, 2000), chemotherapy-induced peripheral neuropathy (Wong and Sagar, 2006), and dysphagia secondary to an esophageal neoplasm (Feng, 1984). Although observational studies by Filshie *et al.* (1996) showed that acupuncture may improve cancer-associated dyspnoea, this was not supported by a later randomized controlled study using semi-permanent acupuncture studs (Vickers *et al.*, 2005). Suppression of anxiety by acupuncture may be associated with an increase in the pain threshold (Widerstrom-Noga *et al.*, 1998). Acupuncture may also play a role in the treatment of fatigue and malignant cachexia through the modulation of cytokines and hormones (Lissoni *et al.*, 1996; Campbell and Murphy, 1998; Glaus, 1998; Stone *et al.*, 1998). A Phase II study of acupuncture for post-chemotherapy fatigue (average of two years) showed a mean improvement of 30% on the Brief Fatigue Inventory (Vickers *et al.*, 2004). This met the research group's pre-specified criterion of clinical importance that has prompted the initiation of a randomized sham acupuncture controlled trial.

Patients who are in remission from their cancer may still continue to suffer from late treatment side effects with reduced quality of life. Radiation-induced xerostomia (dry mouth) is one of the distressing late side effects seen in patients who received radiation treatment that involved the parotid glands. The presence of this condition renders patients with loss of taste and difficulty in speaking and swallowing. Recently, acupuncture treatment has been found to increase blood flow to the parotid glands and may stimulate tissue regeneration in parotid glands damaged by radiotherapy (Blom *et al.*, 1992 and 1993; Talal *et al.*, 1992). A randomized controlled trial of 38 patients with radiation xerostomia was reported from the Karolinska Institute (Sweden) (Blom *et al.*, 1996). Subjects were randomized to either deep acupuncture treatment or superficial acupuncture treatment. The latter group was used as the control, despite previous evidence that superficial acupuncture treatment can have a certain degree of effectiveness and should not be used as a control in acupuncture treatment trials. In this study it was found that in both groups, there was more than a 20% increase in saliva flow rate in more than 50% of patients. In the deep acupuncture group, 68% of patients demonstrated an increase in salivary flow rate. Changes in the control group were smaller and appeared after a longer latency phase. Moreover, patients in the treatment group reported less dryness, less hoarseness and improved taste. In another study, 70 patients with xerostomia due to either Sjögren's syndrome or irradiation were treated with acupuncture (Blom and Lundeberg, 2000). A statistically significant increase in unstimulated and stimulated salivary flow rates (SFR) was found in all patients immediately after acupuncture treatment, and up to six months follow-up. After a review at three years, those patients who chose to be treated with additional acupuncture demonstrated a consistently higher median SFR, compared to those not having additional acupuncture. Despite, some limitations in the study design, both studies provide evidence suggesting acupuncture can be effective in treating radiation-induced xerostomia, with minimal side effects. In a prospective single cohort, visual analogue assessed study of acupuncture in palliative care patients with xerostomia, there was a highly significant alleviation of subjective xerostomia (Rydholm and Strang, 1999). Other studies are confirming the clinical use of acupuncture for relief of radiation-induced xerostomia (Johnstone *et al.*, 2001).

At the Hamilton Regional Cancer Centre (Canada), a Phases I and II study of AL-TENS in the treatment of radiation-induced xerostomia has been completed (Wong *et al.*, 2003). Forty-five patients were randomized into three treatment groups with AL-TENS stimulation using the Codetron™ to three different sets of acupuncture points: Group A — CV 24, St 36, Sp 6, LI 4; Group B — CV 24, St 36, Sp 6, P6; and Group C — CV 24, St 5, St 6, Sp 6, P6. The goal of this study was to determine the optimum pattern of stimulation (based on TCM theory) prior to designing a placebo-controlled study. AL-TENS treatment was administered twice a week for a total of 12 weeks. Unstimulated and stimulated salivary flow rates before, during and after treatment were measured, and a survey of the patients' quality of life was assessed during a follow-up of one year. There was an improvement in xerostomia symptoms with a mean increase in the visual analogue score at three and six months after treatment completion. All patients demonstrated a significant increase in the mean basal and citric acid primed saliva production. The results suggest that Codetron™ treatment improves saliva production and related symptoms in patients suffering from radiation-induced xerostomia. Treatment effects are sustained at least six months after completion of treatment. A recent fMRI study showed activation of the insula region of the brain, the location associated with gustatory function (Deng *et al.*, 2006).

Acupuncture can reduce the hot flushes associated with anti-cancer hormone therapy. Three prospective uncontrolled cohort studies have been done, one in men castrated for prostate cancer, and two others in women taking tamoxifen for breast cancer. They all demonstrated a reduction in vasomotor symptoms (Hammar *et al.*, 1999; Tukmachi, 2000; Cumins and Brunt, 2001). Long-term administration using semi-permanent studs or with needles, especially at SP6 appears to be associated with more long-term relief of symptoms (Filshie *et al.*, 2005).

(4) Improved Function and Quality of Life Through Psycho-Spiritual Integration

Psycho-spiritual philosophy plays an important role in Chinese medicine. It is a complex philosophy beyond the scope of this chapter. Corresponding concepts between Eastern and Western philosophies include the mind or shen (in the Heart meridian), the intellect or *yi* (in the Spleen meridian), the will power or *zhi* (in the Kidney meridian), the corporeal soul or *po* (in the Lung meridian), and the ethereal soul or *hun* (in the Liver meridian). Balancing of the Five Elements, associated with these psycho-spiritual concepts, through herbs and acupuncture, may improve psychological and spiritual well-being. The philosophy is well described in the literature (Hammer, 1990), but no scientific studies have addressed the interaction of herbs and acupuncture with psycho-spiritual adaptation. However, we previously quoted studies of acupuncture being effective for some patients with depressive-anxiety states, and treatment of these symptoms may have a positive effect on psycho-spiritual transformation and transcendence (Han, 1986; Roschke *et al.*, 2000).

Both Eastern and Western cultures have evolved different forms of "hands-on-healing", prayer, and intention to heal through altered states of mind. The philosophy of Chinese medicine encourages an appropriate state of mind, such as compassion and healing intent, to accompany a practical procedure such as acupuncture (Rapgay *et al.*, 2000). Meditation is important for both the practitioner and the patient. It induces beneficial physiological adaptations. For example, meditation can restore a balance between the sympathetic and parasympathetic nervous systems (Benson, 1975). It can also increase melatonin levels that can relieve insomnia, and may have an anti-neoplastic effect (Massion *et al.*, 1995). There are currently multiple hypotheses that scientifically support the rationale of healing through influencing the patient's body-mind memory and information system. These include manipulation of the systemic memory system (Schwartz and Russek, 1999), electromagnetic entrainment (Zimmerman, 1990; Seto *et al.*, 1992; Walleczek, 1992; Sisken and Walder, 1995; Cuzick *et al.*, 1998; Benford *et al.*, 1999; Childre and Cryer, 1999), interaction with subtle energy (Childre and Cryer, 1999), and non-local positive intention through compassion and centering (Grinberg-Zylberbaum *et al.*, 1994; Tiller and Pecci, 1997; Nadeau and Kafatos, 2000). Clinical trials of the effect of intent through prayer have shown efficacy in reducing side-effects and complications (Dossey, 1995; Harris *et al.*, 1999), and a recent systematic review and meta-analysis has confirmed the positive effects of "distant healing" (Astin *et al.*, 2000).

A similar process is seen in the practice of Reiki (from Japan), external Qigong (from China), Polarity Therapy and Therapeutic Touch. There is some evidence that they can all reduce the side effects of cancer and its treatment, and possibly even help to inhibit neoplastic cells (Macek, 1984; Feng *et al.*, 1988; Quizi and Li, 1988; Cohen, 1997; Olson and Hanson, 1997; Shah *et al.*, 1999).

These practices involve the practitioner laying-on her hands at a short distance from the patient, with a positive and loving intent to heal. The patient's "energy field" is assessed for the presence of any disturbance, which may be detected over areas of the body involved by disease processes. If an area of disturbance is detected, the practitioner will "smooth" the disturbance with her hands and channel "external energy" to heal the patient's disturbed somatic energy field.

Many studies have been done to evaluate the usefulness of this practice. Therapeutic touch can reduce anxiety and pain in dying cancer patients. It can be associated with an objective reduction of biochemical and biophysical indicators (Cox and Hayes, 1999). A meta-analysis has also suggested that therapeutic touch has a low to moderate positive effect size with an average effect ratio of 0.39 (Winstead-Fry and Kijek, 1999). Although there are still a lot of controversies regarding the effectiveness of therapeutic touch (Rosa *et al.*, 1998), particularly with respect to technique, end points and controls, the patients' subjective experience should be considered as important since it influences quality of life and immunological status (Engebretson and Wardell, 2000; Wardell and Weymouth, 2004). A recent randomized controlled trial of polarity therapy demonstrated a reduction of fatigue associated with radiotherapy (Roscoe *et al.*, 2005).

Qi gong, tai chi and awareness meditation are scientifically demonstrated to affect physiological processes, including electromagnetic changes that may represent the flow of *qi* (Tiller and Pecci, 1997; Syldona and Rein, 1999). These techniques encourage a personal sense of control, improve mood, reduce side effects of treatment, increase immunity, and may be associated with an improved outcome from cancer treatment (Meares, 1978; Young *et al.*, 1999). Tai chi is a simple exercise for cancer survivors that deserves further investigation. It is a widely practiced movement exercise combining characteristics of meditative practice and aerobic exercise. Cancer survivors may benefit most from a mind-body intervention such as tai chi. While studies previously have compared changes of physiologic parameters comparing tai chi and aerobic exercise, representing the "body" aspect of tai chi, studies are lacking that may demonstrate differential effects of a mind-and-body activity compared to aerobic exercise programs. As the concept of the human being as a mental-spiritual-physical entity is widely held and fundamental to many health systems, there is a need to establish ways of investigating the mind and body effects, as well as their benefits for disease and well-being. A review of published randomized trials of tai chi suggests benefits in the elderly and in cardiovascular diseases (Mansky *et al.*, 2006). It is also likely to help cancer survivors and to contribute to their rehabilitation.

1.7 Conclusions

There is emerging scientific evidence that Chinese medicine can play an important role in the supportive care of cancer patients. There is enough preliminary evidence to encourage good quality clinical trials to evaluate the efficacy of integrating Chinese medicine into Western cancer care (Fontanarosa and Lundberg, 1998; Sagar, 1998 and 1999; Tagliaferri *et al.*, 2001). Currently, the evidence for the utility of TCM in cancer care is promising, but prospective randomized clinical trials for specific clinical scenarios are necessary to obtain reliable and generalizable data. Appropriate stratification and individualization according to TCM diagnostic criteria is possible within the context of a randomized controlled trial (Bensoussan *et al.*, 1998). We believe that an evidence-based approach can be integrated into an individualized therapeutic plan and that there is still a major role for individual belief-systems and psycho-spiritual experience. Assessment and measurement of coping strategies, maintenance of function, quality of life, and patient satisfaction is important. We are hopeful that future integration of different models of health, such as TCM, may lead to further improvement of cancer patients' survival and quality of life (Sagar, 2001).

Acknowledgments

Christina M. Garchinski for administrative assistance.

References

Adlercreutz, H., Mazur, W., Bartels, P., *et al.* (2000) Phytoestrogens and prostate disease. *J. Nutr.* **130**, 658S–659S.

Ahn, J.-Y., Choi, I.S. and Shim, J.-Y. (2006) The immunomodulator ginsan induces resistance to experimental sepsis by inhibiting Toll-like receptor mediated inflammatory signals. *Eur. J. Immunol.* **36**, 37–45.

Ahn, A.C., Wu, J., Badger, J., Hammerschlag, R. and Langevin, H.M. (2005) Electrical impedance along connective tissue planes associated with acupuncture meridians. *BMC Complement. Altern. Med.* **5**, 10.

Alavi, A., LaRiccia, P.J., Sadek, A.H., *et al.* (1997) Neuroimaging of acupuncture in patients with chronic pain. *J. Altern. Complement. Med.* **3**(Suppl 1), S47–S53.

Alimi, D., Rubino, C., Pichard-Leandri, E., *et al.* (2003) Analgesic effect of auricular acupuncture for cancer pain: A randomized, blinded, controlled trial. *J. Clin. Oncol.* **21**, 4120–4126.

Al-Sadi, M., Newman, B. and Julious, S.A. (1997) Acupuncture in the prevention of postoperative nausea and vomiting. *Anaesthesia* **52**, 658–661.

Amkraut, A. and Solomon, G.F. (1972) Stress and murine sarcoma virus (Moloney)-induced tumors. *Cancer Res.* **32**, 1428–1433.

Andersen, B.L., Farrar, W.B., Golden-Kreutz, D., *et al.* (1998) Stress and immune responses after surgical treatment of regional breast cancer. *J. Natl. Cancer Inst.* **90**, 30–36.

Aronson, W.J., Tymchuk, C.N., Elashoff, R.M., *et al.* (1999) Decreased growth of human prostate LNCaP tumors in SCID mice fed a low-fat, soy protein diet with isoflavones. *Nutr. Cancer* **35**, 130–136.

Astin, J.A., Harkness, E. and Ernst, E. (2000) The efficacy of "distant healing": A systematic review of randomized trials. *Ann. Intern. Med.* **132**, 903–910.

Atsuyuki, I., Kodama, N. and Nanba, H. (2002) Effect of maitake (*Grifola frondosa*) D-fraction on the control of the T lymph node Th-1/Th-2 proportion. *Biol. Pharm. Bull.* **25**, 536–540.

Bang, S., Kim, H.-S., Choo, Y.S., *et al.* (2006) Differences in immune cells engaged in cell-mediated immunity after chemotherapy for far advanced pancreatic cancer. *Pancreas* **32**, 29–36.

Baniyash, M. (2006) Chronic inflammation, immunosuppression and cancer: New insights and outlook. *Semin. Cancer Biol.* **16**, 80–88.

Barlas, P., Ting, S.L., Chesterton, L.S., Jones, P.W. and Sim, J. (2006) Effects of intensity of electroacupuncture upon experimental pain in healthy human volunteers: A randomized, double-blind, placebo-controlled study. *Pain* **122**, 81–89.

Baxter, L.T. and Jain, R.K. (1989) Transport of fluid and macromolecules in tumors. 1. Role of interstitial pressure and convection. *Microvasc. Res.* **37**, 77–104.

Benford, M.S., Talnagi, J., Doss, D.B., Boosey, S. and Arnold, L.E. (1999) Gamma radiation fluctuations during alternative healing therapy. *Altern. Ther. Health Med.* **5**, 51–56.

Benson, H. (1975) *The Relaxation Response*. Harper Collins Publisher, New York, NY, USA.

Bensoussan, A., Talley, N.J., Hing, M., *et al.* (1998) Treatment of irritable bowel syndrome with Chinese herbal medicine: A randomized controlled trial. *JAMA* **280**, 1585–1589.

Berczi, I., Chow, D.A., Baral, E. and Nagy, E. (1998) Neuroimmunoregulation and cancer (review). *Int. J. Oncol.* **13**, 1049–1060.

Beuth, J., Ko, H.L. and Schirrmacher, V., *et al.* (1988) Inhibition of liver tumor cell colonization in two animal tumor models by lectin blocking with D-galactose or arabinoglactan. *Clin. Exp. Metastasis* **6**, 115–120.

Bianchi, M., Jotti, E., Sacerdote, P. and Panerai, A.E. (1991) Traditional acupuncture increases the content of beta-endorphin in immune cells and influences mitogen induced proliferation. *Am. J. Chin. Med.* **19**, 101–104.

Bigler, D., Gulding, K.M., Dann, R., Sheabar, F.Z., Conaway, M.R. and Theodorescu, D. (2003) Gene profiling and promoter reporter assays: Novel tools for comparing the biological effects of botanical extracts on human prostate cancer cells and understanding their mechanisms of action. *Oncogene* **22**, 1261–1272.

Blom, M. and Lundeberg, T. (2000) Long-term follow-up of patients treated with acupuncture for xerostomia and the influence of additional treatment. *Oral Dis.* **6**, 15–24.

Blom, M., Dawidson, I. and Angmar-Mansson, B. (1992) The effect of acupuncture on salivary flow rates in patients with xerostomia. *Oral Surg. Oral Med. Oral Pathol.* **73**, 293–298.

Blom, M., Lundeberg, T., Dawidson, I. and Angmar-Mansson, B. (1993) Effects on local blood flux of acupuncture stimulation used to treat xerostomia in patients suffering from Sjögren's syndrome. *J. Oral Rehabil.* **20**, 541–548.

Blom, M., Dawidson, I., Fernberg, J.-O., Johnson, G. and Angmar-Mansson, B. (1996) Acupuncture treatment of patients with radiation-induced xerostomia. *Oral Oncol. Eur. J. Cancer* **32B**, 182–190.

Boik, J. (1996) *Cancer and Natural Medicine: A Textbook of Basic Science and Clinical Research*. Oregon Medical Press, Princeton, MN, USA.

Boik, J. (1997) Emerging trends in cancer research: Development of a mechanism-based approach. *Protocol J. Bot. Med.* **2**, 5–9.

Bone, M.E., Wilkinson, D.J., Young, J.R., McNeil, J. and Charlton, S. (1990) Ginger root — a new antiemetic: The effect of ginger root on postoperative nausea and vomiting after major gynaecological surgery. *Anaesthesia* **45**, 669–671.

Boucher, Y. and Jain, R.K. (1992) Microvascular pressure is the principle driving force for interstitial hypertension in solid tumors: Implications for vascular collapse. *Cancer Res.* **52**, 5110–5114.

Brizel, D.M., Sibley, G.S., Prosnitz, L.R., *et al.* (1997) Tumor hypoxia adversely affects the prognosis of carcinoma of the head and neck. *Int. J. Radiat. Oncol. Biol. Phys.* **38**, 285–289.

Bucinskaite, V., Theodorsson, E., Crumpton, K., *et al.* (1996) Effects of repeated sensory stimulation (electro-acupuncture) and physical exercise on open-field behaviour and concentrations of neuropeptides in the hippocampus in WKY and SHR rats. *Eur. J. Neurosci.* **8**, 382–387.

Cai, Y., Luo, Q., Sun, M. and Corke, H. (2004) Antioxidant activity and phenolic compounds of 112 traditional Chinese medicinal plants associated with anti-cancer. *Life Sci.* **74**, 2157–2184.

Campbell, S.S. and Murphy, P.J. (1998) Extraocular circadian phototransduction in humans. *Science* **279**, 396–399.

Cao, G.W., Yang, W.G. and Du, P. (1994) Observation of the effects of LAK/IL-2 therapy combining with *Lycium barbarum* polysaccharides in the treatment of 75 cancer patients. *Chunghua Chung Liu Tsa Chih* **16**, 428–431.

Cao, Y. and Cao, R. (1999) Angiogenesis inhibited by tea. *Nature* **398**, 381.

Chan, A.S., Yip, E.C., Yung, L.Y., *et al.* (2005a) Immuno-regulatory effects of CKBM on the activities of mitogen-activated protein kinases and the release of cytokines in THP-1 monocytic cells. *Biol. Pharm. Bull.* **28**, 1645–1650.

Chan, W.L., Lam, D.T., Law, H.K., *et al.* (2005b) *Ganoderma lucidum* mycelium and spore extracts as natural adjuvants for immunotherapy. *J. Altern. Complement. Med.* **11**, 1047–1057.

Chao, D.M., Shen, L.L., Tjen-A-Looi, S., *et al.* (1999) Naloxone reverses inhibitory effect of electroacupuncture on sympathetic cardiovascular reflex responses. *Am. J. Physiol.* **276**, H2127–H2134.

Chang, R. (2002) Bioactive polysaccharides from traditional Chinese medicine herbs as anti-cancer adjuvants. *J. Altern. Complement. Med.* **8**, 559–565.

Chen, J.Z. (1990) Clinical effect of chemotherapy combined with Chinese herbs and Western drugs on leukocytes of gastric cancer patients. *Chung His I Chieh Ho Tsa Chih* **10**, 717–719.

Cheng, J.H. (1994) Clinical study on prevention and treatment of chemotherapy caused nephrotoxicity with jian-pi yi-qi li-shui decoction. *Chung Kuo Chung Hsi I Chieh Ho Tsa Chih* **14**, 331–333.

Cheung, N.K., Modak, S., Vickers, A., *et al.* (2002) Orally administered betaglucans enhance anti-tumor effects of monoclonal antibodies. *Cancer Immunol. Immunother.* **51**, 57–64.

Childre, D. and Cryer, B. (1999) *From Chaos to Coherence*. Butterworth-Heinemann, Boston, MA, USA.

Cho, Z.H., Chung, S.C., Jones, J.P., *et al.* (1998) New findings of the correlation between acupoints and corresponding brain cortices using functional MRI. *Proc. Natl. Acad. Sci. USA* **95**, 2670–2673.

Clinical Trials (2006) http://www.clinicaltrials.gov/ct/gui/show/NCT00087009 (accessed August 2006).

Coffey, D.S. (1998) Self-organization, complexity and chaos: The new biology for medicine. *Nat. Med.* **4**, 882–885.

Cohen, K.S. (1997) *The Way of Qigong*: *The Art and Science of Chinese Energy Healing*. Ballantine, New York, NY, USA.

Collins, L., Zhu, T., Guo, J., *et al.* (2006) Phellinus linteus sensitises apoptosis induced by doxorubicin in prostate cancer. *Br. J. Cancer* **95**, 282–288.

Cox, C. and Hayes, J. (1999) Physiologic and psychodynamic responses to the administration of therapeutic touch in critical care. *Complement. Ther. Nurs. Midwifery* **5**, 87–92.

Cui, Y., Shu, X.-O., Gao, Y.-T., Cai, H., *et al.* (2005) Association of ginseng use with survival and quality of life among breast cancer patients. *Am. J. Epidemiol.* **163**, 645–653.

Cumins, S.M. and Brunt, A.M. (2001) Does acupuncture influence the vasomotor symptoms experienced by breast cancer patients taking tamoxifen? *Acupunct. Med.* **18**, 28–29.

Cuzick, J., Holland, R., Barth, V., *et al.* (1998) Electropotential measurements as a new diagnostic modality for breast cancer. *Lancet* **352**, 359–363.

Dardik, I.I. (1996) The origin of disease and health. Heart waves: The single solution to heart rate variability and ischemic preconditioning. *Universal Cycles* **46**, 67–77.

Davis. J.N., Kucuk, O. and Sarkar, F.H. (1999) Genistein inhibits NF-kappa B activation in prostate cancer cells. *Nutr. Cancer* **35**, 167–174.

Davis JN, Muqim, N., Bhuiyan M *et al.* (2000) Inhibition of prostate specific antigen by genistein in prostate cancer cells. *Int. J. Oncol.* **16**, 1091–1097.

Dawidson, I., Blom, M., Lundeberg, T. and Angmar-Mansson, B. (1997) The influence of acupuncture on salivary flow rates in healthy subjects. *J. Oral Rehabil.* **24**, 204–208.

Demaria, S., Bhardwaj, N., McBride, W.H. and Formenti, S.C. (2005) Combining radiotherapy and immunotherapy: A revived partnership. *Int. J. Radiat. Oncol. Biol. Phys.* **63**, 655–666.

Deng, G., *et al.* (2006) Randomized controlled trial of fMRI changes associated with acupuncture at a point used to treat xerostomia versus sham acupuncture or gustatory stimulation. In: *Proceedings of the Third International Conference of the Society for Integrative Oncology*, Boston, USA (Abstract).

DiPaola, R.S., Zhang, H., Lambert, G.H., *et al.* (1998) Clinical and biologic activity of an estrogenic herbal combination (PC-SPES) in prostate cancer. *N. Engl. J. Med.* **339**, 785–810.

Dossey, L. (1995) *Healing Words: The Power of Prayer and the Practice of Medicine*. Harper Collins, San Francisco, USA.

Dundee, J.W., Chestnutt, W.N., Ghaly, R.G. and Lynas, A.G.A. (1986) Traditional Chinese acupuncture: A potentially useful antiemetic? *Br. Med. J.* **293**, 583–584.

Dundee, J.W., Ghaly, R.G., Fitzpatrick, K.T.J. Abram, W.P. and Lynch, G.A. (1989) Acupuncture prophylaxis of cancer chemotherapy-induced sickness. *J. R. Soc. Med.* **82**, 268–271.

Engebretson, J. and Wardell, D.W. (2002) Experience of a Reiki session. *Altern. Ther. Health Med.* **8**, 48–53.

Ernst, E. and White, A.R. (1998) Acupuncture for back pain: A meta-analysis of randomized controlled trials. *Arch. Intern. Med.* **158**, 2235–2241.

Ernst, E. and White, A.R. (1999) Acupuncture as a treatment for temporomandibular joint dysfunction: A systematic review of randomized trials. *Arch. Otolaryngol. Head Neck Surg.* **125**, 269–272.

Ezzo, J., Vickers, A., Richardson, M.A., *et al.* (2005) Acupuncture-point stimulation for chemotherapy-induced nausea and vomiting. *J. Clin. Oncol.* **23**, 7188–7198.

Farrell, M.P. (2003) Ph I/IIA randomized study of PHY906 as a modulator of chemotherapy in patients with advanced colorectal cancer. *Clin. Colorectal Cancer* **2**, 253–256.

Fawzy, F.I., Fawzy, N.W., Arndt, L.A. and Pasnau, R. (1995) Critical review of psychosocial interventions in cancer care. *Arch. Gen. Psychiatry* **52**, 100–113.

Fawzy, F.I. (1999) Psychosocial interventions for patients with cancer: What works and what doesn't. *Eur. J. Cancer* **35**, 1559–1564.

Feng, L., Juqing, Q. and Shugine, C. (1988) A study of the effect of the emitted qi of Qigong on human carcinoma cells. In: *First World Conference for Academic Exchange of Medical Qigong*, Beijing (Abstract).

Feng, P.F., Liu, L.M. and Shen, Y.Y. (1995) Effect of Shenmai injection on s-IL-2R, NK and LAK cells in patients with advanced carcinoma. *Chung Kuo Chung His I Chieh Ho Tsa Chih* **15**, 451–453.

Feng, R. (1984) Relief of oesophageal carcinomatous obstruction by acupuncture. *J. Tradit. Chin. Med.* **4**, 3–4.

Filshie, J., Penn, K., Ashley, S., *et al.* (1996) Acupuncture for the relief of cancer-related breathlessness. *Palliat. Med.* **10**, 145–150.

Filshie, J. and Redman, D. (1985) Acupuncture and malignant pain problems. *Eur. J. Surg. Oncol.* **11**, 389–394.

Filshie, J. (1984) Acupuncture for malignant pain. *Acupunct. Med.* **May**, 12–14.

Filshie, J., Bolton, T., Browne, D. and Ashley, S. (2005) Acupuncture and self-acupuncture for long-term treatment of vasomotor symptoms in cancer patients: Audit and treatment algorithm. *Acupunct. Med.* **23**, 171–180.

Fischer-Rasmussen, W., Kjaer, S.K., Dahl, C. and Asping, U. (1991) Ginger treatment of hyperemesis gravidarum. *Eur. J. Obstet. Gynecol. Reprod. Biol.* **38**, 19–24.

Fontanarosa, P.B. and Lundberg, G.D. (1998) Alternative medicine meets science. *JAMA* **280**, 1618–1619.

Fujiki, H., Suganuma, M., Okabe, S., *et al.* (1999) Mechanistic findings of green tea as cancer preventive for humans. *Proc. Soc. Exp. Biol. Med.* **220**, 225–228.

Fyles, A.W., Milosevic, M., Wong, R., *et al.* (1998) Oxygenation predicts radiation response and survival in patients with cervix cancer. *Radiother. Oncol.* **48**, 149–156.

Gadsby, J.G. and Flowerdew, M.W. (1997) Review: Transcutaneous electrical nerve stimulation reduces pain and improves range of movement in chronic low-back pain. *Evid. Based Med.* **July/Aug**, 107.

Gagnier, J.J., Boon, H., Rochon, P., *et al.* (2006) Reporting randomized, controlled trials of herbal interventions: An elaborated CONSORT statement. *Ann. Intern. Med.* **144**, 364–367.

Gao, Y., Zhou, S., Jiang, W., Huang, M. and Dai, X. (2003) Effects of Ganopoly™: A *Ganoderma lucidum* polysaccharide extract) on the immune functions in advanced-stage cancer patients. *Immunol. Invest.* **32**, 201–215.

Ghoname, E.-S., Craig, W.F., White, P.F., *et al.* (1999) Percutaneous electrical nerve stimulation for low back pain: A randomized crossover study. *JAMA* **281**, 818–823.

Glaus, A. (1998) Fatigue and cachexia in cancer patients. *Support Care Cancer* **6**, 77–78.

Grinberg-Zylberbaum, J., Delaflor, M., Attie, L. and Goswami, A. (1994) The Einstein-Podolsky-Rosen paradox in the brain: The transferred potential. *Physics Essays* **4**, 422–428.

Grontved, A., Brask, T., Kambskard, J. and Hentzer E. (1988) Ginger root against seasickness: A controlled trial on the open sea. *Acta Otolaryngol.* **195**, 45–49.

Grontved, A. and Hentzer, E. (1986) Vertigo-reducing effects of ginger root. A controlled clinical study. *J. Otorhinolaryngol. Relat. Spec.* **48**, 282–286.

Guns, E.S., Goldenberg, S.L. and Brown, P.N. (2002) Mass spectral analysis of PC-SPES confirms the presence of diethylstilbestrol. *Can. J. Urol.* **9**, 1684–1688.

Haker, E., Egekvist, H. and Bjerring, P. (2000) Effect of sensory stimulation (acupuncture) on sympathetic and parasympathetic activities in healthy subjects. *J. Auton. Nerv. Syst.* **79**, 52–59.

Hammar, M., Frisk, J. and Grimas, O. (1999) Acupuncture treatment of vasomotor symptoms in men with prostatic carcinoma: A pilot study. *J. Urol.* **161**, 853–856.

Hammer, L. (1990) *Dragon Rises*; *Red Bird Flies*: *Psychology*, *Energy and Chinese Medicine*. Station Hill Press, Barrytown, NY, USA.

Han, J.S. (1986) Electroacupuncture: An alternative to antidepressants for treating affective diseases. *Int. J. Neurosci.* **29**, 79–92.

Han, S.B., Yoon, Y.D., Ahn, H.J., *et al.* (2003) Toll-like receptor-mediated activation of B cells and macrophages by poysaccharide isolated from cell culture of *Acanthopanax senticosus*. *Int. Immunopharmacol.* **3**, 1301–1312.

Han, S.K., Song, J.Y., Yun, Y.S. and Yi, S.Y. (2005) Ginsan improved Th-1 immune response inhibited by gamma radiation. *Arch. Pharm. Res.* **28**, 343–350.

Hanahan, D. and Weinberg, R.A. (2000) The hallmarks of cancer. *Cell* **100**, 57–70.

Hara, A., Iizuka, N., Hamamoto, Y., *et al.* (2005) Molecular dissection of a medicinal herb with anti-tumor activity by oligonucleotide microarray. *Life Sci.* **77**, 991–1002.

Harris, W.S., Gowda, M., Kolb, J.W., *et al.* (1999) A randomized, controlled trial of the effects of remote, intercessory prayer on outcomes in patients admitted to the coronary care unit. *Arch. Intern. Med.* **159**, 2273–2278.

Hayakawa, K., Mitsuhashi, N., Saito, Y., *et al.* (1997) Effect of Krestin as adjuvant treatment following radical radiotherapy in non-small cell lung cancer patients. *Cancer Detect. Prev.* **21**, 71–77.

Heine, H. and Almer, A.J. (2005) Recognition of bacterial products by Toll-like receptors. In: *Mechanisms of Epithelial Defense. Chemical Immunology and Allergy*, Vol. 86 (eds.) Kabelitz, D. and Schröder, J.-M. Karger, Basel, pp. 99–119.

Hejna, M., Raderer, M. and Zielinski, C.C. (1999) Inhibition of metastases by anticoagulants. *J. Natl. Cancer Inst.* **91**, 22–36.

Hoffmann, T.K., Bier, H. and Whiteside, T.L. (2004) Targeting the immune system: Novel therapeutic approaches in squamous cell carcinoma of the head and neck. *Cancer Immunol. Immunother.* **53**, 1055–1067.

Horie, Y., Kato, K., Kameoka, S., *et al.* (1994) Bu ji (hozai) for treatment of postoperative gastric cancer patients. *Am. J. Chin. Med.* **22**, 309–319.

Houghton, J., Stoicov, C., Nomura, S., *et al.* (2004) Gastric cancer originating from bone marrow-derived cells. *Science* **306**, 1568–1571.

Hou, J., Liu, S., Ma, Z., *et al.* (1991) Effects of gynostemma pentaphyllum makino on the immunological function of cancer patients. *J. Tradit. Chin. Med.* **11**, 47–52.

Huali, S., Shaojin, D. and Guiqing, Y. (1994) Free radical mechanism in enhancement of radiosensitization by SRSBR. *J. Tradit. Chin. Med.* **14**, 51–55.

Ikemi, Y. and Ikemi A. (1986) An oriental point of view in psychosomatic medicine. *Psychother. Psychosom.* **45**, 118–126.

Ito, K., Nakazato, H., Koike, A., *et al.* (2004) Long-term effect of 5-fluorouracil enhanced by intermittent administration of polysaccharide K after curative resection of colon cancer. A randomized controlled trial for 7-year follow-up. *Int. J. Colorectal Dis.* **19**, 157–164.

Jacobsen, B.K., Knutsen, S.F. and Fraser, G.E. (1998) Does high soy milk intake reduce prostate cancer incidence? The Adventist Health Study. *Cancer Causes Control* **9**, 553–557.

Jessel-Kenyon, J., Ni, C., Blott, B. and Hopwood, V. (1992) Studies with acupuncture using a SQUID bio-magnetometer: A preliminary report. *Complement. Med. Res.* **6**, 142–151.

Jessop, D.S. (1998) Beta-endorphin in the immune system: Mediator of pain and stress? *Lancet* **351**, 1828–1829.

Jin, R., Wan, L.L., Mitsuishi, T., *et al.* (1994) Effect of shi-ka-ron and Chinese herbs on cytokine production of macrophage in immunocompromised mice. *Am. J. Chin. Med.* **22**, 255–266.

Johnstone, P.A., Peng, Y.P., May, B.C., *et al.* (2001) Acupuncture for pilocarpine-resistant xerostomia following radiotherapy for head and neck malignancies. *Int. J. Radiat. Oncol. Biol. Phys.* **50**, 353–357.

Jovanovic-Ignjatic, Z. and Rakovic, D. (1999) A review of current research in microwave resonance therapy: Novel opportunities in medical treatment. *Acupunct. Electrother. Res.* **24**, 105–125.

Kaegi, E. (1998) Unconventional therapies for cancer: Green tea. *CMAJ* **158**, 1033–1035.

Kamat, A.M. and Lamm, D.L. (1999) Chemoprevention of urological cancer. *J. Urol.* **161**, 1748–1760.

Kanazawa, M., Mori, Y., Yoshihara, K., *et al.* (2004) Effect of PSK on the maturation of dendritic cells derived from human peripheral blood monocytes. *Immunol. Lett.* **91**, 229–238.

Kang, K., Kang, B., Lee, B., Che, J., Li, G., Trosko, J.E. and Lee, Y. (2000) Preventive effect of epicatechin and ginsenoside Rb(2) on the inhibition of gap junctional intercellular communication by TP and H(2)O(2). *Cancer Lett.* **152**, 97–106.

Kawakita, T., Nakai, S., Kumazawa, Y., Miura, O., Yumioka, E. and Nomoto K. (1990) Induction of interferon after administration of traditional Chinese medicine, xiao-chai-hu-tang (shosaiko-to). *Int. J. Immunopharmacol.* **12**, 515–521.

Keating, A. and Chez, R.A. (2002) Ginger syrup as an antiemetic in early pregnancy. *Altern. Ther. Health Med.* **8**, 89–91.

Kebudi, R., Ayan, I., Darendeliler, E., *et al.* (1995) Immunologic status in children with brain tumors and the effect of therapy. *J. Neurooncol.* **24**, 219–227.

Kerbel, R.S. and Kamen, B.A. (2004) The anti-angiogenic basis of metronomic chemotherapy. *Nat. Rev. Cancer* **4**, 423–436.

Kerr, F.W.L., Wilson, P.R. and Nijensohn, D.E. (1978) Acupuncture reduces the trigeminal evoked response in decerebrate cats. *Exp. Neurol.* **61**, 84–95.

Key, T.J., Sharp, G.B., Appleby, P.N., *et al.* (1999) Soya foods and breast cancer risk: A prospective study in Hiroshima and Nagasaki, Japan. *Br. J. Cancer* **81**, 1248–1256.

Kim, H., Peterson, T.G. and Barnes, S. (1998) Mechanisms of action of the soy isoflavone genistein: Emerging role for its effects via transforming growth factor beta signaling pathways. *Am. J. Clin. Nutr.* **68**, 1418S–1425S.

Kleijnen, J. and Knipschild, P. (1992) Gingko biloba. *Lancet* **340**, 1136–1139.

Koda, K., Miyazaki, M., Sarashina, H., *et al.* (2003) A randomized controlled trial of postoperative adjuvant immunochemotherapy for colorectal cancer with oral medicines. *Int. J. Oncol.* **23**, 165–172.

Kodama, N., Asakawa, A., Inui, A., Masuda, Y. and Nanba, H. (2005a) Enhancement of cytotoxicity of NK cells by D-Fraction, a polysaccharide from *Grifola frondosa*. *Oncol. Rep.* **13**, 497–502.

Kodama, N., Murata, Y., Asakawa, A., *et al.* (2005b) Maitake D-Fraction enhances anti-tumor effects and reduces immunosuppression by mitomycin-C in tumor-bearing mice. *Nutrition* **21**, 624–629.

Kodama, N., Komuta, K. and Nanba, H. (2002) Can Maitake MD-fraction aid cancer patients? *Altern. Med. Rev.* **7**, 236–239.

Kodama, N., Komuta, K. and Nanba, H. (2003) Effect of Maitake (*Grifola frondosa*) D-fraction on the activation of NK cells in cancer patients. *J. Med. Food* **6**, 371–377.

Kosko, B. and Isaka, S. (1993) Fuzzy logic. *Sci. Am.* **July**, 76–81.

Koski, G.K. and Czerniecki, B.J. (2005) Combining innate immunity with radiation therapy for cancer treatment. *Clin. Cancer Res.* **11**, 7–11.

Koukourakis, M.I., Ktenidou-Kartali, S., Bourikas, G., Kartalis, G. and Tsatalas, C. (2003) Amifostine protects lymphocytes during radiotherapy and stimulates expansion of the CD95/Fas and CD31 expressing T-cells, in breast cancer patients. *Cancer Immunol. Immunother.* **52**, 127–131.

Kumar, A., Tandon, O.P., Dam, S., Bhattacharya, A. and Tyagi, K.K. (1994) Brainstem auditory evoked response changes following electro-acupuncture therapy in chronic pain patients. *Anaesthesia* **49**, 387–390.

Kuo, M.-C., Weng, C.-Y., Ha, C.-L. and Wu, M.-J. (2006) *Ganoderma lucidum* mycelia enhance innate immunity by activating NF-kappaB. *J. Ethnopharmacol.* **103**, 217–222.

Langevin, H.M. and Yandow, J.A. (2002) Relationship of acupuncture points and meridians to connective tissue planes. *Anat. Rec.* **269**, 257–265.

Langevin, H.M., Churchill, D.L. and Cipolla, M.J. (2001) Mechanical signaling through connective tissue: A mechanism for the therapeutic effect of acupuncture. *FASEB J.* **15**, 2275–2282.

Lao, B.H., Ruckle, H.C., Botolazzo, T. and Lui, P.D. (1994) Chinese medicinal herbs inhibit growth of murine renal cell carcinoma. *Cancer Biother.* **9**, 153–161.

Lebeau, B., Chastang, C., Brechot, J.M., *et al.* (1994) Subcutaneous heparin treatment increases survival in small cell lung cancer. *Cancer* **74**, 38–45.

Lee, A. and Done, M.L. (1999) The use of non-pharmacologic techniques to prevent postoperative nausea and vomiting: A meta-analysis. *Anesth. Analg.* **88**, 1362–1369.

Lee, C.T. and Wei, L.Y. (1983) Spectrum analysis of human pulse. *IEEE Trans. Biomed. Eng.* **30**(6), 348–352.

Lee, H., Schmidt, K. and Ernst, E. (2005) Acupuncture for the relief of cancer-related pain: A systematic review. *Eur. J. Pain* **9**, 437–444.

Lee, K.-T., Johnke, R.M., Allison, R.R., *et al.* (2005) Radioprotective potential of ginseng. *Mutagenesis* **20**, 237–243.

Lee, Y.-N., Lee, H.-Y., Chung, H.-Y., *et al.* (1996) *In vitro* induction of differentiation by ginsenosides in F9 teratocarcinoma cells. *Eur. J. Cancer* **32A**, 1420–1428.

Levy, S.M. and Wise, B.D. (1987) Psychosocial risk factors, natural immunity, and cancer progression: Implications for intervention. *Curr. Psychol. Res. Rev.* **6**, 229–243.

Li, N.Q. (1992) Clinical and experimental study on shen-qi injection with chemotherapy in the treatment of malignant tumor of digestive tract. *Chung Kuo Chung Hsi I Chieh Ho Tsa Chih* **12**, 588–592.

Li, Y., Bhuiyan, M. and Sarkar, F.H. (1999a) Induction of apoptosis and inhibition of c-erbB-2 in MDA-MB-435 cells by genistein. *Int. J. Oncol.* **15**, 525–533.

Li, Y., Upadhyay, S., Bhuiyan, M. and Sarkar, F.H. (1999b) Induction of apoptosis in breast cancer cells MDA-MB-231 by genistein. *Oncogene* **18**, 3166–3172.

Liang, H.L., Xue, C.C. and Li, C.G. (2004) Regression of squamous cell carcinoma of the lung by Chinese herbal medicine: A case with an 8-year follow-up. *Lung Cancer* **43**, 355–360.

Lim, T.S., Na, K., Choi, E.M., Chung, J.Y. and Hwang, J.K. (2004) Immunomodulating activities of polysaccharides isolated from panax ginseng. *J. Med. Food* **7**, 1–6.

Lin, S.Y., Liu, L.M. and Wu, L.C. (1995) Effects of Shenmai injection on immune function in stomach cancer patients after chemotherapy. *Chung Kuo Chung His I Chieh Ho Tsa Chih* **15**, 451–453.

Lin, Z.-B. (2005) Cellular and molecular mechanisms of immuno-modulation by *Ganoderma lucidum*. *J. Pharmacol. Sci.* **99**, 144–153.

Lindequist, U., Niedermeyer, T.H.J. and Julich, W.D. (2005) The pharmacological potential of mushrooms. *Evid. Based Complement. Altern. Med.* **2**, 285–299.

Ling, H.Y., Wang, N.Z. and Zhu, H.Z. (1989) Preliminary study of traditional Chinese medicine-Western medicine treatment of patients with primary liver carcinoma. *Chung Hsi I Chieh Ho Tsa Chih* **9**, 348–349.

Lissoni, P., Paulorossi, F., Tancini, G., *et al.* (1996) Is there a role for melatonin in the treatment of neoplastic cachexia? *Eur. J. Cancer* **32A**, 1340–1343.

Liu, L.J., Guo, C.J. and Jiao, X.M. (1995) Effect of acupuncture on immuno-logic function and histopathology of transplanted mammary cancers in mice. *Chung Kuo Chung His I Chieh Ho Tsa Chih* **15**, 615–617.

Lu, L.J., Cree, M., Josyula, S., Nagamani, M., Grady, J.J. and Anderson, K.E. (2000) Increased urinary excretion of 2-hydroxyestrone but not 16alpha-hydroxyestrone in premenopausal women during a soya diet containing isoflavones. *Cancer Res.* **60**, 1299–1305.

Macek, C. (1984) East meets West to balance immunologic yin and yang. *JAMA* **251**, 433–441.

Maier, H., Daniel, V., Heimlich, S., Frank, C. and Opelz, G. (1995) Cellular immune defect caused by postoperative radiation in patients with squamous epithelial carcinomas of the upper aerodigestive tract. *HNO* **43**, 364–370.

Mansky, P., Sannes, T., Wallerstedt, D., *et al.* (2006) Tai chi chuan: Mind-nody practice or exercise intervention? Studying the benefit for cancer survivors. *Integr. Cancer Ther.* **5**, 192–201.

Massion, A.O., Teas, J. and Hebert, J.R., Wertheimer, M.D. and Kabat-Zinn, J. (1995) Meditation, melatonin and breast/prostate cancer: Hypothesis and preliminary data. *Med. Hypotheses* **44**, 39–46.

McCraty, R., Atkinson, M., Tiller, W.A., Rein, G. and Watkins, A.D. (1995) The effects of emotions on short-term power spectrum analysis of heart rate variability. *Am. J. Cardiol.* **76**, 1089–1092.

McCulloch, M., See, C., Shu, X.J., *et al.* (2006) Astragalus-based Chinese herbs and platinum-based chemotherapy for advanced non-small-cell lung cancer: A meta-analysis of randomized trials. *J. Clin. Oncol.* **24**, 419–430.

McKenna, D.J., Hughes, K. and Jones K. (2000) Green tea monograph. *Altern. Ther. Health Med.* **6**, 61–84.

Meares, A. (1978) Regression of osteogenic sarcoma metastases associated with intensive meditation. *Med. J. Aust.* **2**, 433.

Milosevic, M.F., Fyles, A.W. and Wong, R., *et al.* (1998) Interstitial fluid pressure in cervical carcinoma. Within tumor heterogeneity, and relation to oxygen tension. *Cancer* **82**, 2418–2426.

Minev, B.R. (2002) Melanoma vaccines. *Semin. Oncol.* **29**, 479–493.

Mitomi, T., Tsuchiya, S., Iijima, N., *et al.* (1992) Randomized, controlled study on adjuvant immunochemotherapy with PSK in curatively resected colorectal cancer. The Cooperative Study Group of Surgical Adjuvant Immunochemotherapy for Cancer of Colon and Rectum (Kanagawa). *Dis. Colon Rectum* **35**, 123–130.

Miyazaki, K., Mizutani, H., Katabuchi, H., *et al.* (1995) Activated (HLA-DR+) T-lymphocyte subsets in cervical carcinoma and effects of radiotherapy and immunotherapy with sizofiran on cell mediated immunity and survival. *Gynecol. Oncol.* **56**, 412–420.

Mowrey, D.B. and Clayson, D.E. (1982) Motion sickness, ginger, and psychophysics. *Lancet* **i**, 655–657.

Moyad, M.A. (1999) Soy, disease prevention, and prostate cancer. *Semin. Urol. Oncol.* **17**, 97–102.

Munemoto, Y., Iida, Y., Abe, J., *et al.* (2002) Significance of postoperative adjuvant immunochemotherapy after curative resection of colorectal cancers: Association between host or tumor factors and survival. *Int. J. Oncol.* **20**, 403–411.

Nakazato, H., Koike, A., Saji, S., *et al.* (1994) Efficacy of immunochemotherapy as adjuvant treatment after curative resection of gastric cancer. Study Group of Immunochemotherapy with PSK for Gastric Cancer. *Lancet* **343**, 1122–1126.

Nadeau, R. and Kafatos, M. (2000) *The Non-local Universe: The New Physics and Matters of the Mind*. Oxford University Press, Oxford, UK.

NIH Consensus Development Panel on Acupuncture (1998) Acupuncture. *JAMA* **280**, 1518–1524.

Ning, C.H., Wang, G.M., Zhao, T.Y., Yu, G.Q. and Duan, F.W. (1988) Therapeutic effects of jian piyi shen prescription on the toxicity reactions of postoperative chemotherapy in patients with advanced gastric carcinoma. *J. Tradit. Chin. Med.* **8**, 113–116.

Nutt, D. (1998) Substance-P antagonists: A new treatment for depression? *Lancet* **352**, 1644–1645.

Ogoshi, K., Satou, H., Isono, K., *et al.* (1995) Immunotherapy for esophageal cancer. A randomized trial in combination with radiotherapy and radiochemotherapy. Cooperative Study Group for Esophageal Cancer in Japan. *Am. J. Clin. Oncol.* **18**, 216–222.

Oh, W.K., Kantoff, P.W., Weinberg, V., *et al.* (2004) Prospective, multicenter randomized Phase II trial of the herbal supplement: PC-SPES, and diethylstibestrol in patients with androgen-independent prostate cancer. *J. Clin. Oncol.* **22**, 3705–3712.

Ohwada, S., Ikeya, T., Yokomori, T., *et al.* (2004) Adjuvant immunochemotherapy with oral Tegafur/Uracil plus PSK in patients with stage II or III colorectal cancer: A randomised controlled study. *Br. J. Cancer* **90**, 1003–1010.

Olson, K. and Hanson, J. (1997) Using Reiki to manage pain: A preliminary report. *Cancer Prev. Control* **1**, 108–113.

Ooi, V.E. and Liu, F. (2000) Immunomodulation and anti-cancer activity of polysaccharide-protein complexes. *Curr. Med. Chem.* **7**, 715–729.

Orsi, A.J., McCorkle, R., Tax, A.W., *et al.* (1996) The relationship between depressive symptoms and immune status phenotypes in patients undergoing surgery for colorectal cancer. *Psycho-Oncology* **5**, 311–319.

Page, G.G. and Ben-Eliyahu, S. (1997) The immune-suppressive nature of pain. *Semin. Oncol. Nurs.* **13**, 10–15.

Patel, M., Gutzwiller, F., Paccaud, F. and Marazzi, A. (1989) A meta-analysis of acupuncture for chronic pain. *Int. J. Epidemiol.* **18**, 900–906.

Peigen, K., Yi, T. and Yaping, T. (1996) Radix salviae miltiorrhizae treatment results in decreased lipid peroxidation in reperfusion injury. *J. Tradit. Chin. Med.* **16**, 138–142.

Pennisi, E. (1997) Tracing molecules that make the brain-body connection. *Science* **275**, 930–931.

Pert, C.B., Dreher, H.E. and Ruff, M.R. (1998) The psychosomatic network: Foundations of mind-body medicine. *Altern. Ther. Health Med.* **4**, 30–41.

Petti, F., Bangrazi, A., Liguori, A., Reale, G. and Ippoliti, F. (1998) Effects of acupuncture on immune response related to opioid-like peptides. *J. Tradit. Chin. Med.* **18**, 55–63.

Pomeranz, B. and Niznik, G. (1987) Codetron: A new electrotherapy device overcomes the habituation problems of conventional TENS devices. *Am. J. Electromed.* **2**, 22–26.

Quella, S.K., Loprinzi, C.L., Barton, D.L., *et al.* (2000) Evaluation of soy phytoestrogens for the treatment of hot flashes in breast cancer survivors: A North Central Cancer Treatment Group Trial. *J. Clin. Oncol.* **18**, 1068–1074.

Quizi, S. and Li, Z. (1988) A clinical observation of Qigong as a therapeutic aid for advanced cancer patients. In: *First World Conference for Academic Exchange of Medical Qigong*, Beijing (Abstract).

Rabin, B.S. (1999) *Stress, Immune Function, and Health: The Connection*. Wiley-Liss, New York, USA.

Rafii, S. and Lyden, D. (2003) Therapeutic stem and progenitor cell transplantation for organ vascularization and regeneration. *Nat. Med.* **9**, 702–712.

Ramirez, A.J., Craig, T.K.J., Watson, J.P., *et al.* (1989) Stress and relapse of breast cancer. *Br. Med. J.* **298**, 291–293.

Rao, X.Q., Yu, R.C. and Zhang, J.H. (1991) Sheng xue tang on immunological functions of cancer patients with spleen-deficiency syndrome. *Chung Hsi I Chieh Ho Tsa Chih* **1**, 218–219.

Rapgay, L., Rinpoche, V.L. and Jessum, R. (2000) Exploring the nature and functions of the mind: A Tibetan Buddhist meditative perspective. *Prog. Brain Res.* **122**, 507–515.

Rezaei, N. (2006) Therapeutic targeting of pattern-recognition receptors. *Int. Immunopharmacol.* **6**, 863–869.

Riess, J. and Abbas, J.J. (2000) Adaptive neural network control of cyclic movements using functional neuromuscular stimulation. *IEEE Trans. Rehabil. Eng.* **8**, 42–52.

Rosa, L., Rosa, E., Sarner, L. and Barrett, S. (1998) A close look at therapeutic touch. *JAMA* **279**, 1005–1008.

Roschke, J., Wolf, C., Muller, M.J., *et al.* (2000) The benefit from whole body acupuncture in major depression. *J. Affect. Disord.* **57**, 73–81.

Roscoe, J.A., Matteson, S.E., Mustian, K.M., Padmanaban, D. and Morrow, G.R. (2005) Treatment of radiotherapy-induced fatigue through a non-pharmacological approach. Integr. *Cancer Ther.* **4**, 8–13.

Roscoe, J.A., Matteson, S.E., Morrow, G.R., *et al.* (2005) Acustimulation wrist bands are not effective for the control of chemotherapy-induced nausea in women with breast cancer. *J. Pain Symptom Manage.* **29**, 376–384.

Rosenberg, Z. (1997) Treating the undesirable effects of radiation and chemotherapy with Chinese medicine. *J. Chin. Med.* **55**, 29–30.

Rubik, B. (1995) Energy medicine and the unifying concept of information. *Altern. Ther. Health Med.* **1**, 71.

Rydholm, M. and Strang, P. (1999) Acupuncture for patients in hospital-based home care suffering from xerostomia. *J. Palliat. Care* **15**, 20–23.

Sagar, S.M., Klassen, G.A., Barclay, K.D., *et al.* (1993) Tumour blood flow: Measurement and manipulation for therapeutic gain. *Cancer Treat. Rev.* **19**, 299–349.

Sagar, S.M., Singh, G., Hodson, D.I. and Whitton, A.C. (1995) Nitric oxide and anti-cancer therapy. *Cancer Treat. Rev.* **21**, 159–181.

Sagar, S.M. (1998) Unproven cancer therapies. *Ann. R. Coll. Physicians Surg Can.* **31**, 160.

Sagar, S.M. (1999) Alternative views on alternative therapies. *CMAJ* **160**, 1697–1698.

Sagar, S.M. (2001) *Restored Harmony: An Evidence-Based Approach for Integrating Traditional Chinese Medicine into Complementary Cancer Care.* Dreaming DragonFly Communications, Hamilton, Ontario, Canada.

Sasada, T., Kimura, M., Yoshida, Y., Kanai, M. and Takabayashi, A. (2003) CD4+,CD25+ Regulatory T cells in patients with gastrointestinal malignancies: Possible involvement of regulatory T cells in disease progression. *Cancer* **98**, 1089–1099.

Sato, T., Yu, Y., Guo, S.Y., Kasahara, T. and Hisamitsu, T. (1996) Acupuncture stimulation enhances splenic natural killer cell cytotoxicity in rats. *Jpn. J. Physiol.* **46**, 131–136.

Scambia, G., Mango, D., Signorile, P.G., *et al.* (2000) Clinical effects of a standardized soy extract in postmenopausal women: A pilot study. *Menopause* **7**, 105–111.

Schipper, H., Goh, C.R. and Wang, T.L. (1995) Shifting the cancer paradigm: Must we kill to cure? *J. Clin. Oncol.* **13**, 801–807.

Schlager, A., Offer, T. and Baldissera, I. (1998) Laser stimulation of acupuncture point P6 reduces postoperative vomiting in children undergoing strabismus surgery. *Br. J. Anaesth.* **81**, 529–532.

Schepetkin, I.A. and Quinn, M.T. (2006) Botanical polysaccharides: Macrophage immunomodulation and therapeutic potential. *Int. Immunopharmacol.* **6**, 317–333.

Schwartz, G.E.R. and Russek, L.G.S. (1999) *The Living Energy Universe.* Hampton Roads, Charlottesville, VA, USA.

Sen, G., Khan, A.Q., Chen, Q. and Snapper, C.M. (2005) *In vivo* humoral immune responses to the isolated pneumococcal polysaccharides are dependent on the presence of associated TLR ligands. *J. Immunol.* **175**, 3084–3091.

Sersa, G., Stabuc, B., Cemazar, M., Miklavcic, D. and Rudolf, Z. (2000) Electrochemotherapy with cisplatin: Clinical experience in malignant melanoma patients. *Clin. Cancer Res.* **6**, 863–867.

Seto, A., Kusaka, C., Nakazato, S., *et al.* (1992) Detection of extraordinary large bio-magnetic field strength from human hand. *Acupunct. Electro. Ther. Res. Inst. J.* **17**, 75–94.

Shah, S., Ogden, A.T., Pettker, C.M., *et al.* (1999) A study of energy healing on *in vitro* tumor cell proliferation. *J. Altern. Complement. Med.* **5**, 359–365.

Shao, B.-M., Dai, H., Xu, W., Lin, Z.-B. and Gao, X.-M. (2004a) Immune receptors for polysaccharides from *Ganoderma lucidum. Biochem. Biophys. Res. Comm.* **323**, 133–141.

Shao, B.-M., Xu, W., Dai, H., *et al.* (2004b) A study on the immune receptors for polysaccharides from the roots of *Astragalus membranaceus*, a Chinese medicinal herb. *Biochem. Biophys. Res. Comm.* **320**, 1103–1111.

Shekelle, R.B., Raynor, W.J., Ostfeld, A.M., *et al.* (1981) Psychological depression and 17-year risk of death from cancer. *Psychosom. Med.* **43**, 117–125.

Shen, J., Wenger, N., Glaspy, J., *et al.* (2000) Electroacupuncture for control of myeloablative chemotherapy-induced emesis: A randomized controlled trial. *JAMA* **284**, 2755–2761.

Shin, J.Y., Song, J.Y., Yun, Y.S., *et al.* (2002) Immunostimulating effects of acidic polysaccharides extract of panax ginseng on macrophage function. *Immunopharmacol. Immunotoxicol.* **24**, 469–482.

Shin, H.J., Kim, Y.S., Kwak, Y.S., *et al.* (2004) Enhancement of anti-tumor effects of paclitaxel (taxol) in combination with red ginseng acidic polysaccharide (RGAP). *Planta Med.* **70**, 1033–1038.

Shin, H.-S., Johng, H.-M., Lee, B.-C., *et al.* (2005) Feulgen reaction study of novel threadlike structures (Bonghan Ducts) on the surfaces of mammalian organs. *Anat. Rec. B New Anat.* **284B**, 35–40.

Shoemaker, M., Hamilton, B., Dairkee, S.H., Cohen, I. and Campbell, M.J. (2005) *In vitro* anti-cancer activity of twelve Chinese medicicinal herbs. *Phytother. Res.* **19**, 649–651.

Shu, X., McCulloch, M., Xiao, H., Broffman, M. and Gao, J. (2005) Chinese herbal medicine and chemotherapy in the treatment of heaptocellular carcinoma: A meta-analysis of randomized controlled trials. *Integr. Cancer Ther.* **4**, 219–229.

Sisken, B.F. and Walder, J. (1995) Therapeutic aspects of electromagnetic fields for soft tissue healing. In: Electromagnetic fields: Biological inter-actions and mechanisms, *Advances in Chemistry Series* (ed.) Blank, M. American Chemical Society, pp. 277–285.

Song, L.Z.Y.X., Schwartz, G.E.R. and Russekm, L.G.S. (1998) Heart-focused attention and heart-brain synchronization: Energetic and physiological mechanisms. *Altern. Ther. Health Med.* **4**, 44–62.

Spiegel, D., Bloom, J.R., Kraemer, H.C. and Gottheil, E. (1989) Effect of psychosocial treatment on survival of patients with metastatic breast cancer. *Lancet* **ii**, 888–891.

Stener-Victorin, E., Waldenstrom, U., Andersson, S.A. and Wikland, M. (1996) Reduction of blood flow impedance in the uterine arteries of infertile women with electro-acupuncture. *Hum. Reprod.* **11**, 1314–1317.

Stephens, F.O. (1999) The rising incidence of breast cancer in women and prostate cancer in men. Dietary influences: A possible preventive role for nature's sex hormone modifiers-the phytoestrogens. *Oncol. Rep.* **6**, 865–870.

Stevenson, F.K. (2005) Update on cancer vaccines. *Curr. Opin. Oncol.* **17**, 573–577.

Stone, P., Richards, M. and Hardy, J. (1998) Fatigue in patients with cancer. *Eur. J. Cancer* **34**, 1670–1676.

Sung, W.H., Chun, J.Y., Cho, C.K., *et al.* (1996) Enhancement of radiation effect by *Gingko biloba* in C3H mouse fibrosarcoma. *Radiother. Oncol.* **41**, 163–167.

Syldona, M. and Rein, G. (1999) The use of DC electrodermal potential measurements and healer's felt sense to assess the energetic nature of qi. *J. Altern. Complement. Med.* **5**, 329–347.

Tagliaferri, M., Cohen, I. and Tripathy, D. (2001) Complementary and alternative medicine in early-stage breast cancer. *Semin. Oncol.* **28**, 121–134.

Taixiang, W., Munro, A.J. and Guanjian, L. (2005) Chinese medical herbs for chemotherapy side effects in colorectal cancer patients. *Cochrane Database Syst. Rev.* **1**, CD004540.

Talal, N., Quinn, J.H. and Daniels, T.E. (1992) The clinical effects of electrostimulation on salivary function of Sjögrens syndrome patients: A placebo controlled study. *Rheumatol. Int.* **12**, 43–45.

Temoshok, L. and Dreher, H. (1992) *The Type C Connection.* Random House, New York, NY, USA.

Temoshok, L. (1985) Biopsychosocial studies on cutaneous malignant melanoma: psychosocial factors associated with prognostic indicators, progression, psychophysiology, and tumor-host response. *Soc. Sci. Med.* **8**, 833–840.

Thomas, D., Collins, S. and Strauss, S. (1992) Somatic sympathetic vasomotor changes documented by medical thermographic imaging during acupuncture analgesia. *Clin. Rheumatol.* **11**, 55–59.

Thompson, J.W. and Filshie, J. (1998) Transcutaneous electrical nerve stimulation (TENS) and acupuncture. In: *Oxford Textbook of Palliative Medicine*, 2nd ed. (eds.) Doyle, D., Hanks, G.W.C. and MacDonald, N. Oxford University Press, Oxford, UK.

Tiller, W.A. and Pecci, E.F. (1997) *Science and Human Transformations: Subtle Energies, Intentionality and Consciousness*. Pavior, Walnut Creek, CA, USA.

Tode, T., Kikuchi, Y., Kita, T., Hirata, J., Imaizumi, E. and Nagata, I. (1993) Inhibitory effects by oral administration of ginsenoside Rh2 on the growth of human ovarian cancer cells in nude mice. *J. Cancer Res. Clin. Oncol.* **120**, 24–26.

Tran, V.H., Nguyen, B.H., Pham, M.H. and Nguyen, B.D. (2002) Radioprotective effects of Vitexina for breast cancer patients undergoing radiotherapy with cobalt-60. *Integr. Cancer Ther.* **1**, 38–43.

Tsan, M.-F. (2006) Toll-like receptors, inflammation and cancer. *Semin. Cancer Biol.* **16**, 32–37.

Tsang, K.W., Lam, C.L., Yan, C., *et al.* (2003) *Coriolus versicolor* polysaccharide peptide slows progression of advanced non-small cell lung cancer. *Respir. Med.* **97**, 618–624.

Tukmachi, E. (2000) Treatment of hot flushes in breast cancer patients with acupuncture. *Acupunct. Med.* **18**, 22–27.

Vickers, A.J., Straus, D.J., Fearon, B. and Cassileth, B.R. (2004) Acupuncture for postchemotherapy fatigue: A Phase II study. *J. Clin. Oncol.* **22**, 1731–1735.

Vickers, A.J., Feinstein, M.B., Deng, G.E. and Cassileth, B.R. (2005) Acupuncture for dyspnea in advanced cancer: A randomized, placebo-controlled pilot trial. *BMC Palliat. Care* **4**, 5.

Vucković-Deki, L.J., Susnjar, S., Stanojević-Baki, N., Rajner, L. and Frim, O. (1992) The protective effect of Thymex L against radiotherapeutically-induced cellular immunodepression in lung cancer aptients. *Neoplasma* **39**, 171–176.

Walleczek, J. (1992) Electromagnetic field effects on cells of the immune system: The role of calcium signalling. *FASEB J.* **6**, 3177–3185.

Wang, G.T. (1990) Treatment of operated late gastric carcinoma with prescription of strengthening the patient's resistance and dispelling the invading evil in combination with chemotherapy: Follow-up study of 158 patients and experimental study in animals. *Chung Hsi I Chieh Ho Tsa Chih* **10**, 712–716.

Wang, J.Z., Tsumara, H., Shimura, K. and Ito, H. (1992) Anti-tumor activity of polysaccharide from Chinese medicinal herb, *Acanthopanax giraldii* harms. *Cancer Lett.* **65**, 79–84.

Wardell, D.W. and Weymouth, K.F. (2004) Review of studies of healing touch. *J. Nurs. Scholarsh.* **36**, 147–154.

Watkins, A.D. (1995) Perceptions, emotions and immunity: An integrated homoeostatic network. *Q. J. Med.* **88**, 283–294.

Watkins, A.D. (1996) Intention and the electromagnetic activity of the heart. *Adv. J. Mind-Body Health* **12**, 35–36.

Watson, M., Haviland, J.S., Greer, S., Davidson, J. and Bliss, J.M. (1999) Influence of psychological response on survival in breast cancer: A population-based cohort study. *Lancet* **354**, 1331–1336.

White, P., Lewith, G., Hopwood, V. and Prescott, P. (2003) The placebo needle, is it a valid and convincing placebo for use in acupuncture trials? A randomised, single-blind, cross-over pilot trial. *Pain* **106**, 401–409.

Whiteside, L.T. (2006) Immune suppression in cancer: Effects on immune cells, mechanisms and future therapeutic intervention. *Semin Cancer Biol.* **16**, 3–15.

Wichmann, M.W., Meyer, G., Adam, M., *et al.* (2003) Detrimental immunologic effects of preoperative chemoradiotherapy in advanced rectal cancer. *Dis. Colon Rectum* **46**, 875–887.

Widerstrom-Noga, E., Dyrehag, L.E., Borglum-Jensen, L., *et al.* (1998) Pain threshold responses to two different modes of sensory stimulation in patients with orofacial muscular pain: Psychological considerations. *J. Orofac. Pain* **12**, 27–34.

Winstead-Fry, P. and Kijek, J. (1999) An integrative review and meta-analysis of therapeutic touch research. *Altern. Ther. Health Med.* **5**, 58–62.

Witte, J.S., Ursin, G., Siemiatycki, J., *et al.* (1997) Diet and premenopausal bilateral breast cancer: A case control study. *Breast Cancer Res. Treat.* **42**, 243–251

Wong, C.K., Tse, P.S., Wong, E.L., *et al.* (2004) Immunomodulatory effects of yun zhi and danshen capsules in healthy subjects: A randomized, double-blind, placebo-controlled, crossover study. *Int. Immunopharmacol.* **4**, 201–211.

Wong, C.K., Bao, Y.X., Wong, E.L., *et al.* (2005) Immunomodulatory activities of Yunzhi and Danshen in post-treatment breast cancer patients. *Am. J. Chin. Med.* **33**, 381–395.

Wong, R. and Sagar, S.M. (2000) The treatment of persistent yawning with acupuncture. *Acupunct. Med.* **18**, 124–126.

Wong, R.K.W., Jones, G.W., Sagar, S.M., Fargas-Babjak, A. and Whelan, T. (2003) A Phases I/II study in the use of acupuncture-like transcutaneous nerve stimulation in the treatment of radiation-induced xerostomia in head and neck cancer patients treated with radical radiotherapy. *Int. J. Radiat. Oncol. Biol. Phys.* **57**, 472–480.

Wong, R. and Sagar, S. (2006) Acupuncture treatment for chemotherapy-induced peripheral neuropath: A case series. *Acupunct. Med.* **24**, 87–91.

Wu, B. (1995) Effect of acupuncture on the regulation of cell-mediated immunity in patients with malignant tumors. *Chen Tzu Yen Chiu* **20**, 67–71.

Wu, B., Zhou, R.X. and Zhou, M.S. (1994) Effect of acupuncture on interleukin-2 level and NK cell immunoactivity of peripheral blood of malignant tumor patients. *Chung Kuo Chung His Chieh Ho Tsa Chih* **14**, 537–539.

Wu, B., Zhou, R.X. and Zhou, M.S. (1996a) Effect of acupuncture on immunomodulation in patients with malignant tumors. *Chung Kuo Chung His Chieh Ho Tsa Chih* **16**, 139–141.

Wu, A.H., Ziegler, R.G., Horn-Ross, P.L., *et al.* (1996b) Tofu and risk of breast cancer in Asian-Americans. *Cancer Epidemiol. Biomarkers Prev.* **5**, 901–906.

Wu, M.T., Hsieh, J.C., Xiong, J., *et al.* (1999) Central nervous pathway for acupuncture stimulation: Localization of processing with functional MR imaging of the brain — preliminary experience. *Radiology* **212**, 133–141.

Xu, G.Z., Cai, W.M., Qin, D.X., *et al.* (1989) Chinese herb "destagnation" series I: Combination of radiation with destagnation in the treatment of nasopharyngeal carcinoma (NPC): A prospective randomized trial on 188 cases. *Int. J. Radiat. Oncol. Biol. Phys.* **16**, 297–300.

Yan, L. (1988) Treatment of persistent hiccupping with electro-acupuncture at "hiccup-relieving" point. *J. Tradit. Chin. Med.* **8**, 29–30.

Yance, D.R. and Sagar, S.M. (2006) Targeting angiogenesis with integrative cancer therapies. *Integrat. Cancer Ther.* **5**, 9–29.

Yang, C.S. and Wang, Z.-Y. (1993) Tea and cancer. *J. Natl. Cancer Inst.* **85**, 1038–1049.

Yang, G., Liu, J., Xie, J., *et al.* (1995) Controlling cancerous pain with analgesic powders for cancers. *J. Tradit. Chin. Med.* **15**, 174–177.

Yang, J., Zhao, R., Yuan, J., *et al.* (1994) The experimental study of prevention and treatment of the side-effects of chemotherapy with acupuncture. *Chen Tzu Yen Chiu* **19**, 75–78.

Yin, D., Tuthill, D., Mufson, R.A. and Shi, Y. (2000) Chronic restraint stress promotes lymphocyte apoptosis by modulating CD95 expression. *JEM* **191**, 1423–1428.

Yonghe, H. (2004) Progress in using combination of Chinese drug with chemotherapy to treat cancer. *J. Tradit. Chin. Med.* **24**, 153–157.

Young, D.R., Appel, L.J., Jee, S.H. and Miller, E.R. (1999) The effects of aerobic exercise and T'ai Chi on blood pressure in older people: Results of a randomized trial. *J. Am. Geriatr. Soc.* **47**, 277–284.

Yu, G., Ren, D., Sun, G. and Zhang, D. (1993) Clinical and experimental studies of JPYS in reducing side-effects of chemotherapy in late-stage gastric cancer. *J. Tradit. Chin. Med.* **13**, 31–37.

Yu, R.C., Guan, C.F. and Zhang, J.H. (1990) Immune function of cancer patients with spleen-deficiency syndrome. *Chung Hsi I Chieh Ho Tsa Chih* **10**, 535–537.

Yuan, J. and Zhou, R. (1993) Effect of acupuncture on T-lymphocyte and its subsets from the peripheral blood of patients with malignant neoplasm. *Chen Tzu Yen Chiui* **18**, 174–177.

Yun, T.K. and Choi, S.Y. (1998) Non-organ specific cancer prevention of ginseng: A prospective study in Korea. *Int. J. Epidemiol.* **27**, 359–364.

Zaidman, B.-Z., Yassin, M., Mahajna, J. and Wasser, S.P. (2005) Medicinal mushroom modulators of molecular targets as cancer therapeutics. *Appl. Microbiol. Biotechnol.* **67**, 453–468.

Zeng, F., Hon, C.-C., Sit, W.-H., *et al.* (2005) Molecular characterization of *Coriolus versicolor* PSP-induced apoptosis in human promyelotic leukemic HL-60 cells using cDNA microarray. *Int. J. Oncol.* **27**, 513–523.

Zhang, X., Yuan, Y., Kuang, P., *et al.* (1997) Effect of acupuncture on vasoactive intestinal peptide in ischemic cerebrovascular diseases. *J. Tradit. Chin. Med.* **17**, 289–293.

Zhang, X., Yuan, Y., Kuang, P., *et al.* (1999) Effects of electro-acupuncture on somatostatin and pancreatic polypeptide in ischemic cerebrovascular diseases. *J. Tradit. Chin. Med.* **19**, 54–58.

Zhang, Z. (1987) Effect of acupuncture on 44 cases of radiation rectitis following radiation therapy for carcinoma of the cervix uteri. *J. Tradit. Chin. Med.* **7**, 139–140.

Zhou, J.Q., Li, Z.H. and Jin, P.L. (1999a) A clinical study on acupuncture for prevention and treatment of toxic side-effects during radiotherapy and chemotherapy. *J. Tradit. Chin. Med.* **19**, 16–21.

Zhou, R.F. and Liu, P.X. (2005) Study progress in reversing multidrug resistance to breast cancer with Chinese herbs. *Zhongguo Zhong Yao Za Zhi* **30**, 1797–1800.

Zhou, J.R., Gugger, E.T., Tanaka, T., *et al.* (1999b) Soybean phytochemicals inhibit the growth of transplantable human prostate carcinoma and tumor angiogenesis in mice. *J. Nutr.* **129**, 1628–1635.

Zhou, Y., Wang, Y., Fang, Z., *et al.* (1995) Influence of acupuncture on blood pressure, contents of NE, DA and 5-HT of spontaneously hypertensive rats and the inter-relation between blood pressure and whole blood viscosity. *Chen Tzu Yen Chiu* **20**, 55–61.

Zhu, B.F. (1994) Observation on 17 patients with radio-ulcer with combined traditional Chinese medicine and Western medicine therapy. *Chung Kuo Chung Hsi Chieh Ho Tsa Chih* **14**, 89–91.

Zhu, H. and Zhang, J. (1993) Treatment of stomatological complications in 31 cases of acute leukemia with Chinese herbal drugs. *J. Tradit. Chin. Med.* **13**, 253–256.

Zimmerman, J. (1990) Laying-on-of-hands healing and therapeutic touch: A testable theory. *BEMI Curr. J. Bioelectromagnetics Inst.* **2**, 8–17.

Zonenshayn, M., Mogilner, A.Y. and Rezai, A.R. (2000) Neurostimulation and functional brain imaging. *Neurol. Res.* **22**, 318–325.

Chapter 2

Recent Status and Outlook of Traditional Chinese Medicine in Cancer Treatment

Dai-Han Zhou

Abstract

Traditional Chinese Medicine (TCM) has contributed significantly to the health of the Chinese people; it has participated widely in anti-tumor therapy and has formed a unique field of TCM oncology. This article, which is based on literature review, clinical and basic research, explores the role and efficacy of TCM in cancer treatment, discusses the problems in the development of cancer therapy with TCM, and demonstrates that this field could be developed on the basis of inheritance. In the process of TCM development, the investigation of theory and concept can be divided into stages so as to make it more objective, standardized and quantitative. One should aim at the establishment of an evaluation system to assess the clinical efficacy of TCM cancer therapy by using its own academic characteristics, and TCM oncology could also strive for the combination and integration of TCM with modern technology.

Keywords: Traditional Chinese Medicine; Cancer Treatment; Evaluation.

2.1 Introduction

This article aims at the investigation of the effect and role of traditional Chinese medicine (TCM) in current cancer treatment and explores the development of TCM oncology in the future.

Traditional Chinese medicine has a very long history and because of the concept that "herbal drug and food are of the same origin", many

Chinese food and herbal medicines which are consumed in daily life are also applied in anti-tumor therapies. This wide application of TCM gives a unique pattern of anti-cancer treatment. In China, few people use Western medicine (WM) alone in cancer treatment. A rather large number of patients place their hope on TCM because of the cultural background and, really, quite a few have obtained good clinical results. Clinical practice has proved that TCM has good effects on the delay of tumor growth and for certain cancers, initiates a direct inhibitory effect, improves the quality of life and survival, increases in the effects of radiotherapy or chemotherapy, or decreases their toxic effects. TCM has its advantage in cancer treatment, which has been recognized by both medical practitioners and patients. There is a Chinese folk saying: "The road to happiness is full of hardships." In the clinical practice of cancer treatment or in the medical market, quite a few patients are deceived by inaccurate newspaper articles, medical advertisements or possibly by medical brokers. They encourage people to take functional food or dietary supplementary as chief anti-cancer drugs for long-term use, which results in a waste of a lot of money and delay in proper treatment. Driven by market economy, the "cancer swindlers" (including some so-called scholars, dishonest advertisements, erroneous directions of newspapers and magazines or duplicity with posting of the banner of an academic society) take advantage of the grey region in law, and proceed with illegal sale of "drugs", causing impairment of the reputation of anti-cancer TCM drugs. Medical specialists and academic associations should strengthen popular science education for the public, and the government should strengthen the management according to the regulations, so that TCM in clinical cancer therapy can proceed and develop in the right way.

2.2 Methods

Through literature review, clinical and basic research we use analytical and inductive methods to objectively lay out the present status and inadequacy of TCM in cancer treatment.

TCM treatment of cancer possesses a long history and rich experiences; its academic essence was recorded in the ancient medical books of internal medicine, surgery, gynecology, pediatrics and other specialties.

The clinical diagnosis and treatment guidelines were formed in Han Dynasty and recorded in the book *Treatise on Febrile and Miscellaneous Diseases* (*Shanghan Zabing Lun*); its development was brilliantly displayed by the four famous scholars in the Jin Yuan Dynasty and the surgical specialists in the Ming Dynasty, and its academic characteristics ripened in the Qing Dynasty. Therapeutic techniques on cancer were scattered over the written experiences of surgery, internal medicine, gynecology and of miscellaneous diseases in the folk literature. It was in the mediocre period of the last century that this branch of medicine sprouted from the many clinical fields and formed a new independent clinical branch of TCM. In academic connotations, it requires prompt strengthening and perfection. For thousands of years, the experiences of TCM treatment in cancer were scattered among the vast territory of ancient literatures and in the inheritance among families of herbal practitioners. The wide application of TCM formed a unique pattern of Chinese anti-cancer therapy and promoted the development of TCM oncology. This TCM oncology covers tumor etiology, pathogenesis, early diagnosis, prognostic evaluation, clinical treatment, convalescent therapy, new TCM anti-cancer drug preparation, mechanism research of anti-cancer TCM drugs, research of TCM therapeutic principles, the literature review and study of ancient TCM books and recorded tumor cases. Through the experiences of TCM cancer treatment over several thousand years, we can see that TCM was entrusted with the task of treating tumors and its complications after surgical operations, increasing the effectiveness and lowering of toxicity in chemotherapy and radiotherapy, and the increase of body resistance and consolidation of patients' constitution in the late stages of cancer. However, there are divergent standards of clinical research in China, so the objectives and research methodology of anti-cancer herbs still have to be improved; the problem of having no standard treatment for cancer patients should not be ignored.

2.3 Results

From the recent status of clinical applications, we can see that the majority of our patients prefer the TCM-WM combined therapy or the use of TCM drugs as the chief treatment option. Individualized syndrome differentiation are adopted by most TCM practitioners in the vast rural basic medical units, who prescribe drugs according to different symptoms. Herbal drug decoctions are taken orally, a treatment method that is simple, low in cost and easily accepted by patients. There are TCM treatments that are combined with modern therapeutic measures, but such combination approaches can only be applied in hospitals. Patients usually obtain clinical or pathological diagnosis in hospitals and if they are weak after an operation, physicians give them adequate convalescent treatment. Treatments to increase the effect of radiotherapy or to lower the toxicity of chemotherapy are also available to patients. For patients in the late stages of cancer, TCM therapy can also be administered, especially for the in-patients of hospitals or out-patients whose tumor masses are comparatively large or have shown metastasis. At this stage, these patients are weak and the measures of modern medicine are difficult to suppress the cancer. Treatment, therefore, chiefly aims at alleviating the symptoms, improving quality of life and prolonging the survival time in the presence of tumors. Research on the development of Class I and Class II new anti-cancer drugs or on adjuvant treatment of radiotherapy and chemotherapy with Class III and Class IV new drugs is ongoing. Investigations of new drugs are usually carried in universities, clinical research centers or State clinical research bases for new drug evaluation where well-designed clinical trial and quality of the study medication make the results more reliable. However, for new drug development, the financial input is comparatively greater, and thus no more TCM drugs are developed in this manner. In general, the number of patients who benefited from this pattern of drug development is low.

In China, over 10,000 TCM drugs, over 50,000 TCM compound formulas, over 3000 TCM drugs and nearly 300 TCM formulas were screened and validated in the anti-cancer activities. It was found that some TCM drugs and preparations had confirmed effectiveness in anti-cancer (including single herbal, herbal formulae, oral liquid or parenteral injections) such as *Liu Shen* pill, *Xi Huang* pill, *Pin Xiao* capsule, *Hechan Pian*, *Huai'er Keli*, *Shen Yi* capsule, *Indigo Naturalis*, Mylabris, *Radix Sophorae Flavescentis*, *Fructus seu Radix Camptothecae Acuminatae*, *Ramulus et Folium Cephalotaxi Fortunei*, *Fructus Bruceae*, Arsenic, *Kang Lai Te* (Coixenolide), Elemene Emulsion, *Ai Di* injection, and so on.

Research of natural drugs from natural sources usually includes the following steps: pharmacological studies, tumor inhibition studies, ingredient analysis, mechanism of action and clinical verification. In the recent decades, the research of anti-cancer TCM drugs, in general, did not deviate from this methodology.

In the development of TCM anti-cancer drugs, complete adoption of WM research methods may lead to the retrogression of efforts because the unique characteristics of TCM are ignored. The soul of traditional Chinese medicine lies in its basic principles and theories. The use of TCM drugs cannot depart from the direction of TCM principles. The characters and functions of Chinese herbal medicines is displayed through the four properties and the five flavors, lifting and lowering, floating and sinking of drug actions, and its influence on the *zang*- and *fu*-organs, channel tropism (such as "supplement *qi*", "nourish *yin*", "activate blood", "purgation", etc.). The investigation of anti-cancer TCM usually starts at the effectiveness of a certain herbal formula. If the research results in the formation of one anti-cancer TCM formula, the TCM principle would be neglected and totally forgotten when applied clinically so that the anti-cancer agents originated from TCM formulae become bodies without soul. These problems lead us to think about the connotations of modernization of TCM. The scientific implication of conventional TCM drugs is revealed in its therapeutic effect, but TCM drugs are different from WM drugs, which are chemically pure. A TCM formula is composed of many herbs and these herbs decocted singly or in combination may vary in ingredients as well as in quantity of the contents. One TCM formula may give off a hundred chemical ingredients and this is why TCM drugs have the character of action on multiple sites, multiple levels and multiple targets. Take the research of *Fructus Bruceae* as an example: this drug was used in ancient times and in folk community to treat intestinal cancer, carcinoma of oesophagus and cervical cancer, and now the *Fructus Bruceae* oil is extracted to form *Fructus Bruceae* emulsion injection for intravenous use or for arterial perfusion to treat digestive system cancer or lung carcinoma. The composition of this herb is complicated; it contains brucamarine, bruceantarin, glucosides (brucealin), organic acid, fatty oil and bitter ingredients which are similar to guassin. The *Fructus Bruceae* oil, water extract and alcohol extract all have anti-cancer effects; in the course of extracting *Fructus Bruceae* emulsion, the amaroid, which has four nigakilactone-like monomers, and also has a comparatively good anti-cancer effect, is discarded. That is to say, the now clinically used *Fructus Bruceae* oil injection does not represent entirely the drug effectiveness of the TCM drug *Fructus Bruceae*. The TCM decocta is time-consuming in preparation and difficult to take, while the preparation of herbal instant powder is convenient to consume and is a good exploration in TCM modernization. But in the process from herb extract to the instant powder, some ingredients may be lost such as pigments, starch and protein, and, in this way, maintenance of its effectiveness is questionable. During the preparation process, when the herbal formula decoction is heated, every herbal ingredient may undergo combination, hydrolysis, aggregation, dissociation, oxidation-reduction reactions with other herbal ingredients in the solution so that the component and the contents are different between the separately decocted and the mixed decocted. An ancient herbal formula is formed according to the "principle of sovereignty, minister, assistant and envoy." These ancient formulae had been used for several thousands of years and the efficacy has been validated. A bowl of bitter decocta may be time-consuming to prepare; however, its effectiveness is reliable. Patients accept this kind of herbal preparation and that is why TCM could pass from generation to generation till today.

A prominent problem in cancer therapy is over-treatment, which means that patients have to accept unnecessary, extra-routine and inefficacious treatment. The main direction of tumor treatment has turned from the 20th century "search and destroy" to the new century, "target and control". But, influenced by the old pattern of treatment, physicians in many hospitals still use non-standard, over-aggressive measures in different degrees. For example, it may be harmful to perform surgical operations for patients with late stage cancer and metastases without life-threatening complications. For some patients, chemotherapy had been performed on tumors under proper indications. After several treatments, the tumors may not be under control yet. However, by this time, the patient has become weak, the bone marrow and multiple organs are damaged. Thus, perseverance of chemotherapy at this stage would only aggravate the deterioration. Moreover, some radio-resistant tumors have shown multiple metastases, therefore enforcement of radiotherapy would undoubtedly add suffering to the patient. While over-treatment may not cause much jeopardy in patients with primary cancer of lower malignancy and longer survival time, however, the harm caused is obvious in those with primary cancer of higher degree of malignancy and relatively short survival time like pulmonary carcinoma, liver carcinoma, or adenocarcinoma of pancreas. This is one instance in which the effects of over-treatment are most disastrous. Repeated use of ineffective over-treatment aggravates damage of visceral organs, lowers the quality of life and shortens the survival time. In China, statistics revealed that 15% of the mortality of late stage cancer had been accelerated by over-treatment and irrational treatment. Over-treatment neglects the human body but pays too much attention to the tumor. It is pitiful that patients are illiterate to medicine so that they still expect recovery of health in spite of the suffering imposed, resulting in early death.

2.4 Discussion

TCM oncology is an old but also young field of medicine. For half a century, the Chinese government has made efforts for the protection and development of TCM, explored and examined the special measures of TCM in cancer treatment as well as discovering the secret formulae for eliminating tumors in the folk community. Due to the wide application of TCM, a special pattern of Chinese anti-cancer treatment is formed and the development of Chinese style oncological sciences is promoted. TCM oncology displays its own characteristics, and at the same time, it develops into a condition that is quantitative, standardized and specified with regulations. Its specific features are still the treatment according to syndrome differentiation and the concept of holism — both are the quintessence of TCM. Treatment according to syndrome differentiation is to apply the theoretical concept, method, formula and drug principles to clinical practice and finally to decide the formula and drugs based on four diagnosis methods and syndrome differentiation of eight principles to clarify the cause of disease, pathogenesis and symptoms and signs. Recently, in the field of clinical research, there is a rapidly developing field named evidence-based medicine (EBM), which is medicine based on evidence.

It stresses on individual experience in clinical practice associated with scientific evidence newly obtained in systemic research, making diagnosis and therapeutic means and methods more effective and safe. The simplicity of treatment according to syndrome differentiation in TCM has substantive similarity with EBM. At the end of the previous century, Chinese medical researchers used the TCM drug arsenic, which had been used in practice for thousands of years, to treat acute promyelocytic leukemia (M3 type) and obtained a complete remission rate of over 93%. This drug was acknowledged as the first choice in treating M3 type leukemia. Arsenic is a highly toxic TCM drug and its heavy metal content is seriously over the standard dosage, but EBM research provided reliable laboratory and clinical evidence and under adequate clinical application, it became an effective anti-cancer drug. The concept of holism acknowledges that the human body is integrated: human body is in union with nature. A regional tumor belongs internally to a certain visceral organ, so that treatment of tumor should vary according to the individual, to time and to the living environment. At present, there are a large number of patients suffering from late stage cancer who are not suitable for operation, chemotherapy or radiotherapy, or who are suffering from relapse of tumor. These patients are seeking for help from TCM. TCM stresses on the support of vital energy (resistant power of the body) and, at the same time, elimination of the causative agents (regional tumors) and considers that the methods of eliminating evil such as chemotherapy and radiotherapy would give harm to the body and vital energy. Restoration of *Yin* and *Yang* balance can decrease the damage given by the tumor to the body. The rising and lowering of the resistant power decisively affects the speed of tumor growth; this explains the special phenomenon that some patients carrying tumor can live longer and have a better quality of life. TCM considers that the basic point in tumor is "toxic expulsion of five visual organs", and "the interior displays itself through the exterior" and therefore, a tumor is a local display of a generalized disease. In *Huangdi Neijing* (*Inner Canon of Huangdi or Yellow Emperor*), it was written "Treatment of disease should aim at the fundamental", so besides paying attention to the tumor, a physician should focus on the whole body that grows the tumor. To avoid over-treating tumors, it is important to adopt the concept of "basing on the human body" and apply treatment that is rational, adequate and standardized.

TCM anti-cancer research should follow the line of thinking that is inherited based on evidence and innovation; it should minimize passive imitation of WM and avoid the increasing tendency of breaking away from its own theory and specific clinical system in the development of anti-cancer TCM drugs.

In 1979, WHO laid down standards for solid tumor treatment and effective rate depending on complete remission (CR) and partial remission (PR), but an obvious drawback was that some survival cases not reaching the standard of CR or PR were not grouped in. In 2000, scholars in Europe, America and Canada established a new evaluation standard for solid tumor treatment (RECIST) (Yi, 2003) and proposed that some steady (SD) cases surviving with tumors in a non-progressive state (PFS) should be evaluated as effective. This promoted a fresh setup for the research of gastrointestinal cancer in Europe. The TCM proposal of survival with tumor is similar to the above PFS standard and the establishment of a TCM standard of treatment in solid tumor became an important work in scientific research, objective evaluation and TCM academic development. Scholars in China have proposed "an evaluation standard for solid tumors in traditional Chinese medicine (draft)" in the book named *Clinical Traditional Chinese Medicine Oncology* (Zhou, 2003). Zhou *et al.* (2005a) conducted a prospective multiple center randomized controlled clinical research to investigate 294 patients with stage III and IV pulmonary carcinoma. Patients were divided into the TCM group (99 cases), taking *Hechan Pian*, *Shen Yi* capsule; WM group (92 cases), taking NVB + DDP; and TCM and WM combination group (103 cases), taking *Hechan Pian*, *Shen Yi* capsule plus NVB and DDP. After treatment, the median survival time and one year accumulated survival rate was 292 days and 45.38%, respectively; 236 days and 42.17%; and 355 days and 48.86%. The quality of life was best in the TCM group, better in combination group and least in the WM group. In the study, the TCM group and WM group were evaluated at the same time by using an evaluation standard for solid tumors in TCM and the RECIST standard, and correlation analysis indicated that there was correlation between the two evaluation methods ($P < 0.01$) (Zhou *et al.*, 2005b), suggesting that the evaluation system of TCM treatment effectiveness in solid tumors is better in revelation of TCM treatment effectiveness than the simple tumor remission rate estimation, and thus, it deserves further investigation. TCM drugs have prominent properties in the delay of tumor development, improvement of quality of life and in prolongation of survival time. It also has a supplementary action with modern anti-cancer and molecular target orientated therapy such as TCM treatment in the relapse of tumor at the original site after liver transplantation, the dredging of channels and cooling of blood therapy in serious skin eruptions secondary to the Iressa or Tarceva therapy, and prevention and treatment of hemorrhagic tendency after Avastin infusion, and these measures contain rich scientific implications. The implicative development of TCM oncology has stepped on a scientific road; treatment according to syndrome differentiation has concrete similarity with evidence-based medicine. Understanding survival with tumor with the concept of holism and the tumor non-progressive survival time (PFS) are two things belonging separately to TCM and WM, but they are actually "reaching the same goal through different routes". We can see the road ahead of TCM anti-cancer research is rough and uneven; it requires much effort and has to go a long way, but the future is brilliant.

References

Yi, J.-L. (2003) Assessment of the guideline of solid tumor therapeutic effects. *Foreign Med. Sci. Clin. Radiol. Fascicle* **26**(5), 330–332.

Zhou, D.-H. (2003) *Clinical Traditional Chinese Medicine Oncology*. People's Medical Publishing House, Beijing, pp. 567–590.

Zhou, D.-H., Lin, L.-Z., Zhon, Y.-G., *et al.* (2005a) Effect of Chinese herbal medicine in prolonging median survival time in patients with non-small-cell lung cancer. *J. Guangzhou Univ. Tradit. Chin. Med.* **22**(4), 255–257.

Zhou, D.-H., Lin, L.-Z. and Tao, Z.-G. (2005b) Traditional Chinese Medicale oncologic evaluation system of response to treatment (TCMOES) in advanced non-small-cell lung cancer. *Zhongyi Zhong Lin* **14**(10), 654–657.

Chapter 3

Chinese Medicine and Cancer Treatment in Hong Kong: A General Review

Ping-Chung Leung, Vincent Ooi, Eliza L.-Y. Wong, Wai-Chun Au, Chun-Kwok Wong, Wai-Kei Lam, Sing-Fai Leung & Tony S.-K. Mok

Abstract

Cancer is a pathological condition. Removal of the cancer is a necessity in the treatment process. However, removal has reached its limitations as the cancer could, in the first place, be too extensive, or, in spite of the removal, recurrence still occurs. When the pathological process is not stopped, no matter how effective is the cancer removal, the formation of cancer is going to be repeated. Cancer treatment has therefore gone beyond the stage of cancer removal and other approaches such as controlling the blood supply, initiating apoptosis, and regulating the responsible genes, are considered important. The treatment approach needs to be modified from a single target, eliminative direction towards a multiple target, holistic direction. Chinese medicine lacks a perfect understanding of the causative pathology, hence it follows a multi-target holistic approach. As new systems of cancer treatment are not yet mature, using Chinese medicine as an adjuvant therapy could be an innovative and practical investment, to bring about better results of cancer control.

Keywords: Traditional Chinese Medicine; Cancer.

3.1 Introduction — Cancer and Ancient Chinese Medicine

Although not documented as cancer in the ancient days, this pathological condition should have been in existence for as long as the human race exists. The word "tumor" (瘤) in Chinese, started to appear in prehistoric cave carvings in North-West China, as far back as 1000BC. The word "tumor" probably referred to the appearance of a lump over some parts of the human body (Bao *et al.*, 2006). Another word (癌), which carried the same literal meaning, appeared around 1200AD. This medical term referred to ulcerative lumps, which were often described together with deformities in the limbs, kyphosis in the spine and occurrences of sinuses and fistulae somewhere in the human body (Li, 1996). Descriptions of treatment related to such tumorous conditions have been scattered, neither systematic nor specialized. When the causative pathology was unclear or not known, clinical presentations described would be mixed, and with regards to treatment, the local appearances would invite policies like those used for infection and inflammation, while the general physiological state of the individual sufferer would provide other basis of treatment. Cancerous conditions were likely to initiate general states of anemia or debilitation, and clues relevant to cancer therapy might also be found under the treatment schemes of these clinical states.

The ancient Chinese healers, therefore, formed three main principles of treatment approach to cancerous conditions. The pathological background was thought to be related to:

(i) toxic internal derangement;
(ii) circulatory stagnation; or
(iii) collapse of defence.

Treatment policy therefore followed the alleged pathological background, so that

(i) toxic derangement was balanced with detoxication through the cooling down of heat;
(ii) circulatory stagnation was removed with the activation of blood movements and resolution of bruises; and
(iii) collapse of defence was rebuilt with the promotion of internal strength.

In addition, the clever ancient healers have observed that toxic material could have controlling effects on cancer growth, hence a system of treatment relying on the use of toxic preparations to counteract toxic derangements was also developed.

3.2 Interest Over the Use of Herbs Against Cancer

Since cytotoxic agents after extensive research appeared on the market as powerful drugs to control cancer growth, the search for new cell-killing items has never stopped. Successful examples demonstrated that powerful cytotoxic material could exist within herbs; like flowers, leaves and tree barks are well shown in the examples of Vincristine from Periwinkle flower, artemisinin from qinghao leaves and taxol from yew tree barks (CNRS, 1999; Kaptchuk and Eisenberg, 1998).

As cytotoxic agents were known to be useful but not ideal because of generalized toxic effects and the readiness of developing drug resistance for some items, research on other mechanisms of cancer control flourished. The prevention of drug resistance, the induction of apoptosis, the blockage of cancer cell messages, the restriction of angiogenesis, and the promotion of immunological defence ability, have all gained extensive attention, and explorations for herbal components with specific cancer control abilities were started. *Rhizome chuanxiang*, *radix stephaniae tetrandrae* and *mylabris phalerate pallus* have been identified for the prevention of cytotoxic drug resistance (Yu *et al.*, 2006). For apoptosis, the ancient formula using arsenic trioxide brought on a breakthrough in childhood leukemia (Zhang *et al.*, 1996); after that, other herbs, *viz. Radix miltiorrhizae* and *Radix Trichosanthis* were found to induce apoptosis of cancer in all cell lines in the laboratory (Liu *et al.*, 2000). A number of herbs were found capable of slowing down cancer cell division by blocking cytokine messages; these were: *Radix Astragalus*, *Radix Angelica* sinuses, *Solani Nigri* and *Radix Puerariae* (Liu *et al.*, 2001b). Angiogenesis is an important facilitating factor for cancer growth. Pharmacological agents on anti-angiogenesis have already been developed and are being sold on the market. Herbs like *Herba Scutellariae Barbatae* (半枝蓮) and *Rhizoma Paridis* (七葉一枝花，重樓) were known to possess anti-angiogenetic properties (Kamata *et al.*, 1993). A lot of work had already been done on the broad front of immunological defence, both in the laboratory and biochemically, on preparations of fungal origin (Wong *et al.*, 1994). One of the most popular fungal product being used in South China as an adjuvant agent during and after cancer treatment, is *Coriolus versicolor*. Frameworks on the study of cytotoxicity, anti-angiogenesis and immunomodulation are represented schematically in Figs. 3.1 to 3.3.

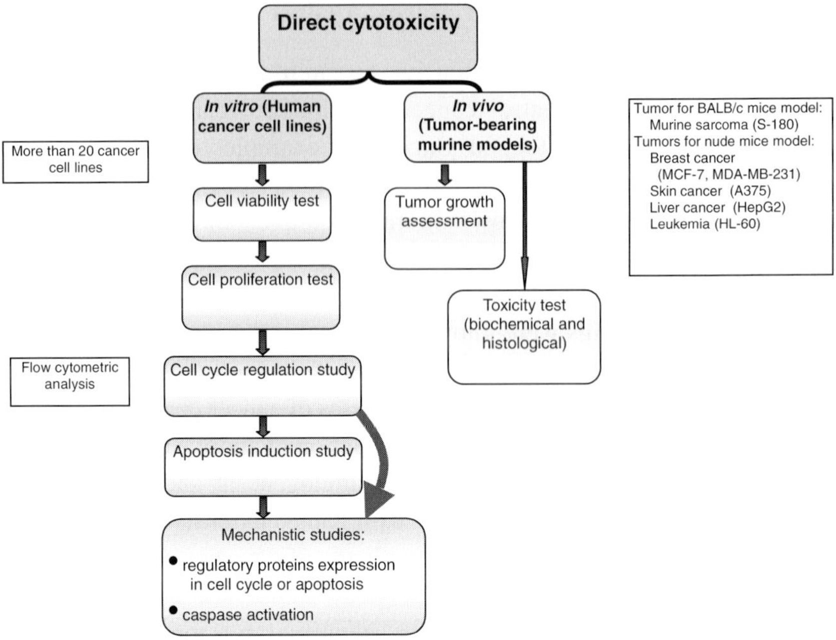

Figure 3.1. Study on cytotoxicity.

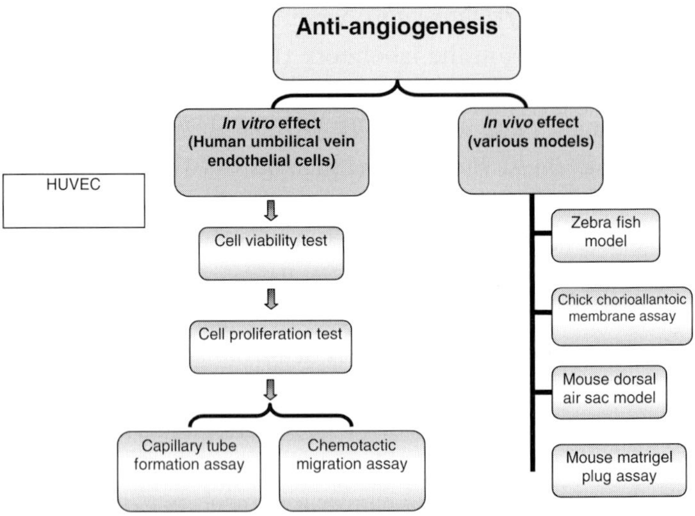

Figure 3.2. Study on anti-angiogenesis.

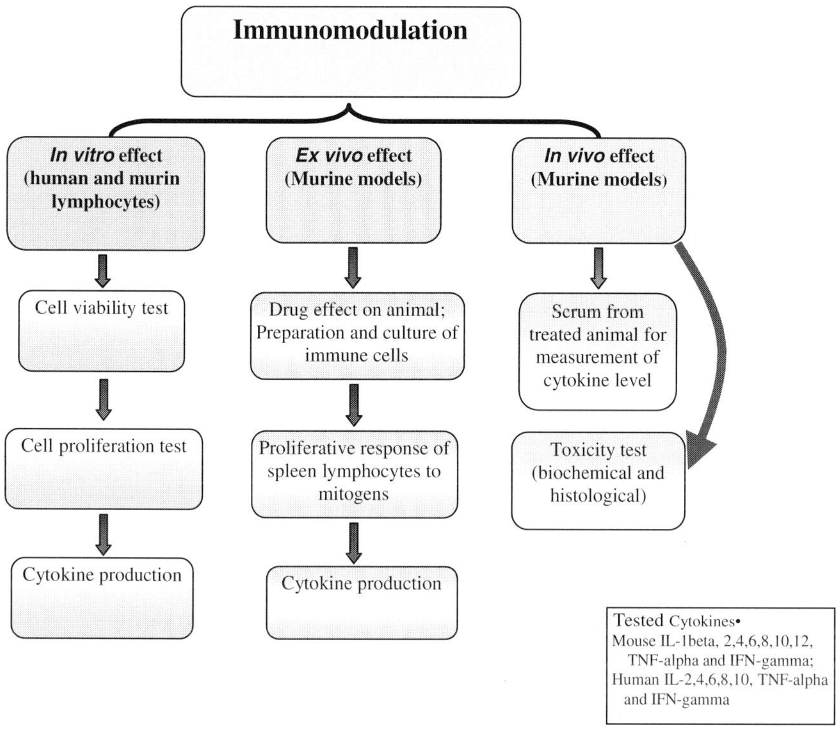

Figure 3.3. Study on immunomodulation.

3.3 A Practical Approach to the Clinical Use of Chinese Herbs for Cancer Patients

While it is realistic to look forward to the production of effective anti-cancer drugs developed from herbs, which may follow new innovative pathways of cancer control, one could choose to start clinical research using herbs of expected promise immediately. The need to look for innovative supplement to the conventional cancer therapy is obvious because of its disappointing limitations and the cytotoxic complications. The current fashion on pharmacological research is aiming at molecular targets with an eventual aim towards drug production.

However, on the practical side, in the Chinese community in Hong Kong, over 90% of cancer patients are receiving supplementary treatments of various natures in an attempt to gain better chances of cancer control and survival (Wong *et al.*, 1993). It is therefore justified to explore the effectiveness of the adjuvant use of the popular herbs through clinical trials. Such efforts should not be viewed as proper endorsement of popular beliefs. But rather, they are practical, responsible plans of clinical study, if well designed according to the modern concepts of good clinical practice, could have a lot to offer in the holistic care of cancer treatment. After all, developing an innovative drug is expensive and time-consuming. The use of herbal supplements could be readily administered and safety is not difficult to ensure.

Of all the possible pathways of action offered by different herbs, since their active components and chemistry are still unknown, the most logical selection would be those that aim at holistic support through nutritional or immunological modulations. Innovative new pharmaceuticals offer specific, immediate effects. Holistic support offers non-specific, slow influences that could be defined as supplementary, palliative or preventive.

A reasonable aim of cancer treatment is not only to remove the tumor mass and the harmful cells, but also to stop the dynamic process that has led to the development of the cancer. The logical expectation is: the holistic support works through complicated, yet unknown indirect pathways, whereby the cancer development process is kept at bay. In the following paragraphs, examples of clinical trials using herbal preparations as adjuvants will be given.

3.4 A Clinical Trial Using Herbal Preparation as Supplements to Chemotherapy for Cancer

A Phase II, randomized, placebo-controlled trial using herbal preparations was done at the Prince of Wales Hospital of Hong Kong in 2002–2004, whereby 60 + 60 patients suffering from advanced cancer of the breast or colon were being treated with cytotoxic chemotherapy. The use of herbal preparations as supplementary support to control pain and other symptoms, tumor size and survival were checked. A qualified, experienced Chinese medicine expert served as the partner of the oncologist in charge. The expert was responsible for the prescription of the herbal preparations given according to the symptom complexes and their individualized indications. The results of this study indicated that symptom control over pain, appetite and diarrhea were improved more with the herbal medicine group compared with the placebo group. The most remarkable improvement was observed with the control of nausea. The important parameters of survival, tumor size and chemotherapy-induced hematological toxicity were not improved in both groups.

This randomized controlled trial was carefully planned to objectively measure the efficacy of herbal supplements in attempts to make chemotherapy more comfortable. Thousands of cancer patients have been relying on the support from traditional Chinese medicine healers who prescribe individualized treatment. This form of individualized treatment was fully respected in the trial. The results might have supported the popular supplementary use of herbal medicine because it did no harm and was alleviating symptoms like nausea. However, the results failed to improve survival and other vital parameters like cytotoxic complications affecting the hematological state (Mok *et al.*, 2007).

3.5 A Clinical Trial Using a Herbal Formula as Supplement to Radiotherapy for Cancer Patients

The second trial was done in the same hospital on nasopharyngeal cancer patients receiving radiotherapy, which was the standard curative treatment for this cancer, common for the male population of South China. It was designed as a small pilot, randomized, placebo-control and double-blinded trial. Apart from general fatigue, the head and neck symptions related to irradiation were well-known and included local skin irritations, muscle tightness and spasm, mouth stiffness, loss of taste, loss of salivation, dry eyes, etc.

For this study, a uniform herbal formula consisting of two herbs was used and the principle of generalization was observed rather than individualization of treatment. This preparation contained a fungal component, *Coriolus*, which had the reputation of immuno-boosting property. For this reason, the immunological state of the 20 + 20 clients was assessed before and after four months of treatment.

Results of the pilot study revealed that fatigue was significantly relieved in the treatment group compared with placebo ($p \leq 0.05$), but the general trend of decline in the quality of life score in both groups after irradiation showed no difference between the two groups. In the immunological assessment, T-lymphocytes suppression was obvious in both groups but the decline was significantly less in the herbal supplement group (Bao *et al.*, 2006).

The objectives on the use of herbal supplement in this study were not confined to the control of symptoms arising from the radiotherapy. Instead, possible positive effects of the herbal preparation in the promotion of immunological defense were explored. Moreover, this cancer is unique in that it possesses a serological marker, the DNA of Epstein-Barr Virus (EBV-DNA), which offers a direct indication of cancer activity. A significant decline indicates a positive control of cancer growth. After radiotherapy, EBV-DNA dropped dramatically. The herbal study tried to look for possible supplementary effects of the *Coriolus* preparation, which might initiate further drops of EBV-DNA. No difference, however, was seen between the herbal and control groups, both of which showed limited changes of the DNA. This observation might indicate that the *Coriolus* preparation did not work through a direct control of the cancer growth, but rather indirectly via the immuno-supportive pathway.

3.6 A Clinical Trial Using Herbal Preparation as a Palliative Agent in the Treatment of Multiple Bone Metastases

This was a clinical trial done in the same hospital in Hong Kong on 46 + 46 patients known to be suffering from multiple bone metastases arising from various types of cancer. It was a randomized, comparative trial using a herbal formula and a bisphosphonate. The assessments included bone mineral density (BMD), control of secondaries, biochemical bone markers, quality of life and adverse effects.

The design was based on observations on the use of bisphosphonates for bone secondaries. Bisphosphonates suppress the bone resorption initiated by osteoclasts without affecting the osteoblasts. The newer bisphosphonate preparations were first used for bone metastases when they were found to be effective in the control of pain arising from bone destruction. Later, it was observed that bisphosphonate also lessened the destruction of bone, hence it might even prevent more secondary deposits. It was therefore deduced that if there were herbal agents which supported bone mineral density, the same agents should have protective effects on bone metastases like bisphosphonates. A herbal preparation active for the support of osteoporosis was therefore compared with a bisphosphonate (clondronate), and the parameters of assessment followed closely those of BMD studies (Wu, 2006).

A total of 46 + 46 patients were recruited randomly into the clondronate and herbal groups. Six months of respective treatment was given, followed by six months of further assessment.

The study was not totally successful because too many (45%) recruited patients died before the completion of treatment. Analyzing the fully treated patients, the herbal group showed some trend of superiority over the bisphosphonate group in pain control and the average quality of life scores.

As some modern drugs non-specific for cancer treatment have started to be used in cancer patients to achieve secondary benefits, such as the control of angiogenesis and the relief of bone pain, many herbal preparations could be studied and developed for similar effects in an attempt to look for practical solutions of symptom control for cancer patients.

3.7 A Clinical Trial Using Herbal Preparation as Preventive Agent for Immuno-Support

Many herbal items are popular among the general public of the Chinese community for use as health promotion agents. These are particularly popular among the elderly, the frail and weak after illnesses, survivors of serious accidents, and those bothered by different forms of derangement. Apart from the large choices of food rarities, well-known energizers and life-supporting herbs include the ginsengs, cordyceps, gonoderma, and other fungi.

A large scale clinical trial using healthy volunteers was designed in 2002 to examine the immuno-modulating effects of a simple preparation consisting of a fungus, *Coriolus*, and another herb. It was a randomized, placebo-controlled, cross-over trial. A group of 50 volunteers given the herbal preparation was tested against 50 others who received placebos. Four months of consumption was required for each group, followed by a cross-over for another four months.

The results showed very convincing immuno-boostering effects of the herbal preparation on all immunological parameters — T-helper cells, T-suppressor cells, T-helper/T-suppressor ratio, B-lymphocyte levels were all increased. Quality of life also showed significant improvement when the volunteers were maintained on the herbal preparation (Wong *et al.*, 2005).

3.8 System Review of Effects of *Coriolus* on the Survival of Cancer patients

This review was done by E. Wong of the Institute of Chinese Medicine at the Chinese University of Hong Kong in 2005. The main outcome measures were set at the survival rate at five years and adverse effects encountered. Fifty-eight potentially eligible trials were identified, of which 12 met the criteria for inclusion in the data-analysis. One trial was split into two sets of comparisons because there were three treatment groups. Therefore, a total of 13 comparisons were included in the meta-analysis. Most trials were of poor to average quality. The overall five-year survival rate was significantly better in patients receiving *Coriolus* than in patients receiving the same conventional cancer treatment without *Coriolus* RR = 1.11 (95% CI, 1.07–1.16), but sub-group analysis showed that the significant effect was restricted to poor quality trials. Among patients randomized to receive *Coriolus*, there was a 6–12% absolute reduction in the five-year mortality. There was no significant difference in the risk of adverse events in the groups treated with and without *Coriolus*. The benefit remained after possible publication bias was corrected. It was therefore concluded that *Coriolus* had a beneficial effect on the survival of cancer patients. This seemed to be particularly evident when *Coriolus* was used in conjunction with chemotherapy (Wong *et al.*, 2007).

Many other clinical trials have been done on the immuno-modulating effects of various herbs, particularly those of the fungal family (Chen *et al.*, 2002; Wong *et al.*, 2001; Liu and Xu, 1985). The clinical observation from volunteers further support these past reports. Nevertheless, in spite of the positive evidences of immunological boostering effects, how that translates to the direct applicative of cancer control is still not understood.

3.9 Conclusion

Cancer is a pathological condition. Removal of the cancer is a necessity in the treatment process. Removal has been achieved through surgery, radiotherapy or chemotherapy. However, removal has reached its limitations as the cancer could, in the first place, be too extensive, or, in spite of the removal, recurrence still occurs, an all too frequent occurence.

Cancer is a pathological process in which the cells either grow too much or too rapidly; or the normal programmed cell death (apoptosis) is not functioning properly. When the pathological process is not stopped, no matter how effective is the cancer removal, the formation of cancer is going to be repeated (van de Greef, 2003).

Cancer treatment has therefore gone beyond the stage of cancer removal and other approaches aiming at the causations, such as controlling the blood supply, initiating apoptosis, and regulating the responsible genes have started. The treatment approach needs to be modified from a single target, eliminative direction towards a multiple targets, holistic direction. Chinese medicine lacks perfect understanding of the causative pathology, hence it has followed a multi-target holistic approach. As new systems of cancer treatment are not yet mature, using Chinese medicine as an adjuvant therapy, could be an innovative and practical investment, to bring about better results of cancer control.

References

Bao, Y.X., Wong, C.K., Leung, S.F., *et al.* (2006) Clinical studies of immunomodulatory activities of Yunzhi-Danshen in patients with nasopharyngeal carcinoma. *J. Altern. Complement. Med.* **12**(8), 771–776.

Chen, H.S., Tsai, Y.F. and Liu, S. (2002) Studies on the immuno-modulating and anti-tumor activities of *Gonoderma Lucidum* polysaccharides. *Bioorg. Med. Chem.* **12**, 5595–5601.

Kamata, K., Iisukat, T., Nagai, M. and Kasuya, Y. (1993) Endothelium dependent vasodilation effects of the extract from Solviae miltiorrhizae. *Gen. Pharmacol.* **24**, 977–981.

Kaptchuk, T.T. and Eisenberg, D.M. (1998) The persuasive appeal of alternative medicine. *Ann. Intern. Med.* **129**, 1061–1065.

Li, P.W. (1996) *Clinical Oncology for Chinese and Western Practitioners*. Chinese Medicine Publisher, Beijing, p. 254.

Liu, G.T. and Xu, R.L. (1985) Immuno-pharmacologic activity of Cordyceps sinensis. *J. Integr. Med.* **5**, 622–624.

Liu, J., Shen, H.M. and Ong, C.N. (2000) Salvia miltiorrhiza inhibits cell growth and induces apoptosis in human hepatoma cells. *Cancer Lett.* **153**, 85–93.

Liu, J., Yang, C.F. and Wasser, S. (2001) Protection of salvia miltiorrhiza against aflatoxin B induced hepatocarcinogenesis in Fisher 344 rats. *Life Science* **69**, 309–326.

Mok, S.K., Yeo, W., Johnson, P.J., *et al.* (2007) A double-blind placebo-controlled randomized study of Chinese herbal medicine as complementary therapy for reduction of chemotherapy-induced toxicity. *Ann. Oncol.* **18**, 768–774.

National Centre for Scientific Research of France. (1999) *Report on the Successes of Development of Drugs from Botanical Plants.* Special Report, CNRS, France.

Nei Jing Chinese Medicine Old Class, New Edition. (1993) Chinese Medicine Publisher, Beijing.

van de Greef, J. (2003) The role of analytical science in medical systems biology. *Curr. Opin. Clin. Biol.* **8**, 944–954.

Wong, C.K., Leung, K.N. and Fung, K.P. (1994) Immunomodulatory and anti-tumor polysaccharides from medicinal plants. *J. Int. Med. Res.* **22**, 299–312.

Wong, C.K., Bao, Y.X. and Wong, E.L. (2005) Immunomodulatory activities of Yunzhi and Danshen in post-treatment breast cancer patients. *Am. J. Chin. Med.* **33**, 381–395.

Wong, E.L.Y., Cheng, K.F., Tse, Y.K., Tang, J.L. and Leung, P.C. (2007) Effect of Yun Zhi (*Coriolus versicolor*) on survival of cancer patients, systematic review and meta-analysis. *Am. J. Chin. Med.* (in press).

Wong, J.W., Wong, S.L. and Donnan, S. (1993) Traditional Chinese medicine and Western medicine in Hong Kong. *J. Hong Kong Med. Assoc.* **45**, 278–284.

Wong, K., Wu, G. and Dai, S.M. (2001) Study on the immunological effects of the aqueous extract of Gonoderma in the mice. *J. Guangxi Med. Univ.* **20**, 871–874.

Wu, K. (2006) *Clinical Observation and Pharmacological Study of the Efficacy of a Chinese Medicine Formula on Malignant Tumor Bone Metastasis.* PhD thesis, Graduate School, The Chinese University of Hong Kong.

Yu, C.W., Li, K.W. and Pang, S.K. (2006) Anti-cancer activity of a series of platinum complexes integrating denethylcautharidin with isomers of 1,2-diaminocydohexane. *Bioorg. Med. Chem. Lett.* **16**, 1686–1691.

Zhang, P., Wang, S.Y. and Wu, L.K. (1966) Arsenic compound treatment for acute granular leukaemia. *Chin. J. Heamatol.* **17**(2), 58–68.

Chapter 4

Advancements of Ayurveda in Cancer Management with Special Focus on Hepatocellular Carcinoma

Premalatha Balachandran

Abstract

In recent decades, the incidence of hepatocellular carcinoma (HCC) has been found to be increasing. In China, HCC ranked second of cancer mortality since 1990s, which accounted for around 53% of the total HCC deaths in the world. With clinical advances made in the modern medicine, though there has been small improvement in survival, the outlook for HCC remains generally dismal (median, eight months). As alternative or complementary therapy, ayurveda, the most ancient traditional system of Indian medicine has been emerging with scientific advancements in the treatment of cancer. Rapidly growing knowledge of anti-cancerous ayurvedic herbs in basic science appears at biochemical and molecular level. Although such research reports provide scientific basis, well-designed case studies are needed for more clear evidence in many anti-cancer treatment modalities that are in debate. The outcome of these studies will open new gateways in drug discovery from bench to bedside for anti-cancer drugs of ayurveda. This review focuses on the ayurvedic concept of cancer pathology, especially hepatocarcinoma, the scientific basis for anti-cancer herbs with hepato-protective efficacy, and recommendations for research design towards further advancement of ayurveda in the study of HCC invasiveness.

Keywords: Ayurveda; Hepatocellular Carcinoma; Cancer; Treatment; Herbal Medicine.

4.1 Introduction

According to a recent report on worldwide incidence of primary liver cancer, it remains the fifth most common cancer in men and the eighth in women (Bosch *et al.*, 2004). In the United States, liver cancer ranks eighth as a cause of cancer mortality in men and age-adjusted incidence have doubled over the past two decades (El-Serag, 2004). Similar increases worldwide have affected the mortality and hospitalization rates. Multidisciplinary scientific investigations are making impressive efforts towards combating this disease, but a sure-shot, perfectly curative remains elusive. Although there has been a small recent improvement in survival, the outlook remains generally dismal (median, eight months) (El-Serag, 2004). This dreadful condition has generated great concern in the minds of ayurvedic practitioners from the very early times with an aim of preventing or suppressing it from angles of treatment and management.

The aim of this chapter is to provide a general outline on ayurvedic description of cancers, and in particular, discuss cancer pathology and treatment with a special focus on hepatocellular carcinoma from the ayurvedic practitioners' perspective, underlying its scientific principles involved in treating these conditions with the use of naturally available plant products. This article reviews the efficient and effective therapies for liver cancer based on an extensive literature search of ayurvedic texts and research reports on hepatoprotective herbs with anti-cancerous property. It is written with an intention to raise awareness and encourage implementation of ayurvedic therapies in hepatocellular carcinoma; it also recommends research design for the further advancement of ayurveda in liver cancer treatment.

4.2 Cancer Definition

Ayurvedic classics namely *Charaka* (Sharma, 1981) and *Sushruta* (Bhishagratha, 1991) samhitas, describe cancer as *Granthi* or *Arbuda*, which can appear in any tissue or organ of the body, whose characteristic symptoms vary according to their function of the affected organ.

Granthi or minor neoplasm is a gland like abnormal growth of localized small swelling within the subcutaneous fat or muscular tissues. *Granthi*

Table 4.1. Characteristics of different types of *granthi.*

Granthi	Characteristics
Vatika granthi	Black colored swelling characterized by contacting, stinging, puncturing, exploding, twisting and incising types of pain, and when opened up, releases a transparent clear discharge.
Paittika granthi	Red or yellow colored swelling with blood mixed discharge and characterized by different types of pain like burning, fumigating, sucking, suppurating, heating with fire, etc.
Kaphaja granthi	Characterized by painless, massive, stony hard, cold swelling with white and dense pus discharge.
Medaja granthi	Characterized by large, painless growth associated with itching. Fat-like oily discharge occurs.
Siraja granthi (*Angioma*)	Occurs when vayu gets vitiated and afflicts the net work of vessels by contraction, pressure and dryness as a result of which round and elevated tumors are formed. It is mobile with painful symptoms and is almost incurable (Sankaran, 1976; Dash and Rashyap, 1987).

has been classified into five types according to their characteristics (Table 4.1) (Sankaran, 1976; Dash and Kashyap, 1987).

Arbuda or major neoplasm is an abnormal, spherical, stable, massive, painless swelling occurring at one site and expand slowly with deeper roots (Bhishagratha, 1991; Sankaran, 1976). These uninfectious and non-suppurative nature of abnormal growths composed of fatty substances secreted from mucous membranes (Bhishagratha, 1991) which could be due to stability and rigid confinement of the *doshas* in a particular place (Parkin *et al.*, 1984). Arbuda can also be divided into different types like *Vataja*, *Pittaja*, *Kaphaja*, *Raktaja* (*leukemia*), *Mamsa* and *Medoja* (Bhishagratha, 1991). Immobile recurrence of *arbuda* at the site of previous swelling is called *Ashyarbuda*. When two arbudas appear simultaneously, the condition is known as *dvirarbuda*, which indicates their malignant nature (Bhishagratha, 1991; Sankaran, 1976).

4.2.1 *Benign versus malignant tumors*

Among three body control systems namely the nervous (*Vata* or air), the venous (*Pitta* or fire), and the arterial (*Kapha* or water), in benign tumor, one or two of these three systems are out of control. This abnormal growth in any part of the body cannot be very harmful because there is still coordination among the systems, which to some extent controls the damage (Bhishagratha, 1991). The word "*Vataja*" or "*Pittaja*" or "*Kaphaja*" or a combination of any two of them is used to signify a benign neoplasm. The study carried out by Parmer (1983) on 50 cases of different types of *arbuda* suggests that *Kaphaja* and *Medhaja Arbudas* could be closely correlated with different benign growths.

Malignant tumor has been indicated as "*Tridosaja*" neoplasm, in which all the three major bodily control systems are out of control, losing mutual coordination and cannot prevent damage to tissues resulting in a deadly morbid condition (Bhishagratha, 1991), e.g. The malignant lesions *viz.*, *Mansaj* and *Raktaj arbudas*, show the features of squamous cell carcinoma, and *kaphaj* shows adenoma and *medaj* shows lipoma.

4.2.2 *Classification*

According to ayurvedic texts, the cancer related diseases could be classified as follows (Prasad, 1987):

Group I: Disease that can be labeled as clear malignancy. Diseases falling under this category include *arbuda*, *granthi*, e.g. *mamsarbuda* (melanoma) and *raktarbuda* (leukemia), *mukharbuda* (oral cancer).

Group II: Diseases that can be considered as cancer, e.g. *tridosaj Gulmas* (abdominal tumors like carcinoma of the stomach and liver, or lymphomas).

Group III: Disease with the possibilities of malignancy. These diseases are *visarpa* (erysipelas), *Asadhya kamala* (incurable jaundice), *tridosha* and *Nadi vrana* (sinusitis) (Prasad, 1987; Singh, 2002).

4.2.3 *Etiology*

Cancer is ultimately the result of interplay between environmental (exogenous) and genetic (host) factors. Ayurveda explains *arbuda* as a disease resulting from the derangement of *doshas* due to dietary constituents (chemical carcinogenesis). Hence, the diseases in each person differ according to different person's *doshas* (pathogens, exogenous) and constitutions (genetic, *bijadosha*).

Table 4.2. Causative factors responsible for the vitiation of doshas (Sastry, 2001).

Aggrevating factors	Food factors	Behavioral factors
Vata prakopa karanas (*Vata* aggrevating factors)	Excessive intake of bitter, pungent and astringent foods; dry foods.	Stress and strain conditions.
Pitta prakopa karanas (*Pitta* aggrevating factors)	Excessive intake of sour and salty and fried food.	Excessive anger.
Kapha prakopa karanas (*Kapha* aggrevating factors)	Excessive intake of sweet, sour and salty diet; oily food.	Sedentary nature.
Rakta prakopa karanas (Blood aggrevating factors)	Excessive intake of acidic or strong alkalis containing food, e.g. fried roasted food, sour or over-ripened fruits, alcoholic beverages, rotten, greasy or stale foods.	Improper behaviors like excessive anger or severe emotional upset, sunbathing or working under scorching sun or too close to fire or hot conditions, etc. are some of the additional causes.
Mamsa prakopa karanas (Muscle aggrevating factors)	Excessive use of exudative foods like meat, fish, yogurt, milk and cream.	Behaviours leading to exudation, like sleeping during the day and overeating are some other causes for pathogens invading the muscular tissues (Sharma, 1981).
Medo prakopa karanas (Fat aggrevating factors)	Excessive intake of oily foods, sweets, alcohol.	Lazy attitude (Sastry, 2001).

Sushruta called the sixth layer of the skin as "*Rohini*", (represents epithelium) where the *granthi* and the *arbuda* manifest their abnormal growth (Bhishagratha, 1991). Pathogenic injuries to the inner layer of the dermis (*Rohini*) in muscular tissues or blood vessels can be caused by lifestyle errors, such as unhealthy foods, poor hygiene, or poor behavior, physical trauma, or imbalances of *vata*, *pitta* and *kapha*, and such damage often cause ulcerous conditions. Because of the rapidly growing nature of the *rohini*, which have a tendency to form poorly vascularized tissue during repair, the process of healing often leaves behind some tiny scars. These slow healing ulcers would develop into early *granthis* or *arbudas*, which are complicated and difficult to cure (Bhishagratha, 1991; Sankaran, 1976). Causative factors responsible for the vitiation of *doshas* are detailed in Table 4.2.

4.3 Ayurveda's Special Focus on Liver Diseases

Although, cancer can develop from any organ, the clinical significance depends on the tissue of origin, prevalence and the ability of the medical world to accomplish complete cure. Among several types, liver cancer represents 4% of all malignant cancers and is the seventh most common cancer in man worldwide (Parkin *et al.*, 1984). Treatment of liver cancer is one of the several gray areas in modern medicine, which evade complete cure.

4.3.1 *Description of liver*

In ayurvedic texts, the liver is mentioned as *Yakrut* or *Yakrit*. "*Ya*" denotes "activity" and "*krut*" denotes "to breakdown or disintegrate." Hence *yakrut* is continuously engaged in the activity of breaking down various stimuli and is instrumental in sustaining life process (Nanal, 2001). Ayurveda describes that the liver has a *Mula sthana* (prime center) of the "*Raktavaha srotas*" (circulatory system) and the role of liver is explained in relation with *dosha* (pathogens), *dhatu* (tissues), *rakta* (blood), *mamsa* (muscle), *mala* (stool), *pranavaha srotas* (respiration) and *hridroga* (heart) (Tilay, 2001) and this is helpful for understanding the pathophysiology of liver disorders and for designing treatment protocols.

Therefore, the maintenance of a healthy liver is vital to overall health and well-being, but unfortunately, this vital organ is often abused by environmental toxins, poor eating habits, alcohol consumption and unprescribed drug use, which can damage the liver, and consequently there is an overall decline in metabolic functions of the liver. This hepatotoxicity eventually leads to dreadful diseases like hepatitis, cirrhosis, alcoholic liver disease, and ultimately resulting in hepatocarcinoma (liver tumors).

4.4 Neoplasm of the Liver

Liver cell cancer (hepatocellular carcinoma) and carcinoma of the biliary epithelium (cholangiocarcinoma) are most common primary malignant hepatic tumors.

4.4.1 *Hepatocellular carcinoma*

Hepatocellular carcinoma (HCC), a fatal malignancy, is regarded as the most aggressive tumor with poor prognosis that affects half a million people worldwide (El-Serag, 2004). It accounts for 90% of all primary liver cancers.

4.4.1.1 Epidemiology

Estimates from the year 2000 indicate that 564,000 new cases occurred worldwide, including 398,364 cases in men and 165,972 in women (Bosch *et al.*, 2004). It is the fourth most common cause of death from cancer, the highest age-standardized mortality is in China (34.7/10), the second cancer killer since 1990s), which alone accounts for 53% of all liver cancer deaths worldwide (Pisani *et al.*, 1999). HCC once thought to be limited to Eastern countries, is now on the increase even in low and medium risk countries (Saracci and Repetto, 1980). According to recent statistics in the US, there have been more than 8500–11,500 new cases of HCC and mortality rates increased from 2.7 per 100,000 persons in 1997 to 4.7 per 100,000 persons in 2001 (El-Serag, 2004).

4.4.1.2 Pathogenesis and diagnosis

In ayurveda, on the basis of *tridoshas* (*vata*, *pitta* and *kapha*), the *pitta* (fire) present in each cell is responsible for digestion and metabolism and its decrease is inversely proportional to the related tissue, and *vice versa*. In *arbuda*, the decreased state of *dhatwagni* (deranged metabolism) will result in the excessive tissue growth. *Vata* can be correlated to the anabolic phase and *kapha* to the catabolic phase. Cancer is the metabolic crisis where anabolic phase exceeds the catabolic phase, resulting abnormal growth. It has got a parallelism with the aggravation of *vata* forces and suppression of *kapha* forces interacting with one another to produce proliferation. In liver cancer, there is excessive growth at a particular site (*Eka Desa Vriddhi*), i.e. liver enlargement accompanied by deficit on other parts of the body (*Anya Sthaniya Kshaya*), i.e. body weight loss (Sastry, 2001).

Sushruta has proposed six stages of pathogenesis of all the diseases but his concept is more appropriate towards the pathology of neoplasms, especially liver tumors:

(1) *Sanchaya* — early stages of localized neoplastic changes;
(2) *Prakopa* — transformation into metastatic tumors;
(3) *Prasara* — metastasis;
(4) *Sthana samsraya* — complete metastasis and secondary growth;
(5) *Vyakti* — stage where clinical signs and symptoms of neoplasms are expressed; and
(6) *Bheda* — the stage where differentiation of growths is made into specific groups on the basis of histopathology (Sastry, 2001).

Since liver tumors develop from advanced stages of chronic hepatic ailments like hepatitis and cirrhosis, all these symptoms have to be correlated for accurate diagnosis. All these hepatic diseases have the symptoms of increased serum bilirubin (*Pittaviridhi*), decreased hepatic uptake (*Yakruta Dhatwagni Manya*), decreased hepatic conjugation (*saman vikruti*), hepatocellular damage (*yakruta shotha*), biliary stasis (*sang*), steostasis (*medomay, yakrut medoj siragranthi*) and cirrhosis (*yakrut shosh*) (Mali and Kulkarni, 2001).

Although a description about the diagnosis of liver pathology is available in old literature, an ayurvedic physician uses modern technology to understand the underlying mechanisms of the diseases. Various imaging modalities *viz.* several conventional radiography methods and scanning methods are widely used for proper and speedy diagnosis of hepatic diseases.

4.4.1.3 Treatment modalities in modern medicine

HCC is an important cause of morbidity and mortality worldwide. What makes this neoplastic cell stop growing is the question still unanswered in the medical world. The course of clinically apparent disease is rapid and if untreated, most patients die within three to six months of diagnosis. Individual prognostic factors such as the extent of the disease, the site of metastasis, the particular histological condition of the tumor, the functional status of other vital organs, the nutritional status and the biochemical abnormalities have to be considered in selection of a therapy. Based on these factors, treatment modalities can be divided into either local therapies consisting of radiotherapy and surgery, or systematic therapies like chemotherapy. Alkylating agents, antimetabolites, and antibiotics are widely used in chemotherapy, but assessed response rates are in the 5%–25% range (O'Reilly *et al.*, 2001). Few or, arguably, no chemotherapeutic agents have been shown to have any significant impact on survival and HCC also been resistant to current chemotherapeutic regimes (Okada, 1998; Peng *et al.*, 2000). Other approaches includes hepatic artery embolization, ultrasound-guided cryoablation, immunotherapy with monoclonal antibodies tagged to cytotoxic agents, and gene therapy with retroviral vectors containing cytotoxic agents (Isselbacher and Dienstay, 1998), but all these methods have some limitations.

To summarize conventional treatment modalities for HCC: surgery is seldom of value for hepatic metastases and in radiotherapy, the clinical benefits are of modest value. Although chemotherapy is an essential component of an effective multidisciplinary cancer treatment program, current systematic therapies for hepatic cancers are less effective and responses are incomplete and short-lived (WHO, 1994). Liver transplantation may be considered as another therapeutic option, but again, the recurrence of tumor or metastases after transplantation has limited its usefulness. The major problem with the treatment of HCC is that it has a significant propensity to develop metastases with major sites of spread to other parts of the liver, lymph nodes, lungs, bones, adrenal glands, and peritoneal cavity (Okada *et al.*, 1977; Lee and Gheere, 1987). Thus, multi-focal HCC is a very difficult neoplasm and WHO categorized hepatic cancers under group 3 tumors for which there are no effective drugs (WHO, 1994; Venook, 1994; Colombo, 1995).

These indicate that there is still a long way to go in modern medicine in conquering HCC. An alternative solution to this problem is the use of medicinal plant preparations and many herbs have been evaluated in pre-clinical and clinical studies and are currently being investigated phytochemically to better understand their actions in revitalizing the liver and treating liver dysfunction and disease. Reports also show that the traditional Chinese medicinal herbs were also used in China since long time for the effective treatment of primary liver cancers (Campbell, 1984).

4.4.1.4 Basis for ayurvedic therapy

The therapeutic approaches such as *sodhana chikitsa* using *pancha karma* procedures (purification and elimination of vitiated *doshas*), *somana chikitsa* (pacification of *doshas*), *dhatwagni chikitsa* (correction of metabolic defects), *rasayana prayoga* (immunotherapy), *vyadhipratyanika chikitsa* (anti-cancerous drugs), *lakshanika chitkitsa* (symptomatic treatment), *sastra chikitsa* (surgical treatment), *prakritisthapani chikitsa* (health maintenance), *roganashani chikitsa* (cure of disease), and *naishthiki chikitsa* (spiritual therapy) are widely used in cancer management (Thatte and Dhahanukar, 1991; Sonata, 1986). Surgery is considered only as a last resort.

Alchemic drugs containing poisonous plants, mercury-like minerals and animal products which were rendered non-toxic by process of alchemy were used for rejuvenation. Blood-letting, and cauterization with alkalis and acids and other surgical procedures were also performed with the help of herbal and mineral medicines. Arbuda is excised completely from its deep root seat and cauterization done to destroy any of the remaining cell particles left. If this is not done thoroughly the remaining cancerous cells will flare up again to develop *Adhyarbuda* and *Dviarbuda*, which could have poor prognostic value and usually results in fatality (Sonata, 1986). Additionally, a greater emphasis on health promotion forms an integral part of ayurvedic cancer treatment. Ayurvedic health enhancement approaches includes stress management, spirituality and meaning issues, dietary and nutritional counseling, exercise and fitness, addiction or habit management, especially for tobacco and alcohol use. The classical treatment protocols for *Granthi* and *Arbuda* and list of herbs used by ayurvedic practitioners were previously tabulated previously (Balachandran and Govindarajan, 2005).

4.4.1.5 Ayurvedic treatment modalities

Although specific treatment protocols for liver cancer were not described well in classical ayurvedic texts, the herbal treasure chest of ancient ayurveda offers a host of new phytochemicals that can be used both preventively and clinically to manage a spectrum of liver related imbalances including hepatocarcinoma. Hence during liver cancer management, ayurvedic practitioners are taking the advantage of available knowledge of treatment on *arbuda* from the old classical texts and combining them with their experience and scientific basis of hepatoprotective formulations and are applying those methods in practicing modern ayurvedic therapy. They are utilizing the recent research outcomes on anti-cancer herbs, which also show hepatoprotective properties, and are designing their own appropriate drug formulations. For treating liver disorders, herbal decoctions of ayurvedic drugs that consist of multiple herbs, each possessing tremendous potential for a cure, are commonly used. These formulations are reported to work on multiple biochemical pathways and are capable of influencing several organ systems simultaneously. The benefit of an herbal decoction is that one can nourish the body as a whole by supporting various organ systems, yet its main focus will be on nourishing the liver and its functions (Treadway, 1998).

4.5 Anti-cancer Drugs of Ayurveda Meets Modern Science

Recently, a greater emphasis has been given towards the researches on ayurvedic plant products that have anti-cancer potency. A series of studies have been conducted on folklores under ethnobotanical researches. For example, J. Hartwell L. (Loydia, 1967–1971) has collected data on about 3000 plants that possess anti-cancer properties, and these plants products have subsequently become potential anti-cancer drugs (Pandey, 2002).

4.5.1 *Andrographis paniculata* (*Kalmegh*)

Andrographolide, the active constituent isolated from *Andrographis paniculata*, was found to be more potent than silymarin, a standard hepatoprotective agent, and it significantly increases the viability percentage of the hepatocytes and antagonizes the toxic effects of paracetamol (Visen *et al.*, 1993), CCl_4 and galactosamine, through stimulation of hepatic regeneration, activation of reticuloendothelial system and inhibition of protein biosynthesis (Handa and Sharma, 1990). Additionally, andrographiside and neoandrographolide isolated from this plant showed anti-lipoperoxidative activity (Kapil, 1993), and have proved to be beneficial against hepatic tumorigenesis (Trivedi and Rawal, 1998). The hydroalcoholic extract of *A. paniculata* enhances carcinogen detoxification by the regulation of antioxidant defense system and microsomal drug metabolism (Trivedi and Rawal, 2001; Singh *et al.*, 2001). Thus, *A. paniculata* is clearly known to possess anti-hepatocarcinogenic properties.

4.5.2 *Annona atemoya / muricata* (*Sitaphala*)

Bullatacin, an acetogenin isolated from *Annona atemoya*, was studied by Chih *et al.* (2001) for its cytotoxic activity in 2.2.15 cells, a hepatocarcinoma cell line. From microscopical studies, these authors found that bullatacin-induced cell death is preceded by cell blebbing, chromatin margination and condensation, and that most of the cell death was due to apoptosis and not due to cell necrosis. The efficacy of anti-tumor treatment has been assessed with the intrinsic ability of tumor cells to respond by apoptosis. It acts as a potent inhibitor of mitochondrial electron transport (Ahammadsahib *et al.*, 1993) and NADH oxidase activity (Morre *et al.*, 1995). It arrests abnormal cell growth by inhibiting oxidative phosphorylation and lowering ATP levels. The new acetogenins *viz.* muricins A–G, and muricatetrocin A and B, longifolicin, corossolin, and corossolone, isolated from *Annona muricata*, showed significantly selective *in vitro* cytotoxicities toward the human hepatoma cell lines HepG(2) and 2.2.15 (Chang and Wu, 2001). These observations proves Annona species as anti-hepatocarcinogenic.

4.5.3 *Boerhavia diffusa* (*Punarnava*)

An alcoholic extract of *Boerhavia diffusa* given orally exhibited hepatoprotection against CCl_4 toxicity in rats and mice by increasing normal bile flow, suggesting a strong choleretic activity (Chandan *et al.*, 1991). Rawat *et al.* (1997) showed from their studies that the roots of plants of diameter 1–3 cm, and raw material collected during summer exhibited very high hepatoprotective effect as assessed by liver function tests.

4.5.4 *Eclipta alba* (*Bhringaraj*)

The hydroalcoholic extract of *E. alba* reduces GSH depletion, regulates the drug metabolizing enzymes and restores the activities of lysosomal acid and alkaline phosphatases during hepatic damage in CCl_4-induced toxicity in rats (Saxena *et al.*, 1993). It is also used as a cholagogue and as a deobstruent in hepatic enlargement and in other hepatic ailments, and has been shown to down-regulate HBSAg (Thyagarajan *et al.*, 1982). Wedelolactones from this plant source showed significant stimulatory effects on liver cell regeneration and anti-hepatotoxic activity in cultured rat hepatocytes (Balachandran and Govindarajan, 2005; Wagner *et al.*, 1986).

4.5.5 *Phyllanthus niruri* /*amarus* (*Bhumyamalaki*)

In a clinical study conducted on 55 patients with chronic viral hepatitis B, all the 30 patients under *P. amarus* treatment were cured within three months (Wang *et al.*, 2001) with remarkable recovery of liver functions as well as with inhibition of HBV replication. In another study (Mehrotra *et al.*, 1991), 59% of the *P. amarus* treated patients become HBsAg-negative.

The aqueous extract of *P. amarus* increases the life-span of the HCC bearing rats (33 to 52 weeks) and normalizes serum HCC marker activities (Rajeshkumar and Kuttan, 2000a and b). The ethanolic extract exhibited a hepatoprotective effect on alcohol induced liver damage in non-/partially hepatectomized rats and in CCl_4 and galactosamine-induced cytotoxicity in primary cultured rat hepatocytes (Prabhakar, 2002).

P. amarus extract has the ability to down-regulate HBV mRNA transcription in the Alexander, HCC-derived cell line by specific mechanisms involving interactions between HBV enhancer I and C/EBP transcription factors (Ott *et al.*, 1997; Lee *et al.*, 1996). *P. amarus* also inhibited HBV polymerase activity, decreased episomal HBV DNA content and suppressed virus release into culture medium (Lee *et al.*, 1996). Thus, it plays a major role in the disruption of HBsAg mRNA transcription and post-transcription, which could be beneficial against hepatitis mediated hepatic cancers.

4.5.6 *Picrorrhiza kurroa* (*Katuki*)

P. kurroa has been used traditionally in ayurveda for centuries as a general liver tonic for liver cleansing, liver poisoning (Nadkarni, 1994), hepatitis and alcohol-induced hepatotoxicity (Rastogi *et al.*, 1996). In a randomized, placebo-controlled trial in patients with acute viral hepatitis, *P. kurroa* led to a rapid fall in serum bilirubin and other LFT parameters towards normal range with quicker clinical recovery without side effects (Vaidya *et al.*, 1996a and b). Clinical and biochemical clearance was 100% on treatment (Rajalakshmi *et al.*, 1992). It acts as a direct viricidal agent and induces a state of non-specific increase in resistance in animals, which may also contribute to its anti-viral activity (Singh *et al.*, 1982).

Picroliv is a standardized preparation of active constituents of *P. kurroa viz.*, picroside-1 and kutkoside, iridoid glycoside mixtures. Picroliv pre-treatment prevented the hepatotoxic effects of paracetamol, galactosamine, ethanol and CCl_4 (Singh *et al.*, 1992; Anandan *et al.*, 1999; Visen *et al.*, 1996; Santra *et al.*, 1998), which could be due to an alteration in the bio-transformation of the toxic substances (Ramesh *et al.*, 1997) and its ability to inhibit the uncoupling between respiration and oxidative phosphorylation. It also showed antioxidant property against enhanced lipid peroxidation induced by aflatoxin B_1, a powerful hepatocarcinogenic mycotoxin (Rastogi *et al.*, 2001). This drug has the ability to regulate lipid metabolism by reactivating lipolytic enzymes, resulting in a normal level of circulatory lipoproteins and reversal of low-density lipoprotein binding to hepatocytes during hepatic damage

(Singh *et al.*, 1992; Ramesh *et al.*, 1997). As an effective inhibitor of hepatocarcinogenesis, Picroliv causes reduction in liver enlargement and hepatic nodular formation, and reduces the elevated levels of bilirubin and other marker levels in *N*-nitrosodiethylamine induced hepatocarcinoma conditions (Rajeshkumar and Kuttan, 2000a).

4.5.7 *Podophyllum hexandrum* (*Giriparpata*)

P. hexandrum is a potent hepatic stimulant, a blood purifier and anti-cancer drug and is prescribed in liver disorders. Podophyllotoxin, its active principle, is known for its cytotoxic effects by virtue of its properties of mitotic arrest, nuclear fragmentation and impaired spindle formation dispersing the chromosomes, and it affects both dividing and non-dividing cells. The mechanism of action has been suggested as necrosis and is a direct consequence of its cytotoxic effect on tumor tissues and a rapid and a marked reduction of the cytochrome oxidase was also observed in animal tumors (Pandey, 2002).

In Western medicine, chemically modified podophyllotoxins are proved to be potent anti-tumor agents and are used in cancer therapy. VP-16, a semi-synthetic derivative of podophyllotoxin has been used for more than 15 years against HCC and tested both *in vitro* and *in vivo* (Cavalli *et al.*, 1977). Pallavacini *et al.* (1997) have done a phase II study on the anti-cancer effectiveness of etoposide (VP-16) in combination with epirubicin, one of the anti-cancer agents used in HCC chemotherapy (Nerenstone *et al.*, 1988). Out of 36 HCC patients studied, 3% achieved complete response, 36% had partial response and 31% exhibited stable disease, while in the remaining 31%, the disease progressed. Thus this combination appears to be an active and tolerable therapeutic option for HCC patients. Pharmacokinetic studies on etoposide showed that this drug is safer even for the above therapeutic doses and is without hepatotoxic effects (Aita *et al.*, 1999). P-glycoprotein, an energy-dependent drug efflux pump which reduces intracellular concentration of drugs in tumor cells seems to be less effective in reducing VP-16 concentration in hepatoma cell lines, and hence this drug is found to be more efficient in hepatocarcinoma (Park *et al.*, 1994).

4.5.8 *Tinospora cordifolia* (*Guduchi*)

In a clinical study treating malignant obstructive jaundice, none in the *T. cordifolia* treated group developed blood poisoning, and amazingly, 92.4% survived after surgery as compared to 40% survival in a conventionally treated group (Rege *et al.*, 1993). In another clinical trial on infective hepatitis, all of the 20 patients treated with this plant extract showed symptomatic relief, improvement in yellow discolorations of urine, sclera, nails and skin. Treatment also reduced bilirubin and serum marker levels with 75% cure and 25% improvement (Prakash and Rai, 1996).

T. cordifolia prevents liver fibrosis, a major complication during HCC, by stimulating regeneration of hepatic tissue mediating through the activation of kupffer cells in CCl_4-induced liver damage in rats (Nagarkatti *et al.*, 1994). During obstructive jaundice, when it is administered in the pre-operative period, there was a decrease in morbidity and mortality due to sepsis and liver failure (Bapat *et al.*, 1995). It appears to improve surgical outcome by strengthening host defenses, normalizing phagocytic and killing capacities of neutrophils (Sohini and Bhatt, 1996).

The active principles from *T. cordifolia* are powerful immunomodulators and significantly enhances the humoral and cell mediated immunity (Sohini and Bhatt, 1996; Kapil and Sharma, 1997). It stimulates proliferation of stem cells and increases WBCs and bone marrow cells. It has the ability to reduce solid tumor volume by 58.8%, which is comparable to a well-known anti-cancer drug cyclophosphamide (Matthew and Kuttan, 1999). These beneficial properties can be used in the prevention of tumor progression and hence could be a drug choice for HCC therapy where immunosuppression is a major complication.

4.5.9 *Semecarpus anacardium* (*Bhallataka*)

An extensive review describes the phytochemical and pharmacological especially anti-cancerous properties of *S. anacardium*. The chloroform extract of the *S. anacardium* nut possesses anti-tumor action against L1210, P388 and advanced P388 leukemia, B16 melanoma and glioma 26, and increase in life-span of affected individuals after treatment was observed in all these cases (Cassady *et al.*, 1981; Chitinis *et al.*, 1980).

In our earlier *in vivo* studies on this plant product against Aflatoxin B_1-induced HCC in rats, this drug produced regression of HCC by decreasing abnormal nucleic acid content in tissues (Premalatha and Sachdanandam, 1999a) and normalizing serum bilirubin. The activities of liver tumor marker enzymes were brought back to normal on drug treatment (Premalatha *et al.*, 1999) with the dramatic reduction of Alpha-fetoprotein, a specific marker for HCC (Premalatha and Sachdanandam, 1999b). The drug was able to correct the immunosuppression that occurs in this type of cancer. The extract acted as an immune stimulant (Premalatha and Sachdanandam, 1998a), stabilized the lysozomes and normalized the glycoprotein content (Premalatha and Sachdanandam, 2000a) and regulated the abnormal mineral metabolism (Premalatha and Sachdanandam, 1998b). It cured hypoglycemia (Premalatha *et al.*, 1997b) and controlled abnormal lipid peroxidation (Premalatha *et al.*, 1997a) by its free radical quenching property and maintenance of antioxidant defense status of the host (Premalatha and Sachdanandam, 1999c). In the microsomes, the nut extract acts as a bifunctional inducer and induces both phase I and phase II biotransformation enzymes. This property helps in detoxification of carcinogens in liver and prevents their accumulation (Premalatha and Sachdanandam, 2000b). In addition to detoxification, the nut extract also inhibits the metabolic activation of carcinogens to its ultimate state and thus prevents tumor initiation (Premalatha and Sachdanandam, 2000c). Histologically, after treatment with the extract, the tumor nodules become completely regressed and necrotic tissues are replaced by newly regenerated hepatocytes (Premalatha and Sachdanandam, 1999a).

Anacartin forte, an ayurvedic preparation from *Semecarpus anacardium*, exhibited not only a broad spectrum of anti-cancer properties in clinical and animal studies but also a wide margin of safety in therapeutic dosage even when used for longer periods, giving subjective and objective improvement, alleviation or disappearance of troublesome symptoms and clinical benefit with extension of survival time in various types of cancers like oesophageal cancer, chronic myeloid leukemia, urinary bladder and liver cancer. A case report shows the complete regression of the early stages of hepatocarcinoma after the treatment with *S. anacardium* drug (Vad, 1973). The patient gained weight and liver abnormalities reverted to normal. There was marked clinical improvement with normal blood count and L.F.T was within normal limits.

Another ayurvedic drug containing *Semecarpus anacardium* nuts, *Amura rohitaka*, *Glycyrrhiza glabra*, and copper powder has been subjected to clinical trials; 250 cancer patients with different types and stages of cancer were divided into the following groups:

(1) chemotherapy (Vincristine, Cyclophosphamide, 5-flurouracil) and adriablastin + radiotherapy (4000–6000v) + above-mentioned ayurvedic drug;
(2) chemotherapy + radiotherapy;
(3) chemotherapy + ayurvedic drug;
(4) chemotherapy alone; and
(5) ayurvedic drug alone.

The response of patients to different kinds of therapy is in the following order: Group 1 > Group 3 > Group 5 > Group 2 > Group 4. The estimation of γ-aminobutyric acid levels and glutamic acid decarboxylase activities at different time intervals clearly suggest the anti-cancer efficiency of ayurvedic drug without toxic manifestation. It also reduces the toxic effects of other chemotherapeutic agents, prolongs the drug efficiency and increases the body's resistance to cancer (Prasad and Deshpande, 1968).

4.5.10 *Hepatoprotective ayurvedic formulations*

A comparative hepatoprotective efficacy of four different ayurvedic formulations was studied by Nair *et al.* (1998). These drugs are Gudapippali (includes *Embelia ribes*, *Piper longum*, *Zingiber officinale*, *Piper nigrum*, *Plumbago rosea*, *Nigella sativa*, salt and mineral additives), *Vasagulu chyadi arkom* (consists of *Adhatoda vasica*, *T. cordifolia*, *Glycyrrhiza glabra*, *Strychnos potatorum*, *Melia azadirachta*), *Patolakaturohinyadi arkom* (includes *Trichosanthus cucumarina*, *Picrorrhiza kurroa*, *Santalum album*, *T. cordifolia*, *Chonemopha fragrans*) and *Draksnadi arkom* (includes *Vitis vinifera*, *Madhuca latifolia*, *Glycyrrhiza glabra*, *Symplocos racemosa*, *Cyperus rotundus*). Of these four drugs, *Patolakaturohinyadi arkom* was found to be highly effective and has the highest potential in the treatment of liver diseases (Table 4.3).

Table 4.3. Beneficial ayurvedic formulations in hepatic diseases.

Name of the ayurvedic formulation	Composition
Arogyavardhini (Antarkar *et al.*, 1980)	Mercury — 2 mg, Sulfur — 2 mg, Lohabhasma — 2 mg, Tamrabhasma — 2 mg, Abhrakbhasma — 2 mg, Triphala churna — 4 mg, Shilajit — 6 mg, Guggul — 8 mg, Chitrakamal Churna — 8 mg, Kutaki churna — 36 mg, decoction of *A. indica* — 128 mg (total approx 200 mg). In the case of moderate hepatitis, *Arogyavardhini* is used in combination with viricidal and virechaka drugs. In the case of severity, minerals like *Tapyadi lauha* and *srothoshodhaka* drugs like *shilajithu, nirgundi, bhallataka, guduchi* and *shallaki* are additionally used (Shripathi, 2002).
Hepax (500 mg) (Dange *et al.*, 2001)	*Plumbago zeylanica* (*Chitraka*) — 30 mg; *Picrorrhiza kurroa* (*kali kutki*) — 30 mg; *Piper nigrum* (*kali Miri*) — 30 mg; *Zingiber officinalis* (*Suntha*) — 30 mg; *Carbonate of soda* (*Sajikhar*) — 30 mg; *Phyllanthus emblica* (*Amla*) — 25 mg; *Calcium hydroxide* (*Chuna*) — 25 mg; *Pearlash* (*Papadkhar*) — 275 mg.
ov valiliv (250 mg) (Dange *et al.*, 2001)	*Arogyavardhini* — 60 mg; *Picrorrhiza kurroa* — 15 mg; *Terminalia chebula* — 15 mg; *Eclipta alba* — 30 mg; *Solanam nigrum* — 15 mg; *Kanthloh bhasma* — 15 mg; *Caparis spinosa* — 15 mg; *Fumaria parviflora* — 15 mg; *Tamarix gallica* — 10 mg; *Embelica ribes* — 15 mg; *Somnathi tamra* — 15 mg.
Kamalahar forte (250 mg) (Dange *et al.*, 2001)	*Chichorium intybus* — 25 mg; *Solanum nigrum* — 50 mg; *Mineral salts* — 75 mg; *Mandur bhasma* — 20 mg; *Terminalia arjuna* — 20 mg; *Achyaranthes aspera* — 15 mg; *Tinospora cordifolia* — 10 mg; *Tephrosia purpurea* — 12 mg; *Boerhavia diffusa* 5 mg; *Emblica officinalis* — 5 mg; *Terminalia chebula* — 3 mg; *Andrographis paniculata* — 3 mg; *Berberis aristata* — 3 mg; *Plumbago zeylanica* — 3 mg.

Table 4.3. (*Continued*)

Name of the ayurvedic formulation	Composition
Liv. 52 (275 mg) (Dange *et al.*, 2001)	*Capparis spinosa* — 65 mg; *Cichorium intybus* — 65 mg; *Solanum nigrum* — 32 mg; *Cassia occidentalis* — 16 mg; *Terminalia arjuna* — 32 mg; *Achillea millefolium* — 16 mg; *Tamarix gallica* — 16 mg; *Mandur Bhasma* — 33 mg.

Two reviews have been published so far on hepatoprotective ayurvedic drugs: (1) Vaidya *et al.* (1996b) have reviewed the experimental and clinical research of hepatoprotective effects of medicinal plants and their preparations; and (2) Bhatt and Bhatt (1996) have compiled the information on various studies on these plant medicines.

A combination of the following herbs *viz.*, *Aegle marmelos*, *Andrographis paniculata*, *Bacopa monnieir*, *Citrullus lanthus*, *Eclipta alba*, *Phyllanthus niruri*, *Phyllanthus asperulatus*, *Piper longum*, *Picrorrhiza kurroa*, *Plumbago zeylanica*, *Sphaeramthus indicus*, and *Tephrosia purpurea* may give rise to a potent drug formulation effective against hepatic disease. These herbs possess one or more properties such as hepatoprotective, antiviral, cholerectic, regeneration of hepatocytes, antifibrotic, etc. (Vaidya *et al.*, 1996b)

4.6 Benefits and Risks of Ayurvedic Medicine in Cancer Care

Among the several potential benefits of ayurvedic medicine, relief of cancer symptoms is especially valuable. This medicine also results in a total healing process, reduces unnecessary side-effects and the cost of care. Each herbal product contains multiple chemical agents as active principles that may operate synergistically, producing therapeutic benefits and lowering risks on adverse effects. It also avoids unnecessary supplemental therapy. This treatment promotes health rather than just focusing on disease by carefully attending to illness and suffering. Empowerment, participation in the healing process, time and personal attention are essential elements in cancer treatment. This kind of orientation toward self-healing and health promotion makes ayurvedic treatment approach to liver cancer especially attractive.

Despite the presence of above said benefits in liver cancer treatment, the extent of research on this disease condition and practice is minimal. The anti-cancer products available in the market greatly vary in the method of their preparations. Thus, even if one drug is proven safe and effective, other similar products on the market may have quite different effects that preclude consistent dosing. Some of the medicines in this system and methods of treatment needs new observations, hypothesis-driven testing, innovations and peer-review.

4.7 Recommended Research Design

The clinical efficacy and extent of toxicity of many of the natural anti-cancer agents are largely unknown. Research on majority of ayurvedic hepatoprotective drugs is in the pre-clinical phase or is not being actively pursued. Ayurvedic practitioners and researchers in medical sciences can help to improve this medicine by increasing their involvement and contribution. Although the word "research" may inspire images of large and expensive clinical trials, a multitude of research design exist that are less complicated and less expensive.

The case study is a research design particularly suited to the ayurvedic practitioners. These studies form the basis for the future directions in research and provide valuable contributions to the body of knowledge on a subject. Case studies have been suggested by the Office of Alternative Medicine at NIH as a means to determine whether a complementary anti-cancer therapy demonstrates potential efficacy against particular cancer and whether clinical development of the therapy should continue. The essential elements of a best case series are suggested in Table 4.4 (OAM, 1994; Boik, 1996). Such case studies on ayurvedic drugs will help to identify safe and effective drug for dreadful hepatic disorders and will further the understanding of the mechanism of their action.

Table 4.4. Essential elements of case study (OAM, 1994).

Treatment protocols	Details of records to be maintained
Diagnosis records	• A record about confirming the disease by tissue biopsy technique during patient diagnosis and about other diagnosis tools used. • A note about the date of identification of the primary tumor site and further metastasis. • A record of nature and sites of metastasis.
Pre-treatment records	• Details of cancer treatment given to the patients before this trial. • Details of disease status at the onset of therapy and also the progress during treatment.
Treatment schedules	• Maintenance of each patient's health records and examination schedules. • Details of the treatments employed.
Response	• A record on the measures used to examine the extent of tumor reduction during treatment. • A definition of the objective response criteria used. • A description of each patient's overall clinical status during therapy and medical condition. • A criteria such as abnormal clinical observations or treatment associated toxicities which was made to modify the proposed original treatment protocol.

4.8 Conclusion

A complete cure of HCC is one of the biggest challenges to human kind and the medical world. The future therapy for liver cancer will rest on a better understanding of the molecular pathology of the disease and the development of non-cytotoxic therapies. Although much progress has been made in the study of ayurvedic anti-cancer herbs, the increasing promise of targeted drug therapy needs to be particularly pursued in the treatment of HCC. These issues stress the need for the multi-angled scientific research in ayurveda in order to find out a perfect remedy for this most dreadful disease.

References

Ahammadsahib, K.I., Hollingworth, R.M., McGovern, J.P., *et al.* (1993) Mode of action of bullatacin: A potent antitumor and pesticidal annonaceous acetogenin. *Life Sci.* **53**, 1113–1120.

Aita, P., Robieux, I., Sorio, R., *et al.* (1999) Pharmacokinetics of oral etoposide in patients with hepatocellular carcinoma. *Cancer Chemother. Pharmacol.* **43**, 287–294.

Anandan, R., Prabhakaran, M. and Devaki, T. (1991) Biochemical studies on the hepatoprotective effect of *Picrorrhiza kurroa* on changes in liver mitochondrial respiration and oxidative phosphorylation in D-galactosamine induced hepatitis in rats. *Fitoterapia* **70**, 548–551.

Antarkar, D.S., Vaidya, A.B., Joshi, J.C., *et al.* (1980) A double blind clinical trial of Arogyavardhini in Ayurvedic drug in acute viral hepatitis. *Indian J. Med. Res.* **72**, 588–590.

Balachandran, P. and Govindarajan, R. (2005) Cancer — an ayurvedic perspective. *Pharmacol Res.* **51**, 19–30.

Bapat, R.D., Rege, N.N., Koti, R.S., *et al.* (1995) Can we do away with PTBD? *HPB Surg.* **9**, 5–11.

Bhatt, A.D. and Bhatt, N.S. (1996) Indigenous drugs and liver disease. *Indian J. Gastroenterol.* **15**, 63–67.

Bhishagratha, K.L. (1991) *Sushruta Samhita.* Choukhama Orientalia, Varanasi.

Boik, J. (1996) Conducting research on natural agents. In: *Cancer and Natural Medicine* (ed.) Boik, J. Oregon Medical Press, Minnesota, pp. 176.

Bosch, F.X., Ribes, J., Diaz, M. and Cleries, R. (2004) Primary liver cancer: Worldwide incidence and trends. *Gastroenterology* **127**, S5–S16.

Campbell, P.N. (1984) Alternative medicine. *Arogya-J. Health Sci.* **X**, 1–8.

Cassady, J.M., Chang, C.J. and McLaughlin, J.L. (1981) Recent advances in the isolation of structural elucidation of antineoplastic agents of higher plants. In: *Natural Products as Medicinal Agents* (eds.) Beal, J.L. and Reinhard, E. Hippokrates, Verlag, pp. 93.

Cavalli, F., Tschopp, L., Gerber, A., *et al.* (1997) Therapiersultate mit VP 16.213 allein oder kombiniert mit 5-fluorouracil beim leberzell karzinom (hepatoma). *Schweiz. Med. Wochenschr.* **107**, 1960–1964.

Chandan, B.K., Sharma, A.K. and Anand, K.K. (1991) *Boerhavia diffusa*: A study of its hepatoprotective activity. *J. Ethnopharmacol.* **3**, 299–307.

Chang, F.R. and Wu, Y.C. (2001) Novel cytotoxic annonaceous acetogenins from *Annona muricata. J. Nat. Prod.* **64**, 925–931.

Chih, H., Chiu, H.F., Tang, K.S., *et al.* (2001) Bullatacin, a potent antitumor annonaceous acetogenin, inhibits proliferation of human hepatocarcinoma cell line 2.2.15 by apoptosis induction. *Life Sci.* **69**, 1321–1331.

Chitinis, M.P., Bhatia, K.G., Phatak, M.K., *et al.* (1980) Antitumor activity of the extract of *Semecarpus anacardium* L. nuts in experimental tumor models. *Indian J. Exp. Biol.* **18**, 6–8.

Colombo, M. (1995) Hepatocellular carcinoma. *J. Hepatol.* **15**, 2255–2336.

Dange, S.V., Patki, P.S., Pawar, S.S., *et al.* (2001) Comparative efficacy of five indigenous compound formulations in patients of acute viral hepatitis. In: *Ayurved and Hepatic Disorders* (ed.) Kulkarni, P.H. Sri Satguru Publications, Delhi, pp. 155.

Dash, B. and Kashyap, L. (1987) *Diagnosis and Treatment of Galaganda, Gandamala, Apaci, Granthi and Arbuda in Diagnosis and Treatment of Diseases in Ayurveda.* Concept Publishing Company, New Delhi, pp. 437–466.

El-Serag, H.B. (2004) Hepatocellular carcinoma: Recent trends in the United States. *Gastroenterology* **127**, S27–34.

Handa, S.S. and Sharma, A. (1990) Hepatoprotective activity of andrographolide against galactosamine and paracetamol intoxication in rats. *Indian J. Med. Res.* **92**, 284–292.

Isselbacher, K.J. and Dienstay, J.L. (1998) Tumors of the liver and biliary tract. In: *Harrisons Principles of Internal Medicine* (eds.) Fauci, J.B., Braunwald, E. and Isselbacher, K.J. Mc-Graw-Hill, New York, pp. 579–580.

Kapil, A. (1993) Antihepatoxic effects of major diterpenoid constituents of *Andrographis paniculata. Biochem. Pharmacol.* **46**, 182–185.

Kapil, A. and Sharma, S. (1997) Immunopotentiating compounds from *Tinospora cordifolia. J. Ethnopharmacol.* **58**, 89–95.

Lee, C.D., Ott, M., Thyagarajan, S.P., *et al.* (1996) *Phyllanthus amarus* down-regulates hepatitis B virus mRNA transcription and replication. *Eur. J. Clin. Invest.* **26**, 1069–1076.

Lee, Y.T. and Gheere, D.A. (1987) Primary liver cancer: Pattern of metastasis. *J. Surg. Oncol.* **36**, 26–37.

Mali, M.D. and Kulkarni, P.H. (2001) Clinical interpretation of LFT with ayurvedic point of view. In: *Ayurved and Hepatic Disorders* (ed.) Kulkarni, P.H. Sri Satguru Publications, Delhi, pp. 59–66.

Matthew, S. and Kuttan, G. (1999) Immunomodulatory and antitumor activities of *Tinospora cordifolia. Fitoterapia* **70**, 35–43.

Mehrotra, R., Rawat, S., Kulshreshtha, *et al.* (1991) *In vitro* effect of *Phyllanthus amarus* on hepatitis B virus. *Indian J. Med. Res.* **93**, 71–73.

Morre, J.D., Cabo, R., Farley, C., *et al.* (1995) Mode of action of bullatacin, a potent antitumor acetogenin: Inhibition of NADH oxidase activity of HeLa and HL-60, but not liver, plasma membranes. *Life Sci.* **56**, 343–348.

Nadkarni, A.K. (1994) *Indian Materia Medica*, Vol. 1. Popular Prakashan, Bombay.

Nair, R.B., Pillai, R.P., Nair, K.V., *et al.* (1998) Hepatoprotective effect of Gudapippali, Vasagulu chyadi arkom, Patolakaturohinyadi arkom, Draksnadi arkom and Madantha decoction on rats — a comparative study. *J.R.A.S.* **19**, 49–58.

Nagarkatti, D.S., Rege, N.N., Desai, N.K., *et al.* (1994) Modulation of kupffer cell activity by *Tinospora cordifolia* in liver damage. *J. Postgrad. Med.* **40**, 65–67.

Nanal, V. (2001) Liver disorders and their ayurvedic management. In: *Ayurved and Hepatic Disorders* (ed.) Kulkarni, P.H. Sri Satguru Publications, Delhi, pp. 142–154.

Nerenstone, S.R., Ihde, D.C. and Friedman, M.A. (1988) Clinical trials in primary hepatocellular carcinoma: Current status and future directions. *Cancer Treat. Rev.* **15**, 1–31.

OAM (1994) *Office of Alternative Medicine Workshop on the Collection of Clinical Research Data Relevant to Alternative Medicine and Cancer*. Office of Alternative Medicine, Bethesda.

Okada, S. (1998) Chemotherapy in hepatocellular carcinoma. *Hepatogastro-enterology* **45**, 1259–1263.

Okuda, K., Musha, H., Nakajima, Y., *et al.* (1977) Clinicopathologic features of encapsulated hepatocellular carcinoma: A study of 26 cases. *Cancer* **40**, 1240–1245.

O'Reilly, E.M., Stuart, K.E., Sanz-Altamira, P.M., *et al.* (2001) A phase II study of Irinotecan in patients with advanced hepatocellular carcinoma. *Cancer* **91**, 101–105.

Ott, M., Thyagarajan, S.P. and Gupta, S. (1997) *Phyllanthus amarus* suppresses hepatitis B virus by interrupting interactions between HBV enhancer I and cellular transcription factors. *Eur. J. Clin. Invest.* **27**, 908–915.

Pallavacini, E.B., Porta, C., Moroni, M., Bertulezzi, G., Civelli, L., Pugliese, P. and Nastasi, G. (1997) Epirubicin and etoposide combination chemotherapy to treat hepatocellular carcinoma patients: A phase II study. *Eur. J. Cancer* **33**, 1784–1788.

Pandey, G. (2002) *Anticancer Herbal Drugs of India with Special Reference to Ayurveda*. Sri Satguru Publications, Delhi.

Park, J.G., Lee, S.H., Hong, I.G., *et al.* (1994) MDR1 gene expression its effect on drug resistance to doxorubicin in human hepatocellular carcinoma cell lines. *J. Natl. Cancer Inst.* **86**, 700–705.

Parkin, D.M., Stiernward, J. and Muir, C.S. (1984) Estimates of the worldwide frequency of the twelve major cancers, *Bull. WHO* **62**, 163–186.

Parmer, R.K. (1983) *Comparative Study of Arbuda in Relation to Neoplastic Lesion and Its Management by Indigenous Drugs*. M.D. (Ay.) Thesis, B.H.U., Varanasi, India.

Peng, D., Qian, C., Sun, Y., *et al.* (2000) Transduction of hepatocellular carcinoma (HCC) using recombinant adeno-associated virus (rAAV) *in vitro* and *in vivo* effects of genotoxic agents. *J. Hepatol.* **32**, 975–985.

Pisani, P., Parkin, D.M., Bray, F. and Ferlay, J. (1999) Estimates of the worldwide mortality from 25 cancers in 1990. *Int. J. Cancer* **83**, 18–29.

Prabhakar, S. (2002) Hepatoprotective activity. *Ayurmedline* **7**, 29–35.

Prakash, S. and Rai, N.P. (1996) Role of *T. cordifolia* (WILLD.) MIERS. (Guduchi) in the treatment of infective hepatitis. *J.R.A.S.* **17**, 58–68.

Prasad, G.C. (1987) Studies on cancer in Ayurveda and its management. *J.R.A.S.* **3**, 147–167.

Prasad, G.C. and Deshpande, P.J. (1968) Effect of Rohitaka (*Amura rohitaka*) on leukemia. *J. Res. Indian Med.* **3**, 36–38.

Premalatha, B. and Sachdanandam, P. (1998a) Immunomodulatory activity of *Semecarpus anacardium* Linn. Nut milk extract in Aflatoxin B_1 induced hepatocellular carcinoma in rats. *Pharm. Pharmacol. Commun.* **4**, 507–510.

Premalatha, B. and Sachdanandam, P. (1998b) Regulation of mineral status by *Semecarpus anacardium* Linn. nut milk extract in aflatoxin B_1 induced hepatocellular carcinoma. *J. Clin. Biochem. Nutr.* **25**, 63–70.

Premalatha, B. and Sachdanandam, P. (1999a) Effect of *Semecarpus anacardium* nut extract against aflatoxin B_1 induced hepatocellular carcinoma. *Fitoterapia* **70**, 484–492.

Premalatha, B. and Sachdanandam, P. (1999b) Effect of *Semecarpus anacardium* nut milk extract on rat serum alpha-fetoprotein level in aflatoxin B_1 mediated hepatocellular carcinoma. *Fitoterapia* **70**, 279–283.

Premalatha, B. and Sachdanandam, P. (1999c) *Semecarpus anacardium* L. nut extract administration induces the *in vivo* antioxidant defense system in aflatoxin B_1 mediated hepatocellular carcinoma. *J. Ethnopharmacol.* **66**, 131–139.

Premalatha, B. and Sachdanandam, P. (2000a) Stabilization of lyzosomal membrane and cell membrane glycoprotein profile by *Semecarpus anacardium* Linn. nut milk extract in experimental hepatocellular carcinoma. *Phytother Res.* **14**, 352–355.

Premalatha, B. and Sachdanandam, P. (2000b) Potency of *Semecarpus anacardium* Linn. nut milk extract against aflatoxin B_1 induced hepatocarcinogenesis: Reflection on microsomal biotransformation enzymes. *Pharmacol Res.* **42**, 161–166.

Premalatha, B. and Sachdanandam, P. (2000c) Modulating role of *Semecarpus anacardium* L. nut milk extract on aflatoxin B_1 biotransformation. *Pharmacol Res.* **41**, 19–24.

Premalatha, B., Muthulakshmi, V., Vijayalakshmi, T., *et al.* (1997a) *Semecarpus anacardium* nut extract induced changes in enzymic antioxidants studied in aflatoxin B_1 caused hepatocellular carcinoma bearing Wistar rats. *Int. J. Pharmacog.* **35**, 1–6.

Premalatha, B., Sujatha, V. and Sachdanandam, P. (1997b) Modulating effect of *Semecarpus anacardium* Linn. nut extract on glucose metabolizing enzymes in aflatoxin B_1 induced experimental hepatocellular carcinoma. *Pharmacol. Res.* **36**, 187–192.

Premalatha, B., Muthulakshmi, V. and Sachdanandam, P. (1999) Anticancer potency of the milk extract of *Semecarpus anacardium* Linn. nuts against aflatoxin B_1 mediated hepatocellular carcinoma bearing Wistar rats with reference to tumor marker enzymes. *Phytother Res.* **13**, 183–187.

Rajalakshmi, S., Sivanandam, G. and Veluchamy, G. (1992) Effect of Kadugurchini (*P. kurroa*) in the treatment of viral hepatitis — a double blind study with placebo control. *J.R.A.S.* **13**, 27–34.

Rajeshkumar, N.V. and Kuttan, R. (2000a) Inhibition of *N*-nitrosodiethylamine induced hepatocarcinogenesis by Picroliv. *J. Exp. Clin. Cancer Res.* **19**, 459–465.

Rajeshkumar, N.V. and Kuttan, R. (2000b) *Phyllanthus amarus* extract administration increases the life span of rats with hepatocellular carcinoma. *J. Ethnopharmacol.* **73**, 215–217.

Ramesh, C., Khanna, A.K. and Dhawan, B.N. (1997) Picroliv regulates lipid metabolism in *Plasmodium berghei* induced liver damage in *Mastomys caucha*. *Indian J. Pharmacol.* **29**, 39.

Rastogi, R., Saxsena, S., Garg, N.K., *et al.* (1996) Picroliv protects against alcohol induced chronic hepatotoxicity in rats. *Planta Med.* **62**, 283–285.

Rastogi, R., Srivastava, A.K. and Rastogi, A.K. (2001) Long term effect of aflatoxin B_1 on lipid peroxidation in rat liver and kidney: Effect of Picroliv and silymarin. *Phytother Res.* **15**, 307–310.

Rawat, A.K., Mehrotra, S., Tripathi, S.C., *et al.* (1997) Hepatoprotective activity of *Boerrhavia diffusa* roots — a popular Indian ethnomedicine. *J. Ethnopharmacol.* **56**, 61–66.

Rege, N., Bapat, R.D., Koti, R., *et al.* (1993) Immunotherapy with *Tinospora cordifolia*: A new lead in the management of obstructive jaundice. *Indian J. Gastroenterol.* **12**, 5–8.

Sankaran, P.S. (1976) Swellings. In: *Susruta's Contribution to Surgery* (eds.) Prasad, G.C. and Udupa, K.N. Indological Book House, Varanasi, pp. 99–11.

Santra, A., Das, S., Maity, A., *et al.* (1998) Prevention of carbon tetrachloride induced hepatic injury in mice by *Picrorrhiza kurroa. Indian J. Gastroenterol.* **17**, 6–9.

Saracci, R. and Repetto, F. (1980) Time trends of liver cancer. *J. Natl. Cancer Inst.* **65**, 241–247.

Sharma, P.V. (1981) *Charaka Samhita*. Choukhama Orientalia, Varanasi.

Sastry, J.L.N. (2001) *Introduction to Oncology, Cancer in Ayurveda*. Chaukhambha Orientalia, Varanasi, India.

Saxena, A.K., Singh, B. and Anand, K.K. (1993) Hepatoprotective effects of *Eclipta alba* on subcellular levels in rats. *J Ethnopharmacol.* **40**, 155–161.

Singh, R.M. (2002) As assessment of ayurvedic concept of cancer and a new paradigm of anticancer treatment in Ayurveda. *J. Altern. Complement. Med.* **8**, 609–614.

Singh, N., Mishra, N., Singh, S.P., *et al.* (1982) Protective effect of *Picrorrhiza kurroa* against cutaneous vaccinal (viral) infection in guinea pigs. *J.R.A.S.* **3**, 162–171.

Singh, V., Visen, P.K., Patnaik, G.K., *et al.* (1992) Effect of Picroliv on low density lipoprotein receptor binding of rat hepatocytes in hepatic damage induced by paracetamol. *Indian J. Biochem. Biophys.* **29**, 428–432.

Singh, R.P., Bannerjee, S. and Rao, A.R. (2001) Modulatory influence of *Andrographis paniculata* on mouse hepatic and extrahepatic carcinogen metabolizing enzymes and antioxidant status. *Phytother. Res.* **15**, 382–390.

Sohini, Y.R. and Bhatt, R.M. (1996) Activity of a crude extract formulation in experimental hepatic amoebiasis and in immunomodulation studies. *J. Ethnopharmacol.* **54**, 119–124.

Sonata, S. (1986) The efficacy of ayurveda drugs on cancer (Arbuda). *Workshop on Cancer Souvenir*. Central Research Institute for Siddha, Chennai, India, pp. 81.

Thatte, U. and Dhahanukar, S. (1991) Ayurveda, the natural alternative. *Sci. Today* **2001**, 12–18.

Tilay, D. (2001) Role of *Yakrit*: Ayurvediya vivechana. In: *Ayurved and Hepatic Disorders*. (ed.) Kulkarni, P.H. Sri Satguru Publications, Delhi, India, pp. 131–136.

Treadway, S. (1998) An ayurvedic herbal approach to a healthy liver. *Clin. Nutr. Insights* **6**, 1–3.

Trivedi, N. and Rawal, U.M. (1998) Effect of aqueous extract of *Andrographis paniculata* on liver tumor. *Indian J. Pharmacol.* **30**, 318–322.

Trivedi, N.P. and Rawal, U.M. (2001) Hepatoprotective and antioxidant property of *Andrographis paniculata* in BHC induced liver damage in mice. *Indian J. Exp. Biol.* **39**, 41–46.

Thyagarajan, S.P., Thiruneelakantan, K., Subramanian, S. and Sundaravelu, T. (1982) *In vitro* inactivation of HBsAg by *Eclipta alba* Hassk and *Phyllanthus niruri* Linn. *Indian J. Med. Res.* **76**, 124–130.

Vad, B.G. (1973) Study of complete regression in four cases of cancer. *Indian Pract.* **26**, 253–263.

Vaidya, A.B., Antarkar, D.S., Doshi, J.C., *et al.* (1996a) *Picrorrhiza kurroa* Royle ex Benth as a hepatoprotective agent experimental and clinical studies. *J. Postgrad. Med.* **42**, 105–108.

Vaidya, A.B., Sirsat, S.M., Doshi, J.C., *et al.* (1996b) Selected medicinal plants and formulations as hepatobiliary drugs-an overview. *Indian J. Clin. Pharmacol. Ther.* **12**, 7–11.

Venook, A.I. (1994) Treatment of hepatocellular carcinoma: Too many options? *J. Clin. Oncol.* **12**, 1323–1334.

Visen, P.K., Shukla, B., Patnaik, G.K., *et al.* (1993) Andrographolide protects rat hepatocytes against paracetamol-induced damage. *J. Ethnopharmacol.* **40**, 131–136.

Visen, P.K.S., Saraswathi, B., Patnaik, G.K., *et al.* (1996) Protective activity of Picroliv isolated from *Picrorrhiza kurroa* against ethanol toxicity in isolated rat hepatocytes. *Indian J Pharmacol.* **28**, 98–101.

Wagner, H., Geyer, B., Kiso, Y., *et al.* (1986) Coumestans as the main active principles of the liver drugs *Eclipta alba* and *Wedelia calendulacea*. *Planta Med.* **14**, 370–374.

Wang, X.-H., Li, C.-Q., Guo, X.-B. and Fu, L.-C., *et al.* (2001) A comparative study of *Phyllanthus amarus* compound and interferon in the treatment of chronic viral hepatitis B. *Southeast Asian J. Trop. Med. Public Health* **32**, 140–142.

WHO consultation (1994) Essential drugs for cancer chemotherapy. *Bull. WHO* **72**, 693.

Chapter 5

Complementary Approaches to Cancer in Italy

Ralph W. Moss

Abstract

This article contains some observations on cancer and complementary and alternative medicine (CAM) in Italy. Italy does not have a strong tradition of using CAM approaches in the treatment of cancer. While the Italian population is eager to learn more about CAM, the medical profession is largely dismissive of these methods. In 1997–1998 the notorious Luigi Di Bella Affair occurred in Italy, when a professor of physiology at Modena proposed a non-conventional approach to cancer treatment, based around the off-label use of somatostatin. This treatment found champions in the media and general public, but was opposed by most of the medical profession. This affair divided Italian public opinion. Italy no longer has prominent proponents of non-conventional treatments in cancer. However, it continues to have innovative scientists who do work that is consonant with a CAM approach. This article considers the work of three such scientists: Paolo Lissoni, MD, of Monza (Milan), who has carried out numerous clinical trials with the pineal hormone, melatonin; Giancarlo Pizza, MD, of Bologna, who has done extensive work on the use of transfer factor (TF) and other immunomodulators in the treatment of renal cell and other kinds of cancer; and Aldo Mancini, MD, of Naples, who has isolated a mutated form of Mn-SOD-2 from the growth medium of a unique liposarcoma cell line. These scientists have introduced some flexibility into a rigid state-run hospital system by offering patients innovative treatment options in the context of approved clinical trials.

Keywords: Cancer; Italy; Complementary; Alternative; Immunotherapy; Melatonin; Transfer Factor; Somatostatin; Di Bella.

5.1 Introduction

Italy has a long and venerable tradition in medicine. The West's first medical schools were established in Salerno (10th century AD) and Bologna (11th century AD), and during the late medieval period Italy was in the vanguard of medical research. The science of anatomy had its origins in Renaissance Italy, and its early pioneers — Malpighius, Fallopius, Eustachius and many others — remain as foundational to modern medicine as Michelangelo and Leonardo Da Vinci are to the world of art.

Indeed, as the historian of cancer Michael Shimkin, MD, has pointed out, modern medicine as a whole could claim Italy as its birthplace and 1543 AD as its birth date, since this was the year in which Andreas Vesalius, then a professor at the university of Padua, wrote the first complete textbook of human anatomy, *De Humani Corporis Fabrica* (Shimkin, 1979).

Italian physicians were among the first to document the ravages of cancer and to devise plausible treatments for it: the first descriptions of stomach cancer came from Antonio Benivieni (1443–1502 AD) of Florence, and Gabriele Fallopius (1523–1562 AD) of Pisa and Padua was one of the first to propose the use of arsenic-containing pastes for cancer. Four centuries later, the US Food and Drug Administration approved the use of arsenic as an internal treatment for cancer (FDA, 2000).

This distinguished tradition continues. In the mid-1960s, scientists from an Italian pharmaceutical company, Farmitalia, isolated *Streptomyces peucetius* from a rare species of fungus that was found growing in a ruined tower overlooking the shores of the Adriatic Sea (Sikora and Thomas, 1990). This organism yielded the first anthracycline drugs, daunorubicin and doxorubicin. Because of the seaside location of the original discovery, the latter drug was given the trade name Adriamycin. This compound, and related anthracyclines, are now among the most widely used chemotherapeutic agents in the world, especially for the treatment of metastatic solid tumors (Ratain, 2001). The CMF regimen for breast cancer was also devised in Italy (Nagykalnai, 2002). Altogether, Italy has had a long, proud record in the field of cancer therapy.

However, Italians are not great users of complementary and alternative medicine (CAM) During 1997–1999 only 15.6% of the Italian population used some form of unconventional therapy, i.e. approximately one-third of American usage. Herbal medicine was used by only 4.8%. Although such usage may be increasing, and one sees herbalists and homeopathic pharmacies in all the big cities, Italy still ranks "among the 'light' users [of CAM, ed.] compared with other European countries (Menniti-Ippolito *et al.*, 2002)."

By all accounts, then, the knowledge and utilization of CAM in Italy is low. There are no CAM treatment, education, support or information services listed in an international directory of alternative therapy centers (Fink, 1997). None of the physicians listed in *Alternative Medicine: The Definitive Guide to Cancer*, practices in Italy (Diamond *et al.*, 1997).

5.1.1 *The Di Bella affair*

In modern times, Italy had at least one contentious encounter with alternative cancer treatments. Dr. Luigi Di Bella was a long-time professor of physiology at Modena University who died in July 2003 at the age of 91 (William, 2003). For some years, Dr. Di Bella quietly used an anticancer regimen of his own devising, which consisted of a combination of the drug somatostatin, as well as vitamins, retinoids, melatonin, and bromocriptine (Simini, 1998).

The affair that bears his name was precipitated in December, 1997, by the case of a pediatric cancer patient in Lecce, a town in Puglia, whose parents sought to have him treated by Di Bella's method. The medical authorities refused to administer such an unconventional treatment and the case was brought before the courts. The judges sided with the parents and ordered local oncologists to administer the treatment and the health authorities to pay for it. The case came to the attention of the media and became a national scandal. Although the child died in February 1998, public interest in the Di Bella treatment continued to build. A growing number of patients and their supporters organized demonstrations calling for medical freedom of choice. Various newspapers, magazines and television stations focused intently on the case and its far-reaching implications concerning who should properly make treatment decisions in Italian society (Willan, 2003).

In early July, 1998, the first results of a clinical trial from the Lombardy region were released. Out of 333 evaluable patients, only one (0.3%) showed a partial response, and one-third of patients showed no change. Half the patients had local growth of their tumors, and 14% had new metastatic involvement. Adverse effects (nausea, vomiting, diarrhea, neurological signs) were reported in 23% of patients, and 3.3% had to stop the treatment because of adverse effects.

Such results were understandably interpreted as proving that the Di Bella treatment had failed. But Dr. Di Bella was quoted in the *New York Times* as saying that the clinical trials had been rigged by oncologists jealous of his success. Many ordinary Italians agreed with him: 67% of Italian adults continued to have faith in the Di Bella treatment.

The Di Bella affair demonstrated both a pent-up interest in non-traditional cancer treatments on the part of the Italian public as well as an unsuspected degree of cynicism over the "cancer establishment."

On the positive side, the affair raised to prominence the issue of non-conventional treatments in a country that until then had had little exposure to such ideas. But in the aftermath of this affair, with its polarizing effect, proponents of unusual but scientifically reputable treatments became more fearful of speaking out about their own treatments. Each was afraid of becoming "the next Di Bella."

5.2 Methods

In November 2003, I visited Italy to speak at a conference on cancer prevention at the Santa Famiglia Hospital in Rome. I also toured the country to visit with clinicians doing innovative work in the field of cancer treatment. What follows are some of my observations on cancer and complementary and alternative medicine (CAM) in this ancient country.

5.3 Results

The first of these was the New San Gerardo Hospital (Ospedale S. Gerardo dei Tintori) in Monza, an industrial suburb of Milan. Dr. Paolo Lissoni, the head of oncology, is the author of over 250 peer-reviewed,

PubMed-listed articles, 33 of which are randomized controlled trials (RCTs). I will focus on a few of the most provocative RCTs of the past dozen years.

Non-Small Cell Lung Cancer: In 1992, Lissoni found that adding melatonin to chemotherapy in metastatic non-small cell lung cancer had a beneficial effect on survival. In addition, not only was no drug-related toxicity noted but, on the contrary, treated patients "showed a significant improvement in performance status (Lissoni *et al.*, 1992)."

Solid Tumors Other Than Renal Cell and Melanoma: Lissoni published an article in the *British Journal of Cancer* in which they showed that melatonin added to the standard immune stimulant interleukin 2 increased survival, even in cancers in which IL-2 was not thought to be effective (Lissoni *et al.*, 1994a).

Brain Metastases: In a study that appeared the same year in *Cancer*, Lissoni *et al.* showed that the outcome for patients with unresectable brain metastases could also be improved by administration of melatonin. The authors concluded that "the pineal hormone melatonin may be able to improve the survival time and the quality of life in patients with brain metastases due to solid tumors (Lissoni *et al.*, 1994b)."

Colorectal Cancer: In 1995, Lissoni published a study on the effects of immunotherapy with IL-2 and melatonin versus supportive care alone in the treatment of patients with metastatic colorectal cancer that was no longer responsive to the standard 5-fluorouracil-based chemotherapy of the time (Barni *et al.*, 1995). No complete response was observed. However, a partial response (PR) was achieved in two out of 16 patients treated with CPT-11 alone versus five out of 14 patients also treated with melatonin (MLT). Moreover, stable disease (SD) was obtained in five out of 16 patients treated with CPT-11 alone but in seven out of 14 patients treated with CPT-11 plus MLT.

Metastatic Colon Cancer: According to Lissoni, melatonin was able to amplify the effects of IL-2, which allowed it to be given at lower, and therefore less toxic, doses. Lissoni's group performed a clinical trial to evaluate the impact of low-dose IL-2 plus melatonin on the survival time in metastatic colon cancer, which had progressed following treatment with 5-FU plus folates. The study included 50 patients. Patients were randomized to receive either supportive care alone or else low-dose subcutaneous IL-2 (three million IU/day for six days/week for four weeks) plus melatonin (40 mg/day orally).

A partial response was achieved in three out of 25 (12%) of patients treated with combined immunotherapy.

5.3.1 *A visit to Bologna*

I also visited the Immunotherapy Module, Department of Urology and Nephrology, S. Orsola-Malpighi Hospital, in Bologna, Italy. The director of that unit is Giancarlo Pizza, MD. For his long career he has been affiliated with this 1500-bed hospital. He is presently the chief of the Immunodiagnosis and Immunotherapy Unit in the hospital's First Division of Urology.

Dr. Pizza's protocol for metastatic renal cell carcinoma (MRRC) consists of one monthly intralymphatic injection of interleukin-2 (IL-2) and lymphocyte-activated killer (LAK) cells. This comes after three consecutive days of IL-2 inhalation. Patients also receive i.m. injections of transfer factor (TF) monthly and interferon (INF)-α biweekly. The initial treatment cycle lasts six months, with restaging at three and six months. If the disease is put into complete remission then an additional six-month cycle is initiated as a preventive measure. Similarly, persistent disease is also followed by an additional six-month cycle in an attempt to initiate a response. In cases of progression, however, the treatment is discontinued, unless the patient expresses a desire to pursue it, in which case he/she is given an additional cycle. All patients are included in the ongoing statistical analysis (Pizza *et al.*, 2001).

The results from April 1986 to September 2000 were as follows: 122 MRCC patients were treated. Adverse effects were negligible. There were complete responses in 11 and partial responses in 13 patients, for a total response rate of 19.7%. Of the 24 responding patients, 17 resumed progression, whereas seven remained in remission 11–69 months later. The overall median survival of treated patients (28 months) was 3.5-fold higher than the median survival of historical controls (7.5 months). A

Kaplan-Meier curve showed 25% survival 11 years after the beginning of immunotherapy. The addition of IL-2 by inhalation appeared to improve survival.

The authors concluded: "The present immunotherapy protocol appears to be efficacious, safe, devoid of adverse side effects, far less costly than others and able to offer a good quality of life to MRCC patients. If confirmed in a multicenter trial, it could set the basis for developing low-cost immunomodulatory treatments."

5.3.2 *Santa Famiglia conference and LSA-CM*

My final destination was Casa di Cura Santa Famiglia in Rome for a conference entitled "An International Day of Study on Prevention in Oncology: Present and Future Developments" (November 13, 2003). This event was hosted by Massimo Bonucci, MD, chief of the Pathological Anatomy Service at this gynecological diagnosis and treatment center, which is affiliated with the University of Rome. Dr. Bonucci, who is also an oncologist, is an ardent proponent of integrating complementary methods into cancer care.

I would like to focus on the presentation of Aldo Mancini, MD, chief of Experimental Oncology at the Ospedale Pascale, Naples, and an associate of the Fondation Pascale of the Italian National Cancer Institute. His presentation was on certain "cancer proteins" that are being developed as both a therapy and as a preventative. The essential feature is that this is a novel cancer cell line, named LSA, that has been isolated from a human liposarcoma. These cells have both morphological and biochemical features that strongly resemble adipocytes (fat-storing cells found mostly in the abdominal cavity and subcutaneous tissue). When grown in a conditioned cell growth medium (a modification of the standard F12 medium), these liposarcoma cells confer both cytostatic and cytotoxic effects on the medium, which then itself becomes a potential therapeutic agent. In 2006, he and his colleagues published encouraging results with LSA (Mancini *et al.*, 2006).

LSA-CM (i.e. the "culture medium" of LSA cells) appears to induce both apoptosis and cell necrosis, and is also associated with a down-regulation of c-myc and the up-regulation of p53 in several human cancer cell lines (breast, lung, glioblastoma, etc.). A toxicity analysis of LSA-CM, performed in three different animal species, showed that this new therapeutic substance is absolutely free of acute, subacute, and chronic toxicity.

According to a limited amount of published work, the MCF-7 human breast cancer cell line and also glioblastoma cells are killed by LSA-CM in five to six days. However, these same cells are killed in just 30 hours by LSA-CM that has first been co-incubated with low doses of the standard chemotherapeutic drug cisplatin. LSA-CM therefore has promise not only as monotherapy but also as an adjunct to low-dose cisplatin chemotherapy (Mancini *et al.*, 2000).

In animal experiments on mice with mammary tumors (Balb-c-fc3H), Mancini has been able to demonstrate that LSA-CM delivered for 15 days through peritumoral injections resulted in the rapid disruption of existing malignant growths and the prevention of metastases. By contrast, in untreated controls, tumor masses were four times larger than the initial lesions, and numerous metastases were found in the lungs.

From the LSA-CM, Mancini and his coworkers isolated a protein that expressed this cytotoxic activity. This protein was specific and selective only for tumor cells that express estrogen receptors. Amino acid sequencing revealed that it was in fact a mutated form of manganese superoxide dismutase (Mn-SOD-2). These results have also been confirmed by using a form of recombinant Mn-SOD-2 that is expressed in *E. coli*. As a free radical scavenger, Mn-SOD-2 may also be useful in the prevention of ischemic injury (Mancini, 2004). Having been patented internationally, the substance is now in toxicological testing by Fidia, Italy's fourth largest pharmaceutical company (Italy Global Nation, 2003).

Although still in an early stage of development, the use of Mn-SOD-2 (with or without chemotherapy) could be an exciting departure from standard toxic treatments. Dr. Mancini is performing *in vitro* and *in vivo* tests and Phases I/II clinical trials have already been approved in Italy. Dr. Mancini is eager to find international colleagues who wish to further develop this exciting concept and, along with Dr. Bonucci, to foster the development of a truly integrative form of oncology in Italy.

5.4 Discussion

Cancer is a problem of considerable gravity in Italy, just as it is in other industrialized countries. There are elements of the Italian lifestyle that are conducive to low cancer incidence and mortality rates, such as the legendary Mediterranean diet, with its outstanding wine and olive oil. However, the country is also pulled in the opposite direction by high tobacco and saturated fat consumption and an increasing reliance on American-style fast food restaurants. It is thus a study in contrasts (Moss, 2004). Similarly, it is divided in its attitude towards CAM. While there is an atmosphere of disapproval of such methods in the official medical system, there is huge public interest, and a few examples of innovative work even in state-run hospitals.

References

Abbott, A. (1998) Controversial cancer drug wins local approval in Italy. *Nature* **391**, 217.

Barni, S., Lissoni, P., Cazzaniga, M., *et al.* (1995) A randomized study of low-dose subcutaneous interleukin-2 plus melatonin versus supportive care alone in metastatic colorectal cancer patients progressing under 5-fluorouracil and folates. *Oncology* **52**, 243–245.

Diamond, W.J., Cowden, W.L. and Goldberg, B. (1997) *Alternative Medicine: The Definitive Guide to Cancer*. Future Medicine Publishing Co., Tiburon, CA, USA.

Fink, J. (1997) *Third Opinion*, 3rd ed. Avery Publishing Group, Garden City Park, NY, USA.

Food and Drug Administration. (2000) FDA *Talk Paper*: FDA approves arsenic trioxide for leukemia treatment in record time for a cancer drug development program. http://www.fda.gov/bbs/topics/ ANSWERS/ANS01040.html

Italy Global Nation. (2003) Testing on anti-free radicals in Naples. October, 2003. http://www.adnkronos.com/news/prod/bolletti/history/2003/ottobre/qviott3.htm

Lissoni, P., Barni, S., Ardizzoia, A., *et al.* (1992) Randomized study with the pineal hormone melatonin versus supportive care alone in advanced nonsmall cell lung cancer resistant to a first-line chemotherapy containing cisplatin. *Oncology* **49**, 336–339.

Lissoni, P., Barni, S., Tancini, G., *et al.* (1994a) A randomised study with subcutaneous low-dose interleukin 2 alone versus interleukin 2 plus the pineal neurohormone melatonin in advanced solid neoplasms other than renal cancer and melanoma. *Br. J. Cancer* **69**, 196–199.

Lissoni, P., Barni, S., Ardizzoia, A., Tancini, G., Conti, A. and Maestroni, G. (1994b) A randomized study with the pineal hormone melatonin versus supportive care alone in patients with brain metastases due to solid neoplasms. *Cancer* **73**, 699–701.

Mancini, A. (2004) Personal communication with author, February 2, 2004.

Mancini, A., Borrelli, A., Masucci, M.T., *et al.* (2000) A conditioned medium from a human liposarcoma-derived cell line induces p53-dependent apoptosis in several tumor cell lines. *Oncol. Rep.* **7**, 629–637.

Mancini, A., Borrelli, A., Schiattarellla, A., *et al.* (2006) Tumor suppressive activity of a variant isoform of manganese superoxide dismutase released by a human liposarcoma line. *Int. J. Cancer* **119**, 932–943.

Menniti-Ippolito, F., Gargiulo, L., Bologna, E., Forcella, E. and Raschetti, R. (2002) Use of unconventional medicine in Italy: a nation-wide survey. *Eur. J. Clin. Pharmacol.* **58**, 61–64.

Moss, R.W. (2004) Is Italy's "Mediterranean Diet" a myth? *CancerDecisions Newsletter*, January 11. http://www.cancerdecisions.com/011104.html

Nagykalnai, T. (2002) Evolution of adjuvant chemotherapy of breast cancer from Bonadonna to the taxanes. *Magy Onkol.* **46**, 307–313.

Pizza, G., De Vinci, C., Lo Conte, G., *et al.* (2001) Immunotherapy of metastatic kidney cancer. *Int. J. Cancer* **94**, 109–120.

Ratain, M.J. (2001) Pharmacology of cancer chemotherapy. In: *Cancer: Principles and Practice of Oncology*, 6th ed. (eds.) DeVita, V.T., Hellman, S. and Rosenberg, S. Williams and Wilkins, Philadelphia, Lippincott, pp. 347.

Shimkin, M. (1979) *Contrary to Nature*. DHEW Publication No. (NIH) 79–720. US Government Printing Office, Washington, DC, pp. 48.

Sikora, K. and Thomas, H. (1990) *Fight Cancer*. BBC Books, London.

Simini, B. (1998) Somatostatin fever mounts in Italy. *Lancet* **351**, 428.

Willan, P. (2003) Obituary: Luigi di Bella. In: *The Guardian*, July 8.

Chapter 6

Kampo Treatment for Cancer

Kenji Watanabe

Abstract

Kampo medicine originated in ancient China and developed uniquely in Japan. More than 70% of Japanese physicians use Kampo medicine in daily practice. As for cancer treatment, Kampo medicine is widely used by surgeons and oncologists. It is used in the regular practice for the treatment of cancer and cancer-related symptoms from the early stage to the terminal care. This paper describes Kampo treatment for cancer, making references to publications in clinical and basic research.

Keywords: Kampo Medicine; Cancer.

6.1 Introduction

Kampo medicine originated in ancient China and developed uniquely in Japan. It has been both taught to, and used by, conventional Western physicians for the last 30 years.

Currently, more than 70% of Japanese physicians (including nearly 100% of Japanese obstetrics and gynaecology (Ob/Gyn) doctors) use Kampo medicine in daily practice including the university hospital, together with high-tech medical treatments like organ transplantation or robotic surgery (Watanabe *et al.*, 2001). Kampo medicine is considered a government-regulated prescription drug and currently 148 formulas are listed on the Japanese national insurance program.

As for cancer treatment, Kampo medicine is widely used by surgeons and oncologists. It is widely used in the regular practice for the treatment of cancer and cancer-related symptoms from the early stage to the terminal care. Because Kampo medicine has been totally integrated into Western medicine in Japan, motivation to promote clinical trials is lacking. On the contrary, basic research concerning cancer treatment have piled over the last 30 years by the physicians and pharmaceutical researchers. Prevention of recurrence or metastasis of cancer cells have been well studied in basic research, however there is little data in the clinical study because it takes time to accomplish.

In this review article, Kampo treatment for cancer will be described based on the clinical and basic research articles.

6.2 Prevention of Cancer

Chemoprevention is one of the topics in cancer treatment since it has been reported that non-steroidal anti-inflammatory drugs (NSAIDs) reduce the prevalence of colon cancer (Thun *et al.*, 1991).

6.2.1 *Shosaikoto* (小柴胡湯) *for the prevention of the hepatocellular carcinoma*

Since *Shosaikoto* was reported to decrease the serum levels of AST and ALT (Fujiwara *et al.*, 1988), it has been widely used for the treatment of chronic hepatitis. Because chronic hepatitis is very common in Japan as well as other Asian countries and no established treatment is available, *Shosaikoto* is widely used for the purpose of liver protection. Oka *et al.* (2002) reported on a five-year follow-up study of liver cirrhosis patients. The subjects were 260 patients and randomly divided into two groups, one treated with *Shosaikoto* and the other without. Onset of the hepatocellular carcinoma and survival rate were evaluated. The results revealed that the onset of hepatocellular carcinoma decreased and longevity improved in the group with *Shosaikoto* especially in the group of liver cirrhosis by non-B viruses. In the US, the effectiveness of *Shosaikoto*, *Hochuekkito* and *Ninjinyoueito* as well as glycirrhizine are listed as the effective treatment for chronic hepatitis (Shiota *et al.*, 2002). However the mechanism is not obvious, it is assumed that oxidative stress plays an important role in hepatocarcinogenesis. Shiota *et al.* (2002) investigated the anti-oxidative actions of *Shosaikoto*, and found that, *Shosaikoto* inhibited the 8-hydroxy-2′- deoxyguanosine (8-OHDG) formation, which is a DNA adduct by reactive oxygen species and known to be a genetic risk for hepatocarcinogenesis (Seeff *et al.*, 2001).

6.2.2 *Shoseiryuto* (小青竜湯) *for the prevention of lung cancer*

In the basic research, there are several reports. One is the *Shoseiryuto* (小青竜湯) for the prevention of lung cancer (Konoshima *et al.*, 1994). Lung cancer was induced in the mouse model by 4-nitroquinolone-N-oxide (4NQO) s.c. followed by the glycerol intake. This treatment induced the lung tumor in 93.3% of mice without *Shoseiryuto*, and 33.3% with *Shoseiryuto*. This data showed the reduction of the onset of lung cancer with *Shoseiryuto*.

6.2.3 *Shosaikoto* (小柴胡湯) *for the prevention of melanoma*

Another study was done by Kato *et al.* (1998). He established a *RET*-transgenic mouse line (304/B6) in which stepwise development of a skin melanocytic benign tumor and malignant melanoma can be observed. In this mouse model, he demonstrated that the herbal medicine *Shosaikoto* has anti-tumor and anti-metastatic effects on malignant melanoma through regulation of protein expression levels of matrix metalloproteinase (MMP) and its inhibitor. This study was followed by additional evidence showing that Ret protein expression levels of tumors in *Shosaikoto*-treated mice were higher than those of tumors in untreated mice at benign, malignant, and terminal stages of the tumors. The reduced Ret expression at the terminal stage was partially restored. From this experiment, it was concluded that the anti-tumor effect of *Shosaikoto* involves the promoted preparation of Ret protein as a tumor transplantation antigen, which probably overcomes its potentially increased oncogenic activity (Kato *et al.*, 2005).

6.3 Treatment with Surgical Operation

6.3.1 *Daikenchuto* (大建中湯) *for the prevention of post-surgical ileus*

Daikenchuto has been shown to be effective in preventing the post-surgical ileus and widely used to prevent ileus after abdominal surgeries in the field of not only gastrointestinal but also gynecology (Itoh *et al.*, 2002). *Daikenchuto* also prevents post-surgical intestinal adhesion by gastroprokinetic and anti-inflammatory effects. Motilin, one of the neuro-peptides which is a powerful inducer of motor activity in the gastro-intestine, was elevated in the blood after the administration of *Daikenchuto* in humans (Nagano *et al.*, 1999). In addition, *Daikenchuto* has been shown to induce production of vasoactive intestinal peptide (VIP) and 5-hydroxytryptamine (serotonin) in human plasma (Nakamura *et al.*, 2002). These neuropeptides may play a role to induce the motility of the gastro-intestine. Also, Sanshol in *Zanthoxylum piperitum* binds to the vaniloid receptor and stimulates the peristalsis (Satoh *et al.*, 2001). [6]-shogaol is an important component in dried ginger and produces an increase in the gastrointestinal blood flow, which is medicated by calcitonine gene-related peptide (CGRP), and explains why *Daikenchuto* is useful in the treatment of intestinal ischemia-related diseases (Murata *et al.*, 2001; Hashimoto *et al.*, 2001). This action is observed only when steamed ginger is used and not the dry ginger. Steam manipulation is observed in converting the Gingerol to Shogaol in the ginger and this Shogaol is important in secreting CGRP leading to the increase of blood flow of the gut as a result.

Prolonged paralytic ileus occurring in the hepatectomized patients may induce hyperammonemia. *Daikenchuto* is used to suppress the elevation of serum ammonia in hepatectomized patients (Kaiho *et al.*, 2005). Presumably, *Daikenchuto* stimulates the peristalsis and does not allow the growth of the intestinal bacteria producing ammonia. Imazu *et al.* (2006) showed this hypothesis with a different Kampo formula, *Juzentaihoto*. He showed that the change of the intestinal flora is the main resource of the serum ammonia elevation and this is suppressed by *Juzentaihoto*, because with *Juzentaihoto*, the change of the intestinal flora was suppressed.

6.4 Treatment with Chemotherapy

There are many reports that Kampo treatment reduces the side-effects of chemotherapy. *Juzentaihoto* alleviates the side-effect of UFT (Uracil-Tegafur, anti-cancer drug). Six months follow-up study of gastric cancer patients with UFT after curative operation revealed that suppressor T cell function was lower and cytotoxic/killer cell function higher in the group with *Juzentaihoto* (Yamada *et al.*, 1993). This study also showed that subjective and objective adverse symptoms caused by UFT were less with *Juzentaihoto*.

6.4.1 *Saireito* (柴苓湯) *alleviates the side-effects of CDDP*

Another study examined 26 cases of lung cancer, which was divided into 2 groups, one with *Saireito* (n = 10) and the other without (n = 16) (Okimoto *et al.*, 1991). Nephrotoxicity with cis-diamminedichloroplatinum (CDDP) was evaluated. Serum levels of BUN increased in the group without *Saireito*, while serum BUN levels were not elevated in the group with *Saireito*. Also, creatinin clearance became lower and N-acetyl-D-glucosaminidase increased, while those markers stayed as normal in the group with *Saireito*. This study showed that *Saireito* is effective in alleviating the nephrotoxicity of CDDP.

6.4.2 *Juzentaihoto* (十全大補湯) *alleviates the side-effects of CDDP*

Sugiyama *et al.* screened 11 Kampo formulae to evaluate the protection of nephrotoxicity induced by CDDP (Sugiyama *et al.*, 1993a and 1994). Among the 11 Kampo formulae, nine formulae showed significant reduction of nephrotoxicity. Although Flosemide also reduced the nephrotoxicity, it also diminished the effectiveness of CDDP. Among nine Kampo formulae that reduced the nephrotoxicity, *Juzentaihoto* was the most effective. *Juzentaihoto* also protected the liver and suppressed the liver injury. Among the herbs in *Juzentaihoto*, *Angelicae radix* showed the most effectiveness in liver and kidney protection (Sugiyama *et al.*, 1993b). Sodium malate in *Angelicae radix* was responsible for protecting the liver and kidney functions. The mechanism of action of sodium malate was that this compound binds to CDDP and forms the diammino-platinum(II) malate, which has a similar chemical structure to the CDDP-derived chemical, Carboplatin (CBDCA). This CBDCA is used clinically and it has less toxicity against the kidney, however, the effect is weaker. Also, this sodium malate did not increase bone toxicity; *Juzentaihoto* protected the bone marrow and blood cell count was not decreased with *Juzentaihoto*.

6.4.3 *Hangeshashinto* (半夏瀉心湯) *alleviates the side-effects of CPT-11*

Another good example that showed the reduction of the side-effects of chemotherapy is *Hangeshashinto*. Irinotecan hydrochloride (CPT-11), a semi-synthetic derivative of camptothecin, is an anti-cancer drug which inhibits nucleic acid synthesis by topoisomerase I inhibition. CPT-11 possesses a wide anti-tumor spectrum and is widely used for the treatment of lung cancer, colon cancer and malignant lymphoma. Diarrhea is the main side-effect that occurs in the early stage and causes the discontinuation of the drug administration. *Hangeshashinto* is used to stop the irinotecan-induced diarrhea. Mori *et al.* (2003) reported the result of RCT of *Hangeshashinto* and CPT-11. Of the 41 patients with advanced lung cancer, 18 took *Hangeshashinto* and 23 did not. Among 41 patients, 39 experienced diarrhea. Although there were no differences of diarrhea frequency and duration, severe diarrhea (grades 3 and 4) was reduced in the group with *Hangeshashinto* (one among 18 patients) as compared to the group without *Hangeshashinto* (nine among 23 patients). This study showed that *Hangeshashinto* is recommended for use with CPT-11. The mechanism of action is also well studied (Takasuna *et al.*, 1995). CPT-11 is changed to 7-ethyl-10 hydroxy-camptotecin (SN-38) in the liver and SN-38 undergoes glucronate conjugation changing into inactive SN-38 glucronide. Later, it is excreted into the bile, and is then deconjugated by β-glucronidase, which was contained in the intestinal bacteria to become SN-38 again. This SN-38 induces delayed diarrhea. *Hangeshashinto* contains baicalin, which serve as another resource of β-glucronidase. This competitive action of baicalin against SN-38 glucronide inhibited the formation of active form of SN-38 without glucronide. As a result, the delayed diarrhea caused by deconjugated SN-38 was alleviated by *Hangeshashinto*.

6.5 Treatment with Irradiation

There is a report that the irradiation with Kampo improved the survival rate in the progressive uterus cervical cancer. Treatment was the combination of low dose *in situ* irradiation and external irradiation. Kampo formulae were *Juzentaihoto* (十全大補湯), *Ninjinyoueito* (人參養栄湯) and *Hochuekkito* (補中益気湯). Irradiation only survival rate is higher in the group treated with Kampo formulae. Five- and ten-year survival rates were 65.6% and 49.1% in the irradiation only group (total number was 119; stage IIb, 64 cases and stage IIIb, 55 cases). On the other hand, these were 75.6% and 65.9% in the irradiation with Kampo group (total number was 82; stage IIb, 43 cases and stage IIIb, 39 cases). This study showed that the combination of Kampo formula and irradiation improved the survival rate of progressive uterus cancer patients (Takekawa *et al.*, 2000).

6.5.1 *Juzentaihoto for the hematopoiesis after irradiation*

Effects of *Juzentaihoto* on the recovery of hemopoietic systems from radiation injury are analyzed (Ohnishi *et al.*, 1990). Colony-forming unit-spleen (CFU-S) are hematopoietic colonies formed in the spleen of recipient mice that have been lethally irradiated and injected with donor bone marrow cells. Day-14 CFU-S represents primitive hematopoietic stem cells (HSCs) and day-9 CFU-S represents more mature HSCs. The mice injected with *Juzentaihoto*-treated bone marrow cells showed better general condition, heavier spleens with larger and more numerous colonies than the control mice on day 14. On the other hand, there was no difference in the number of CFU-S between *Juzentaihoto*-treated and control groups on day 9. Since the day-14 CFU-S assay is thought to reflect the most primitive progenitor cells in the hematopoietic system, these results strongly suggested that *Juzentaihoto* acts on stem cells in the G0 phase to manifest recovery-enhancing effects from radiation injury. After this study, the same group fractionated *Juzentaihoto* to obtain oleic acid and found that linolenic acid in *Juzentaihoto* was the responsible compound (Hisha *et al.*, 1997).

6.6 Prevention of Recurrence and/or Metastasis

This is one of the very interesting points with Kampo treatment. There are a lot of basic research studies and several clinical studies currently ongoing. The mechanism is also being studied.

6.6.1 *Juzentaihoto for the prevention of colon cancer metastasis*

Oral administration of *Juzentaihoto* before tumor inoculation resulted in the dose-dependent inhibition of liver metastasis of colon 26-L5 carcinoma cells and significant enhancement of survival rate compared to the untreated control (Ohnishi *et al.*, 1998). This effect was lost when macrophages and T-cells were eliminated. These data support the fact that immunological function plays a central role in the mechanism of *Juzentaihoto*.

6.7 Palliative Care

Kampo medicine is also used in palliative care. *Ninjinto* (人參湯), *Shikunshito* (四君子湯), *Rikkunshito* (六君子湯) and *Bukuryoshigyakuto* (茯苓四逆湯) were often used to improve patients' appetite and help them recover from the cachexia.

6.7.1 *Daikenchuto for the constipation by morphine*

Morphine is the most effective anti-nociceptive agent and is used to manage pain experienced by terminal cancer patients. However, it induces severe constipation, causing an obvious reduction in quality of life. *Daikenchuto* is evaluated in the mouse model and has been shown to improve the gastrointestinal movement. The mechanism is assumed to enhance the contraction of longitudinal muscle and relax the tonic contraction of circular muscle (Fukuda *et al.*, 2006). This mechanism explains the mechanism of action of *Daikenchuto* for the constipation induced by morphine.

6.8 Conclusion

I introduced a part of the evidences of Kampo medicine for the treatment of cancer. As a matter of fact, Kampo medicine is broadly used for the treatment of cancer from the early stage to the end of life care. *Juzentaihoto* and *Hochuekkito* are the most commonly used; *Juzentaihoto* is investigated to a greater extent than *Hochuekkito*. However, we need to further investigate the indications and mechanism of action and clarify the usefulness of Kampo treatment for cancer.

References

Fujiwara, K., Ohta, H. and Oka, H. (2002) Suppression of the liver function with Shosaikoto and its components. *J. Tradit. Med.* **5**, 238–241.

Fukuda, H., Chen, C., Mantyh, C., Ludwig, K., Pappas, T.N. and Takahashi, T. (2006) The herbal medicine, Dai-kenchu-to, accelerates delayed gastrointestinal transit after the operation in rats. *J. Surg. Res.* **131**, 290–295.

Hashimoto, K., Satoh, K., Kase, Y., Ishige, A., Kubo, M., Sasaki, H., Nishikawa, S., Kurosawa, S., Yakabi, K. and Nakamura, T. (2001) Modulatory effect of aliphatic acid amides from *Zanthoxylum piperitum* on isolated gastrointestinal tract. *Planta Med.* **67**, 179–181.

Hisha, H., Yamada, H., Sakurai, H., *et al.* (1997) Isolation and identification of hematopoietic stem cell-stimulating substances from Japanese herbal medicine, *Juzen-Taiho-to* (TJ-48). *Blood* **90**, 1022–1030.

Imazu, Y., Tsuiji, K., Toda, T., *et al.* (2006) Juzentaihoto reduces post-partial hepatectomy hyperammonemia by stabilizing intestinal microbiota. *J. Tradit. Med.* **23**, 208–215.

Itoh, T., Yamakawa, J., Mai, M., Yamaguchi, N. and Kanda, T. (2002) The effect of the herbal medicine *Dai-kenchu-to* on post-operative ileus. *J. Int. Med. Res.* **30**, 428–432.

Kaiho, T., Tanaka, T., Tsuchiya, S., *et al.* (2005) Effect of the herbal medicine Dai-kenchu-to for serum ammonia in hepatectomized patients. *Hepatogastroenterology* **52**(61), 161–165.

Kato, M., Liu, W., Yi, H., Asai, N., Hayakawa, A., Kozaki, K., Takahashi, M. and Nakashima, I. (1998) The herbal medicine *Sho-saiko-to* inhibits growth and metastasis of malignant melanoma primarily developed in ret-transgenic mice. *J. Invest. Dermatol.* **111**(4), 640–644.

Kato, M., Isobe, K., Dai, Y., Liu, W., Takahashi, M. and Nakashima, I. (2005) Further characterization of the *Sho-saiko-to*-mediated anti-tumor effect on melanoma developed in RET-transgenic mice. *J. Invest. Dermatol.* **114**, 599–601.

Konoshima,, T., Takasaki, M., Kozuka, M. and Tokuda, H. (1994) Anti-tumor promoting activities of *kampo* prescriptions. II. Inhibitory effects of *souseiryu-to* on two-stage carcinogenesis of mouse skin tumors and mouse pulmonary tumors. *Yakugaku Zasshi* **114**(4), 248–256.

Mori, K., Kondo, T., Kamiyama, Y., Kano, Y. and Tominaga, K. (2003) Preventive effect of *Kampo* medicine (*Hangeshashin-to*) against irinotecan-induced diarrhea in advanced non-small-cell lung cancer. *Cancer Chemother. Pharmacol.* **51**(5), 403–406.

Murata, P., Hayakawa, T., Sato, K., Kase, Y., Ishige, A. and Sasaki, H. (2001) The herbal medicine *Dai-kenchu-to* and one of its active components [6]-shogaol increase intestinal blood flow in rats. Effects of *Dai-kenchu-to*, a herbal medicine, on uterine and intestinal motility. *Phytother. Res.* **15**(4), 302–306.

Nagano, T., Itoh, H. and Takeyama, M. (1999) Effects of Dai-kenchu-to on levels of 3 brain-gut peptides (motilin, gastrin and somatostatin) in human plasma. *Biol. Pharm. Bull.* **22**(10), 1131–1133.

Nakamura, T., Sakai, A., Isogami, I., Noda, K., Ueno, K. and Yano, S. (2002) Abatement of morphine-induced slowing in gastrointestinal transit by *Daikenchuto*, a traditional Japanese herbal medicine. *Jpn. J. Pharmacol.* **88**, 217–221.

Ohnishi, Y., Yasumizu, R., Fan, H., Liu, J., *et al.* (1990) Effect of *Juzen-taiho-to* (TJ-48), a traditional Oriental medicine, on hematopoietic recovery from radiation injury in mice. *Exp. Hematol.* **18**, 18–22.

Ohnishi, Y., Fujii, H., Hayakawa, Y., *et al.* (1998) Oral administration of a *Kampo* (*Juzen-Taiho-to*) inhibits liver metastasis of colon 26-L5 carcinoma cells. *Jpn. J. Cancer Res.* **89**, 206–213.

Oka, H., Yamamoto, S., Kuroki, T., Harihara, S., Marumo, T., Kim, S.R., Monna, T., Kobayashi, K. and Thango, T. (2002) Prospective study of chemoprevention of hepatocellular carcinoma with Sho-saiko-to (TJ-9). *Cancer* **76**, 743–749.

Okimoto, J., Kimura, M., Hashiguchi, K., *et al.* (1991) The effect of Saireito on nephrotoxicity incuced by Cisplatin (CDDP). *Diagnos. Ther.* **79**, 1497–1501.

Satoh, K., Hashimoto, K., Hayakawa, T., Ishige, A., Kaneko, M., Ogihara, S., Kurosawa, S., Yakabi, K. and Nakamura, T. (2001) Mechanism of atropine-resistant contraction induced by *Dai-kenchu-to* in guinea pig ileum. *Jpn. J. Pharmacol.* **86**, 32–37.

Seeff, L.B., Lindsay, K.L., Bacon, B.R., Kresina, T.F. and Hoofnagle, J.H. (2001) Complemantary and alternative medicine in chronic liver disease. *Hepatology* **34**, 595–603.

Shiota, G., Maeta, Y., Mukoyami, T., *et al.* (2002) Effects of *Sho-saiko-to* on hepatocarcinogenesis and 8-hydroxy-2′-deoxyguanosine formation. *Hepatology* **35**(5), 1125–1133.

Sugiyama, K., Ueda, H., Suhara, Y., Kajima, Y., Ichio, Y. and Yokota, M. (1993a) Protective effects of *Kampo* medicines against cis-diamminedichloroplatinum (II)-induced nephrotoxicity and bone marrow toxicity in mice. *J. Med. Pharm. Soc.* **10**, 76–85.

Sugiyama, K., Ueda, H., Ichio, Y. and Yokota, M. (1993b) Improvement of cisplatin toxicity and lethality by Juzentaihoto in mice. *Biol. Pharm. Bull.* **18**, 53–58.

Sugiyama, K., Ueda, H., Suhara, Y., Kajima, Y., Ichio, Y. and Yokota, M. (1994) Protective effect of sodium L-malate, an active constituent isolated from *Angelicae Radix*, on cis-diamminedichloroplatinum (II)-induced toxic side effect. *Chem. Pharm. Bull.* **42**, 2565–2568.

Takasuna, K., Kasai, Y., Kitano, Y., Mori, K., Kobayashi, R., Hagiwara, T., Kakihata, K., Hirohashi, M., Nomura, M., Nagai, E. and Kamataki, T. (1995) Protective effects of *Kampo* medicines and baicalin against intestinal toxicity of a new anticancer camptothecin derivative, irinotecan hydrochloride (CPT-11), in rats. *Jpn. J. Cancer Res.* **86**(10), 978–984.

Takekawa, Y., Ikushima, J. and Matsumoto, H. (2000) Irradiation and Kampo. *Gan no Rinsho* **46**, 313–317 (in Japanese).

Thun, M.J., Namboodiri, M.M. and Heath, C.W. Jr. (2002) Aspirin use and reduced risk of fatal colon cancer. *N. Engl. J. Med.* **325**, 1593–1596.

Watanabe, S., Imanishi, J., Satoh, M. and Ozasa, K. (2001) Unique place of kampo (Japanese traditional medicine) in complementary and alternative medicine: A survey of doctors belonging to the regional medical association in Japan. *Tohoku J. Exp. Med.* **194**, 55–63.

Yamada, T., Nabeya, K. and Li, S. (1993) Postoperative combination therapy of chemotherapy and *Juzen-taiho-to* patients with digestive organ (especially gastric) cancer. *Igakuno Ayumi* **167**, 760–764 (in Japanese).

Chapter 7

Risk Management of Complementary Alternative Medicines in Cancer

Ursula Werneke

Abstract

Purpose: Cancer patients widely use complementary alternative medicines. Although some remedies have been shown to be of benefit, there is also a risk of potentially serious interactions with conventional cancer therapies and diagnostic procedures. The aim of this review is to identify the main factors which might make complementary medicines potentially unsafe in cancer.

Method: Systematic review of potential interactions with chemo- and radiotherapy and review of the purported mechanisms of action.

Results: Four factors were identified. These included the potential modification of the clinical course, interaction with the pharmacodynamics and pharmacokinetics of conventional therapies and potential alterations of investigations. Complementary immunostimulants may be contraindicated in lymphomas and other cancers in which suppression of the immune system is desired. Phytoestrogens could stimulate growth of hormone sensitive cancer cells. Antioxidants should not be used in chemotherapies whose mechanisms of action rely on cell damage through oxidative stress. Many remedies can interact with the cytochrome P450 system thereby potentially changing plasma levels of conventional medicines. However, *in vitro* effects or findings from animal studies may not translate into clinically relevant effects. Some remedies may interfere with the membrane transporter proteins thereby contributing to multi-drug resistance. Finally some complementary medicines remedies may interfere with unsealed source radiotherapy or nuclear scans.

Conclusions: Predicting the safety profile of complementary medicines is complex and may depend on personal and genetic factors. In cancer therapy, where the therapeutic margin of chemotherapies is very narrow, potential risks and benefits need to be meticulously evaluated.

Keywords: Cancer; Complementary Alternative Medicines; Chemotherapy; Radiotherapy; CYP; ABC; Multi-Drug Resistance; Antioxidants.

7.1 Introduction

The use of complementary alternative medicines (CAMs) in patients suffering from cancer is well documented. The reported evidence varies widely and may depend on how CAMs are defined. Current estimates suggest that between 7% and 80% of patients may take such treatments (Bernstein and Grasso, 2001; Ernst and Cassileth, 1999). The reasons for using CAMs may be complex. In cancer patients, themes identified evolve around reduction of side effects, reduction of psychological distress, attempts to gain control but also dissatisfaction with conventional care or using CAMs when other treatment options have failed (Lengacher *et al.*, 2006; Verhoef *et al.*, 2005). At the same time, patients may have difficulties indicating why they chose a specific remedy. They may then give more general reasons such as fighting cancer, boosting the immune system and enhance well-being (Humpel and Jones, 2006; Werneke *et al.*, 2004a).

Increasingly, where CAMs are thought to be beneficial, the mechanisms of actions are identified. Anti-cancer mechanisms include anti-proliferative, proapoptotic, antioxidant, anti-angiogenic and endocrine properties. Other remedies can interfere with tumour promoter and suppressor genes. Immunological mechanisms include stimulation of B lymphocytes, modification of leukocyte activity, activation of complement factors and cytokines (Werneke *et al.*, 2004b). However, "proof of principle" studies, often conducted *in vitro* or in animal experiments, need to be followed by systematic clinical testing of efficacy and safety in human beings. This is a time consuming process, and with the rapid expansion of the availability of information and remedies over the Internet patients may be increasingly less willing to wait for scientifically approved results. At the same time they may not be aware of the implications of CAM use for their cancer care (Ernst and Schmidt, 2004; Tascilar *et al.*, 2006). Clinicians need to be aware of CAM-induced side effects or interactions and should be able to identify hazards, advise patients accordingly and avoid uncritical encouragement of potentially harmful use (Werneke *et al.*, 2006). Ignorance in this area, given the independent usage of CAMs, may lead to criticism and possibly litigation (Cohen and Eisenberg, 2002). Equally, patients should be encouraged to disclose information about CAMs to health care professionals.

The aim of this review is to identify the main factors potentially making CAM use unsafe in cancer patients by critically reviewing the evidence base for the mechanism of action of such purported risks.

7.2 Methods

The Medline and Cochrane databases were searched for evidence in regard to the safety of CAMs for the treatment of different cancers and potential interactions with chemo- and radiotherapy. Search terms included the identified CAMs categorised as cancer treatments, immunostimulants, antioxidants, CAMs with endocrine and psychotropic properties and other CAMs identified to be used frequently by cancer patients (Werneke *et al.*, 2004b). These terms were combined with various chemotherapeutical radiopharmaceutical agents. Additional search terms included "side effects", "adverse drug reaction", "interaction", "antioxidants", "ABC cassette proteins", "P-glycoprotein", "BCRP", "MDRP", "multi-drug resistance", "cytochrome" and "CYP". The recovered papers were reviewed for further relevant references. Web-based resources such as Natural Medicines Comprehensive Database (NMCD) 2006 were also accessed for further information on the identified substances. Where available, reviews summarising safety data and the proposed mechanism of action were used, since presenting all the evidence in detail would have been beyond the scope of this paper, duplicating existing work. For clinical studies, meta-analyses and randomised controlled trials were given priority. However, due to the lack of systematic pharmacovigilance for CAMs, case reports, animal studies and *in vitro* evidence were also considered.

7.3 Results

Four potential factors were identified. These are the potential modification of the clinical course of specific tumour types, interaction with the pharmacodynamics and pharmacokinetics of conventional therapies as well as potential alterations of investigations.

7.3.1 *Potential modification of clinical course*

Potential interactions which could modify the clinical course will vary according to cancer type. Haematological cancers including lymphomas and hormone sensitive cancers may be affected. However, some of the findings are conflicting and pharmacological activity may be dependent on type of extract, dose and length of exposure.

7.3.1.1 Haematological cancers

In haematological cancers and lymphomas, abnormal and dysfunctional cell lines are produced with detrimental consequences for the immune system. That is why it comes as no surprise that patients may wish to undo damage to the immune system by using CAM immunostimulants. Remedies which may induce leukocyte proliferation and increase cell survival time include echinacea species, mistletoe, cat's claw and astragalus.

In animal and in *in vitro* experiments, echinacea has been associated with increase of white blood count and increase of mononuclear cells and decrease of granulocytes (Cundell *et al.*, 2003), proliferation of T lymphocytes (Morazzoni *et al.*, 2005; Jurkstiene *et al.*, 2004), and proliferation of B lymphocytes and macrophages (Luettig *et al.*, 1989; Stimpel *et al.*, 1984). However, some studies did not find increase of T cell activity (Stimpel *et al.*, 1984; South and Exon, 2001) and suggested that echinacea may even have immunosuppressant activity (South and Exon, 2001). It is unclear whether these effects are time dependent (Kemp and Franco, 2002). Mistletoe has been tested in clinical experiments and shown to lead to increases in total lymphocyte, monocyte and natural killer cell counts (Dohmen *et al.*, 2004). Mistletoe has also been found to be a potent activator of human neutrophil-induced apoptosis (Lavastre *et al.*, 2002). Induction of tumour proliferation such as in B cell lymphoma has been suggested but *in vitro* evidence has not substantiated this concern (Kelter and Fiebig, 2006; Hugo *et al.*, 2005). In animal experiments, cat's claw has been shown to increase lymphocyte survival time without increasing proliferation rate (Akesson *et al.*, 2003). Astragalus stimulates lymphocyte proliferation in healthy individuals (Sun *et al.*, 1983 and 2006). At the same time, astragalus has been shown to improve T cell function (Chu *et al.*, 1988). The effects of astragalus may be dose dependent, and immunosupression may occur at a higher dose (NMCD, 2006a).

Theoretically, extracts from these plants could boost malignant cell proliferation. Such proliferative effects have to be offset against improved function, for instance through activation of cytokines. However, non-specific stimulation of the immune system not targeted at specific tumour antigens is unlikely to translate into a specific anti-carcinogenic effect (Block and Mead, 2003).

7.3.1.2 Hormone sensitive cancers

Sex steroid sensitive cancers include breast, endometrial ovarian, testicular and prostate cancers. Sex steroid deprivation leading to successful therapy of metastatic cancer has long been known and was first reported in 1896 (Ellis and Swain, 2001). Pharmacological mechanisms of sex steroid deprivation include disruption of the biosynthesis, interference with the hypothalamic-pituitary feedback mechanism targeting luteinising releasing hormone (LRHR), action at end-organ receptors using full or partial antagonists or administration of opposing sex steroids, for instance using oestrogenic agents for the treatment of prostate cancer. Herbal remedies can unfold similar actions, but problems may arise when patients use these remedies to counteract undesired side effects of hormone deprivation. The main concern is that these agents stimulate proliferation of hormone sensitive cancer cells, for instance oestrogenic agents may promote breast cancer growth. These concerns can be difficult to prove clinically, since studies which carry a tangible risk of harm, may not be approved by ethics committees. Thus, most research in this area will rely on *in vitro* and animal experiments.

Oestrogen receptor agonists include panax ginseng (Lee *et al.*, 2003), liquorice (Maggiolini *et al.*, 2002), red clover (Huntley and Ernst, 2003), chaste berry and hops (Liu *et al.*, 2001). Soy with its active ingredient genistein is an oestrogen receptor agonist by itself but may unfold anti-oestrogenic properties in the presence of oestrogen (Messina *et al.*, 2006). Wild yam with its active ingredient diosgenin augments oestrogenic effects (Aradhana *et al.*, 1992). Dong Quai has been also been implicated as a phytoestrogen (Oerter Klein *et al.*, 2003). Black cohosh exerts its activity on the pituitary axis. Black cohosh binds to oestrogen receptors and depresses the luteinising hormone (Duker *et al.*, 1991; Seidlova-Wuttke *et al.*, 2003).

Predicting an effect of these plants on breast cancer cell proliferation is not straightforward. For instance, panax ginseng has many different ingredients, some of which are inhibitors of cell growth and proliferation whilst others are inducers of apoptosis and cell cycle arrest (Wang *et al.*, 2006). Such properties could outweigh a potentially adverse oestrogen-mediated cell proliferative stimulus, but only if such anti-carcinogenic activities were sufficiently tumour specific. Also, oestrogenic activity may depend on the extract chosen. In a recent *in vitro* study on American ginseng, only a methanol but not a water extract was able to elicit oestrogenic activity and stimulate breast cancer cell proliferation at low concentrations (King *et al.*, 2006).

Conversely, plants containing γ-linolenic acid such as evening primrose or borage have anti-oestrogenic properties. These could enhance the therapeutic response to tamoxifen in endocrine sensitive breast cancer through potentiation of the tamoxifen-induced down-regulation of the oestrogen receptor (Kenny *et al.*, 2000 and 2001).

7.3.2 *Potential interactions with pharmacodynamics of conventional therapies*

Cancer chemotherapies exert their function through causation of cell damage, interference with cell metabolism, specific immune responses to tumour antigens and reversal of endocrine activity. CAMs are often used to combat the significant adverse effects of such therapies. However, such improvements may come at the expense of a deterioration of the long term prognosis if the chemotherapeutic effect is attenuated (Labriola and Livingston, 1999).

7.3.2.1 Antioxidants

Chemically, oxidation is defined as the loss of electrons and reduction as a gain of electrons. Loss of electrons can leave the outer shell of an atom unstable producing a free radical. This will try to regain stability by scavenging electrons from another atom, which then becomes unstable. Thus, a chain reaction is started. Free radical production plays a role in many physiological mechanisms at cellular level. Free radicals can lead to cell damage when reactive oxygen species such as superoxide hydrogen peroxides and the hydroxyl radical or reactive nitrogen species such as nitric oxide are involved. For instance, reactive oxygen species can act as secondary messengers in intracellular signaling cascades which induce and maintain the oncogenic phenotype of cancer cells. However, reactive oxygen species can also induce cellular ageing and apoptosis (Volko *et al.*, 2006). Although these properties can be used therapeutically they can also cause organ damage as an unwanted effect.

Antioxidants are substances which can donate free radicals without becoming unstable themselves though electron loss. They come from a variety of sources including metals, minerals and plant products. Commonly used antioxidants include some vitamins and trace elements such as vitamins A, C and E, β-carotene, co-enzyme Q10 and selenium. Many plant extracts also have antioxidant properties such as green tea, grape seed, tomato and tumeric (Werneke *et al.*, 2004b). Other antioxidants include N-acetylcysteine, glutathione and melatonin. Zinc, manganese and copper are considered antioxidants when incorporated into superoxide dismutase and iron when incorporated into catalase (Labriola and Livingston, 1999).

Chemotherapeutic agents relying on oxidative stress include alkylating agents such as cyclophosphamide, anthracycline antibiotics such as doxorubicin, and epipodophyllotoxins such as etoposide (Labriola and Livingston, 1999; Pommier *et al.*, 2001). Essentially, these agents produce reactive oxygen species to target DNA thereby arresting cell cycles and inducing apoptosis. Antioxidants may suppress free radical formation and thus compromise the ability of chemotherapeutic agents to destroy micrometastases. This could translate into higher risk of recurrence. Antioxidants may also promote multi-drug resistance mediated through membrane transporter proteins. Expression of p-glycoprotein may be inhibited by reactive oxygen species (Wartenberg *et al.*, 2005) although the evidence is not consistent. For instance, glutamate has been shown to increase reactive oxygen species formation and enhance expression and activity of p-glycoprotein. This process could be reversed by n-acetylcysteine (Zhu and Liu, 2004). Equally, radiotherapy depends on irradiation-induced free radical formation and antioxidants may potentially compromise radiotherapy results (Agostinelli and Seiler, 2006; D'Andrea, 2005). However, individual antioxidants vary in action and may not necessarily compromise chemo- and radiotherapy (Labriola and Livingston, 1999).

7.3.2.2 Antifolates and folic acid

Probably the best known antifolate is methotrexate (MTX) which interferes with DNA biosynthesis. One mechanism of action is based on the inhibition of dihydrofolate reductase leading to accumulation of inactive folate forms (Messmann and Allegra, 2001). Theoretically, folate supplementation could at least partly reverse the antifolate activity. On the one hand, this could lead to relief of adverse effects including the reduction of treatment related death (Calvert, 2002). On the other hand, this could also adversely affect the effectiveness of chemotherapy. The research evidence remains conflicting (Kelemen, 2006). For instance, one study in children with lymphoblastic leukaemia showed that folic acid could stimulate the bone marrow (Schroder *et al.*, 1986).

7.3.2.3 Endocrine therapies and immune therapies

The most commonly used sex steroid therapies include anti-oestrogenic and anti-androgenic therapies (Table 7.1). Mechanisms of action include direct activity at end organ receptors, interference with the hypothalamic-pituitary feedback mechanism or inhibition of synthesis. Anti-androgens currently used include non-steroidal anti-androgens such as flutamide, ketoconazole and finasteride. Saw palmetto is an herbal anti-oestrogen commonly used in benign prostate hyperplasia (Prager *et al.*, 2002). Anti-oestrogens include tamoxifen, a mixed oestrogen receptor agonist and antagonist and aromatase inhibitors such as anastrozole, which inhibit the production oestrogen through aromatization of adrenal androgens (Ellis and Swain, 2001). As well as increasing oestrogen-sensitive cell proliferation, herbal oestrogens could reverse the endocrine action of anti-oestrogenic therapies. However, clinical experience is limited.

Table 7.1. Examples of common anti-cancer drugs and CYP metabolism.

Drug class	Drug	Pharmaco-logically active	Main CYP enzyme for primary conversion	Metabolite pharmacologically active	MDR resistance gene (Zhou-Pan *et al.*, 1993)
Alkylating agents	Cyclophospha-mide	No	2B6, 3A4	Yes (Scripture *et al.*, 2005; Baumhakel *et al.*, 2001)	
			3A4	Inactivation of primary metabolite (Scripture *et al.*, 2005)	
	Ifophosphamide	No	3A4	Yes (Scripture *et al.*, 2005)	
Camptothecins (Topoisomerase I targeting agents)	Irinotecan	No	N/A	Yes (Scripture *et al.*, 2005)	
			3A4	No (Scripture *et al.*, 2005)	
	Topotecan	Yes	3A	Yes: weaker (Takimoto and Arbruck, 2001)	ABCB1 ABCG2

Table 7.1. (*Continued*)

Drug class	Drug	Pharmaco-logically active	Main CYP enzyme for primary conversion	Metabolite pharmacologically active	MDR resistance gene (Zhou-Pan *et al.*, 1993)
Epidodophyollo-toxins (Topoisomerase II inhibitors)	Etoposide	Yes	3A4, 3A5	Yes (Pommier *et al.*, 2001; Relling *et al.*, 1994)	ABCB1 ABCC1 ABCC3 ABCG2
	Teniposide	Yes	3A4, 3A5	Unclear (Pommier *et al.*, 2001; Relling *et al.*, 1994)	ABCB1
Taxols	Paclitaxel	Yes	2C8, 3A4, 3A5	Yes: weaker (Scripture *et al.*, 2005; Rowinsky and Donehower, 2001)	ABCB1
	Docetaxel	Yes	3A: 3A4, 3A5, 2B, 1A	Yes: weaker (Scripture *et al.*, 2005; Rowinsky and Donehower, 2001)	ABCB1

Table 7.1. *(Continued)*

Drug class	Drug	Pharmaco-logically active	Main CYP enzyme for primary conversion	Metabolite pharmacologically active	MDR resistance gene (Zhou-Pan *et al.*, 1993)
Vinca alkaloids	Vincristine	Yes	3A4, 3A5	Unclear (Baumhakel *et al.*, 2001; Rowinsky and Donehower, 2001; Dennison *et al.*, 2006)	ABCB1 ABCC1
	Vinblastine	Yes	3A, 3A4	Yes (Rowinsky and Donehower, 2001; Zhou-Pan *et al.*, 1993)	ABCB1 ABCC2
Partial oestrogen antagonists	Tamoxifen	Yes	3A4, 2D6	Yes: stronger (Scripture *et al.*, 2005)	

Glucocorticoids have cytotoxic as well immunosuppressant effects. They are integrated into many chemotherapeutic treatment schemes. CAMs stimulating the immune system, such as astragalus, beta-glucans, cat's claw, echinacea and mistletoe could theoretically modify the immunosuppressant effects. Some CAMs can also theoretically interfere with monoclonal antibodies by inducing proliferation in the same cell lines targeted by the antibody. This could either lead to synergistic effects as demonstrated at molecular level for beta-glucans (Yan *et al.*, 2005) or antagonistic effects such as stimulation of B lymphocytes through echinacea (Stimpel *et al.*, 1984).

7.3.3 *Pharmacokinetic interactions*

The pharmacokinetics of most anti-cancer drugs is highly variable between patients and may be genetically modified. For instance, the oxidative metabolism depends on the cytochrome (CYP) system. Several proteins mediating drug transport through cell membranes have been identified in the context of multi-drug resistance (MDR). Finally direct interactions between CAMs and anti-cancer drugs may possibly lead to accumulation of toxic metabolites. Genetics may account for 20% to 95% of the variability in therapeutic response and toxic effects (Scripture *et al.*, 2005).

7.3.3.1 The CYP system

The liver is the most important site of CYP metabolism but other organs can also express these enzymes. About 60% of all clinically used drugs are metabolised through CYP 3A4 including HIV protease inhibitors, HIV non-nucleoside reverse transcriptase inhibitors, warfarin, cyclosporine, ketoconazole, oral contraceptives, some anti-convulsants such as carbamazepine, digoxine and theophylline (CSMMCA, 2000).

In anti-cancer agents, metabolisation through the CYP system may not necessarily lead to a decrease in plasma level or diminution of effect. For instance, cyclophosphamide is an inactive pro-drug, which is transformed to the effective substance by CYP2B. Tamoxifen although pharmacologically active, is metabolised to much more potent anti-oestrogenic metabolites (Scripture *et al.*, 2005). Corticosteroids are mainly metabolised through CYP3A4, but the activity of the metabolites depends on the formulation of the different subtypes. The effects of CYP inducers and inhibitors are essentially differential depending on whether metabolites are more or less active (Table 7.1). If metabolites are less active than the original agent, CYP inhibitors increase whereas inducers reduce therapeutic effectiveness. Conversely, if metabolites are more active than the original agent, CYP inhibitors reduce whereas inducers increase therapeutic effectiveness. However, the pharmacodynamic net effects may change in those drugs whose active metabolites undergo CYP mediated inactivation. For instance, cyclophosphamide metabolites are further inactivated by CYP3A4 (Scripture *et al.*, 2005).

This differential metabolic activity has to be considered when the safety profiles of CAMs are evaluated. Many herbal remedies can modify CYP activity, however activity demonstrated *in vitro* does not always translate into clinical effects (Tables 7.2a–d). Also for some remedies, microsomal activity may be extract dependent (Sparreboom *et al.*, 2004). Given that the expression of the microsomal enzymes is also affected by age, sex, type of tumour, liver function and genetic polymorphisms (Scripture *et al.*, 2005) as well as type of remedy and extract (Sparreboom *et al.*, 2004), the clinical impact on metabolism may be extremely difficult to predict.

7.3.3.2 ABC transporters

The ABC cassette genes represent proteins which bind to ATP and use this energy to drive various molecules through cell membranes. The transport is mostly unidirectional (Sparreboom *et al.*, 2003). This can lead to drug resistance in cancer chemotherapy when drugs are increasingly transported out of the target cells. Multi-drug resistance can occur when a transporter protein is stimulated by one agent but the resulting resistance affects several agents transported by the respective protein. Three ABC genes seem to be responsible for nearly all the drug resistance in cancer chemotherapy: ABCB1 encoding p-glycoprotein (p-GP), ABCC1 encoding multi-drug resistance associated protein 1 (MRP1) and ABCG2 encoding breast cancer resistance associated protein (BCRP) (Sparreboom *et al.*, 2003). However, not all chemotherapies are affected by these transporter

Table 7.2a. CAMs and CYP and MDR activity: anti-cancer, immunostimulant and antioxidant remedies.

Remedy	CYP *in vitro* activity*	CYP *in vivo* activity*	MDR *in vitro*	MDR *in vivo*
Goldenseal	2C9 INH (Chatterjee and Franklin, 2003)	3A4, 3A5, 2D6 INH (Gurley *et al.*, 2005)		
Quercetin	3A4 IND long term or INH short term (Pal and Mitra, 2006) 1A, 2B IND (Rahden-Staron *et al.*, 2001)	3A4 IND in animal model (Choi and Li, 2005)	P-gp† INH (Wang *et al.*, 2005a; Limtrakul *et al.*, 2005)	P-gp INH (animal model) (Choi and Li, 2005; Hsiu *et al.*, 2002)
Echinacea	2C9, 3A4 (weak) INH (Yale and Glurich, 2005)	3A4 INH (weak) (Yale and Glurich, 2005; Gurley *et al.*, 2004) IND or INH depending on extract (Sparreboom *et al.*, 2004)		
Grape seed	2E1 INH (Ray *et al.*, 2001)	3A IND (animal model) (Nishikawa *et al.*, 2004)		
Green tea	1A1, 1A2, 3A4 INH or IND depending on cell lines (Netsch *et al.*, 2006; Yang and Raner, 2005) 1A1, 2A6, 2C19, 2E1, 3A4 INH (Muto *et al.*, 2001)	3A IND in liver and 3A INH in small intestinum (Nishikawa *et al.*, 2004)	P-gp, MRP‡2: no effect (Netsch *et al.*, 2005) P-gp INH (Kitagawa *et al.*, 2004; Mei *et al.*, 2004; Jodoin *et al.*, 2002)	

*INH: Inhibition, IND: Induction.

†P-gp: P-glycoprotein.

‡MRP: Multi-resistance protein.

§BCRP: Breast cancer resistance protein.

Table 7.2b. CAMs and CYP and MDR activity: endocrine remedies.

Remedy	CYP *in vitro* activity	CYP *in vivo* activity	MDR *in vitro*	MDR *in vivo*
Liquorice	3A4, 2C9, 2B6 INH (Kent *et al.*, 2002)	2C9, 3A4 in animal model (Mu *et al.*, 2006)		
	3A, 1A2, 2B1 IND after repeated doses (Paolini *et al.*, 1999)			
Red clover	1A1, 1B1 INH (Roberts *et al.*, 2004) 1A2, 2C8, 2C9, 2C19, 2D6, 3A4 INH (Unger and Frank, 2004)			
Soy	1A1, 1A2, 2E1 INH (Helsby *et al.*, 1998)	3A4: no induction (Sparreboom *et al.*, 2004)	BRCP but not P-gp INH (Imai *et al.*, 2004)	P-gp INH (animal model) (Green *et al.*, 2005)
	Unhydrolysed: 1A2, 2A6, 2D6 INH and 3A4 IND (Anderson *et al.*, 2003) Hydrolysed: 1A2, 2A6, 2C9 2D6, 3A4 INH (Anderson *et al.*, 2003)		P-gp, MRP1, MRP2 INH (Sparreboom *et al.*, 2003)	
Evening primrose	1A2, 2C9, 2C19, 2D6, 3A4 INH (Zou *et al.*, 2002)			
Saw palmetto	2C9, 2D6, 3A4 INH (Yale and Glurich, 2005)	1A2, 2D6, 2E1, 3A4: no significant effect (Gurley *et al.*, 2004) 2D6, 3A4: no significant effect (Markowitz *et al.*, 2003b)		

Table 7.2c. CAMs and CYP and MDR activity: psychotropic remedies.

Remedy	CYP *in vitro* activity	CYP *in vivo* activity	MDR *in vitro*	MDR *in vivo*
Ginkgo	1A1, 1A2, 2B1/2, 3A1 INH (Zhao *et al.*, 2006) 2C9, 3A4 INH (Yale and Glurich, 2005) 2C19 INH (Sparreboom *et al.*, 2004)	2C19, 3A4 INH (Sparreboom *et al.*, 2004) 3A4 INH (weak) (Markowitz *et al.*, 2003c)	cf. Quercetin	
Ginseng	1A1, 1A2, 1B1, 2C9, 2C19, 2D6, 2E1, 3A4 INH or 3A4: no effect (Sparreboom *et al.*, 2004)	2D6 INH (weak) in elderly (Gurley *et al.*, 2005)	BRCP INH (weak) (Jin *et al.*, 2006) P-gp INH of protopanaxatriol ginsenosides in high concentrations (Choi *et al.*, 2003) P-gp INH of Rg (3) ginsenoids (Kim *et al.*, 2003)	Rg (3) increased life span in mice implanted with doxorubicin-resistant leukaemia cells (Kim *et al.*, 2003)
St. John's wort	3A4 IND long term or INH short term (Pal and Mitra, 2006) CYP 1B1 INH (Chaudhary and Willett, 2006) 2D2, 2A2 INH and 2C6 IND (Dostalek *et al.*, 2006)	2E1, 3A4 IND in elderly (Gurley *et al.*, 2005)	P-gp IND (weak) (Weber *et al.*, 2004) P-gp IND (Tian *et al.*, 2005) P-gp INH (Patel *et al.*, 2004)	
Valerian	3A4 INH (Lefebvre *et al.*, 2004)	3A4 INH (weak) (Gurley *et al.*, 2005) 3A4: minimal INH and 2D6 no effect (Donovan *et al.*, 2004)	P-gp INH (Lefebvre *et al.*, 2004)	

Table 7.2d. CAMs and CYP and MDR activity: other remedies.

Remedy	CYP *in vitro* activity	CYP *in vivo* activity	MDR *in vitro*	MDR *in vivo*
Milk thistle	2D6, 2E1, 3A4 INH: not at clinically achievable doses (Sparreboom *et al.*, 2004)	1A2, 2D6, 2E1, 3A4: no significant effect (Gurley *et al.*, 2004)	P-gp INH (Chung *et al.*, 2005) P-gp: no effect (Patel *et al.*, 2004; DiCenzo *et al.*, 2003)	
	2C9, 3A4 INH (Sridar *et al.*, 2004)			
Garlic	CYP2C9*1, 2C19, 3A4, 3A5, 3A7 INH, 2D6: no effect (Sparreboom *et al.*, 2004)	2D6 INH in elderly (Gurley *et al.*, 2005)	P-gp INH and MRP2 IND (Demeule *et al.*, 2004)	
		2E1 INH, 1A, 2B IND long term (animal model) (Sparreboom *et al.*, 2004)	P-gp INH (Patel *et al.*, 2004)	
		2D6, 3A4: no effect (Markowitz *et al.*, 2003a)	p-gp INH (weak) (Foster *et al.*, 2001)	

proteins (Table 7.1). Equally, although many CAMs may also exert such an effect (Tables 7.2a–d), the clinical relevance of such pharmacokinetic interactions remains unclear (Morris and Zhang, 2006).

7.3.4 *Toxic effects*

Toxic effects are a great concern not only in cancer chemotherapy but also in CAMs. Such concern may be even greater in view of compromised liver and kidney function found in many cancer patients. Here three examples are given which have raised clinical concerns and highlight general principles.

7.3.4.1 Vitamin C and methotrexate

Many cancer patients take supplements and over 10% may take doses higher than recommended (Werneke *et al.*, 2004a). However, the combination of high dose vitamin C and methotrexate (MTX) should be avoided since this could lead to kidney damage and increased MTX plasma levels and thus MTX toxicity. Vitamin C acidifies urine. This leads to the precipitation of MTX and its less water soluble metabolites 7-hydroxy-MTX and 4-diamino-N(10)-methylpteroic acid (DAMPA), which cannot be excreted (Sketris *et al.*, 1984).

7.3.4.2 Kava: alcohol or water extracts?

Kava has been withdrawn from the market in many high-income countries due to concerns about liver toxicity. About 78 cases have been reported. Of these, 11 patients required a liver transplant, and four died. Reduction of liver glutathione, an antioxidant which plays a role in hepatic detoxification, has been implicated as mechanism of this adverse reaction (Clouatre, 2004). The glutathione content in a kava extract depends on the mechanism of extraction. Whereas in aqueous extracts the glutathione is extracted along with the kavalactones, in acetone or alcohol solutions glutathione is not extracted. This would explain why the indigenous Polynesian population using water mixture have not developed significant liver problems, whilst medicinal use mostly relying on acetone or alcoholic extracts has led to reports of liver toxicity (Cote *et al.*, 2004). Inhibition of CYP3A4, CYP1A2, CYP2C9, and CYP2C19 may also be more pronounced for the commercial rather that the traditional preparations (Cote *et al.*, 2004). However, this hypothesis still requires confirmation.

7.3.4.3 Pyrrolizidine alkaloids and hepatotoxicity

Many plants of the boraginaca and senecio species contain genotoxic pyrrolizidine alkaloids (NMCD: Borage). The major metabolites of many of these compounds are (+/−) 6,7-dihydro-7-hydroxy-1-(hydroxymethyl)-5H-pyrrolizine (DHP) and pyrrolizidine alkaloid N-oxides (Wang *et al.*, 2005b). DHP can react with DNA to form a set of eight DNA adducts involved in the formation of liver tumours (Xia *et al.*, 2006). Additionally, under hypoxic conditions N-oxides can be converted to DHP and the parent alkaloid, whereas under oxidative conditions this reaction is inhibited (Wang *et al.*, 2005b). CYP 3A4 inhibitors also hinder this reaction (Cote *et al.*, 2004) but conversely CYP3A4 inducers may facilitate DHP production (NMCD, 2006b).

7.3.5 *Potential interaction with nuclear medicine*

Most cancer physicians will be aware of radiopharmaceutical interactions with conventional medicines. For instance the uptake of ^{131}I and ^{123}I MIBG (meta-iodo-benzyl-guanidine) are affected by thyroxin and tricyclic

Table 7.3a. CAMs and nuclear medicine: potential interactions with unsealed source radiotherapy.

Radio-pharmaceutical (RP)/method	Target condition	CAM	Uptake	Other effects
^{131}Iodine	Thyroid cancer	Iodine supplements, kelp, selenium (facilitates T4 → T3), garlic preparation with high selenium contents	↓	
^{123}I MIBG (meta-iodo-benzyl-guanidine)	Phaeochromo cytoma	St. John's wort, ephedra, cholinergic stimulants such as lobelia and areca, ginkgo, ginseng, hydergine	↓	↑ blood pressure
		Grapefruit juice ↑ nifedipine levels through CYP3A4 inhibition	↑	
Somatostatin (SS) analogues ^{111}(In Octreo Scan)	Gastro-entero-pancreatic-neuro-endocrine tumours, neural crest, small cell lung and lymphoma	Licorice, ginger, rhubarb, cannabis: Low dose	↓	
		High dose cannabis, ginkgo, panax ginseng, hydergine, areca	↓	

Source: Werneke and McCready (2004).

Table 7.3b. CAMs and nuclear medicine: potential interactions with diagnostic procedures.

Radio-pharmaceutical (RP)/method	Target condition	CAM	Uptake	Other effects
Glomerular filtration rate (GFR) measurements	Kidney	Chromium		↓ GFR
		Parsley, juniper, L-arginine		↑ GFR
		High dose parsley, high dose vitamin C, Ca oxalate containing plants such as rhubarb		Potentially nephrotoxic
Bone scans	Bone	Iron supplements Vitamin C increasing iron absorption	↓	
		Phytoestrogens		Accumulation of RP in breast tissue
Cholescintigraphy	Gall bladder	Opiate derivatives		Possibly ↑ of common bile duct activity, but effect variable
		Agents enhancing the effect of barbiturates such as valerian and kava		Investigation of neonatal jaundice to increase the accuracy of 99mTc-IDA scintigraphy in differentiating extrahepatic biliary atresia from neonatal hepatitis

Source: Werneke and McCready (2004).

Table 7.3b. (*Continued*)

Radio-pharmaceutical (RP)/method	Target condition	CAM	Uptake	Other effects
Adenosine (perfusion studies)	Heart: perfusion imaging	Methylxanthines (purinergic stimulants) containing caffeine such as green tea or theobromine such as cola and cocoa		↑ myocardial ischemia?
		Feverfew		Vasodilatation of smooth muscle
		Milk thistle		↓ doxorubicin metabolism ↓ doxorubicin plasma level, diffuse uptake?
^{123}I Ioflupane (DaTSCAN)	Brain: Parkinson's disease	Substances binding to dopamine (DA) transporter or DA pre-synaptic receptors, affecting DA release such as iboga, St. John's wort, anise chromium	↓	
Sestamibi (breast imaging, multi-drug resistence, perfusion imaging)	Breast multi-drug resistance, perfusion imaging	P-gp inducers such as St. John's wort, (cf. Tables 7.2a–d)	↓	
		P-gp inhibitors (cf. Tables 7.2a–d)	↑	

Source: Werneke and McCready (2004).

anti-depressants or decongestants, respectively. CAMs can equally compete for uptake targeting the same mechanisms as conventional medicines. This may affect unsealed source radiotherapy such as treatment for thyroid cancer, phaeochromocytoma, some gastro- entero- pancreatic- neuro-endocrine tumours, as well as neural crest, small cell lung cancer and some lymphomas (Table 7.3a). Diagnostic procedures such as glomerular filtration rate (GFR) measurements, bone scans, cholescintigraphy, adenosine perfusion studies and MDR scans may be equally affected (Table 7.3b). Unfortunately at present, the clinical evidence for such potential interactions is extremely limited and prediction depends on the hypotheses of the mechanism of action. In clinical practice, such interactions may go unnoticed and may possibly account for a proportion of unexplained or unexpected results of nuclear scans (Werneke and McCready, 2004).

7.4 Conclusions

Predicting the safety profile of CAMs is extremely complex. Potential interactions may depend on the extract chosen, age, sex, conventional medication and genetic factors. This poses a particular challenge in cancer therapy when the therapeutic margin of chemotherapy is very narrow and interference with conventional therapy could destabilise the course of treatment. Many CAMs are taken to counter side-effects of chemo- and radiotherapy. Although this is intuitively appealing, alleviation or even reversal of side-effects may come at the expense of poorer long term outcomes. For instance, partial deactivation of chemotherapy could facilitate the spread of micro-metastasis (Labriola and Livingston, 1999). Much attention has been given to metabolic effects exerted through the hepatic microsomal system leading to alterations in plasma levels and hence therapeutic efficacy. However, *in vitro* effects or findings from animal studies may not translate into equivalent effects in humans and will require extensive and systematic clinical studies with standardised CAM formulations. The same applies to interference of CAMs with nuclear medicine. Whereas use of iodine containing remedies should be avoided when patients receive ^{131}I, patients undergoing glomerular filtration rate measurements should not change their CAM regimen prior to the investigation because sudden changes in kidney activity could alter the results (Werneke and McCready, 2004). However, clinicians and researchers should consider CAM use as a potential cause when the results or treatments or investigations are unusual and unexpected. At present it remains clinically and legally prudent for health professionals to take a detailed history of CAM use and advise patients on the potential risks and benefits as applicable to their individual clinical case. However, in most cases, CAMs may not have be discontinued if conventional treatments are closely monitored. Pharmacovigilance systems for CAMs, which can be easily incorporated into routine clinical practice, need to be developed. At the same time, increasing efforts to systematise CAM research and produce standardised remedies may expand the evidence of potentially adverse interactions and allow quantification of such risks.

References

Agostinelli, E. and Seiler, N. (2006) Non-irradiation-derived reactive oxygen species (ROS) and cancer: Therapeutic implications. *Amino Acids* **31**, 341–355.

Akesson, C.H., Pero, R.W. and Ivars, F. (2003) C-Med 100, a hot water extract of *Uncaria tomentosa*, prolongs lymphocyte survival *in vivo*. *Phytomedicine* **10**, 23–33.

Anderson, G.D., Rosito, G., Mohustsy, M.A. and Elmer, G.W. (2003) Drug interaction potential of soy extract and Panax ginseng. *J. Clin. Pharmacol.* **43**, 643–648.

Aradhana, Rao, A.R. and Kale, R.K. (1992) Diosgenin — a growth stimulator of mammary gland of ovariectomized mouse. *Indian J. Exp. Biol.* **30**, 367–370.

Baumhakel, M., Kasel, D., Rao-Schymanski, R.A., Bocker, R., Beckurts, K.T., Zaigler, M., Barthold, D. and Fuhr, U. (2001) Screening for inhibitory effects of antineoplastic agents on CYP3A4 in human liver microsomes. *Int. J. Clin. Pharmacol. Ther.* **39**, 517–528.

Bernstein, B.J. and Grasso, T. (2001) Prevalence of complementary and alternative medicine use in cancer patients. *Oncology* (*Huntingt.*) **15**, 1267–1272.

Block, K.I. and Mead, M.N. (2003) Immune system effects of echinacea, ginseng, and astragalus: A review. *Integr Cancer Ther.* **2**, 247–267.

Calvert, H. (2002) Folate status and the safety profile of antifolates. *Semin. Oncol.* **2**(Suppl 5), 3–7.

Chatterjee, P. and Franklin, M.R. (2003) Human cytochrome p450 inhibition and metabolic-intermediate complex formation by goldenseal extract and its methylenedioxyphenyl components. *Drug Metab. Dispos.* **31**, 1391–1397.

Chaudhary, A. and Willett, K.L. (2006) Inhibition of human cytochrome CYP 1 enzymes by flavonoids of St. John's wort. *Toxicology* **217**, 194–205.

Choi, C.H., Kang, G. and Min, Y.D. (2003) Reversal of P-glycoprotein-mediated multi-drug resistance by protopanaxatriol ginsenosides from Korean red ginseng. *Planta Med.* **69**, 235–240.

Choi, J.S. and Li, X. (2005) Enhanced diltiazem bioavailability after oral administration of diltiazem with quercetin to rabbits. *Int. J. Pharm.* **297**, 1–8.

Chu, D.T., Wong, W.L. and Mavligit, G.M. (1988) Immunotherapy with Chinese medicinal herbs. I. Immune restoration of local xenogeneic graft-versus-host reaction in cancer patients by fractionated *Astragalus membranaceus in vitro*. *J. Clin. Lab. Immunol.* **25**, 119–123.

Chung, S.Y., Sung, M.K., Kim, N.H., Jang, J.O., Go, E.J. and Lee, H.J. (2005) Inhibition of P-glycoprotein by natural products in human breast cancer cells. *Arch. Pharm. Res.* **28**, 823–828.

Clouatre, D.L. (2004) Kava kava: Examining new reports of toxicity. *Toxicol. Lett.* **150**, 85–96.

Cohen, M.H. and Eisenberg, D.M. (2002) Potential physician malpractice liability associated with complementary and integrative medicinal therapies. *Ann. Intern. Med.* **136**, 596–603.

Committee of Safety in Medicine and Medicines Control Agency (CSMMCA) (2000) Reminder: St. John's wort (*Hypericum perforatum*) interactions. *Curr. Prob. Pharmacovigilance* **26**, 6–7.

Cote, C.S., Kor, C., Cohen, J. and Auclair, K. (2004) Composition and biological activity of traditional and commercial kava extracts. *Biochem. Biophys. Res. Commun.* **322**, 147–152.

Cundell, D.R., Matrone, M.A., Ratajczak, P. and Pierce, J.D. Jr. (2003) The effect of aerial parts of Echinacea on the circulating white cell levels and selected immune functions of the aging male Sprague-Dawley rat. *Int. Immunopharmacol.* **3**, 1041–1048.

D'Andrea, G.M. (2005) Use of antioxidants during chemotherapy and radiotherapy should be avoided. *CA Cancer J. Clin.* **55**, 319–321.

Demeule, M., Brossard, M., Turcotte, S., Regina, A., Jodoin, J. and Beliveau, R. (2004) Diallyl disulfide, a chemopreventive agent in garlic, induces multidrug resistance-associated protein 2 expression. *Biochem. Biophys. Res. Commun.* **324**, 937–945.

Dennison, J.B., Kulanthaivel, P., Barbuch, R.J., Renbarger, J.L., Ehlhardt, W.J. and Hall, S.D. (2006) Selective metabolism of vincristine *in vitro* by CYP3A5. *Drug Metab. Dispos.* **34**, 1317–1327.

DiCenzo, R., Shelton, M., Jordan, K., Koval, C., Forrest, A., Reichman, R. and Morse, G. (2003) Coadministration of milk thistle and indinavir in healthy subjects. *Pharmacotherapy* **23**, 866–870.

Dohmen, W., Breier, M. and Mengs, U. (2004) Cellular immunomodulation and safety of standardized aqueous mistletoe extract PS76A2 in tumor patients treated for 48 weeks. *Anti-cancer Res.* **24**, 1231–1237.

Donovan, J.L., DeVane, C.L., Chavin, K.D., Wang, J.S., Gibson, B.B., Gefroh, H.A. and Markowitz, J.S. (2004) Multiple night-time doses of valerian (*Valeriana officinalis*) had minimal effects on CYP3A4 activity and no effect on CYP2D6 activity in healthy volunteers. *Drug Metab. Dispos.* **32**, 1333–1336.

Dostalek, M., Pistovcakova, J., Jurica, J., Tomandl, J., Linhart, I., Sulcova, A. and Hadasova, E. (2006) Effect of St. John's wort (*Hypericum perforatum*) on cytochrome P-450 activity in perfused rat liver. *Life Sci.* **78**, 239–244.

Duker, E.M., Kopanski, L., Jarry, H. and Wuttke, W. (1991) Effects of extracts from *Cimicifuga racemosa* on gonadotropin release in menopausal women and ovariectomized rats. *Planta Med.* **57**, 420–424.

Ellis, M.J. and Swain, S.M. (2001) Steroid hormone therapies for cancer. In: *Cancer Chemotherapy and Biotherapy*, 3rd ed. (eds.) Chabner, B.A. and Logo, D. Lippincott, Williams & Wilkins, Philadelphia, PA, USA, pp. 85–138.

Ernst, E. and Cassileth, B.R. (1999) How useful are unconventional cancer treatments? *Eur. J. Cancer* **35**, 1608–1613.

Ernst, E. and Schmidt, K. (2004) "Alternative" cures for depression — how safe are web sites? *Psychiatry Res.* **129**, 297–301.

Foster, B.C., Foster, M.S., Vandenhoek, S., Krantis, A., Budzinski, J.W., Arnason, J.T., Gallicano, K.D. and Choudri, S. (2001) An *in vitro* evaluation of human cytochrome P450 3A4 and P-glycoprotein inhibition by garlic. *J. Pharm. Pharm. Sci.* **4**, 176–184.

Green, A.K., Barnes, D.M. and Karasov, W.H. (2005) A new method to measure intestinal activity of P-glycoprotein in avian and mammalian species. *J. Comp. Physiol.* [*B*]. **75**, 57–66.

Gurley, B.J., Gardner, S.F., Hubbard, M.A., Williams, D.K., Gentry, W.B., Carrier, J., Khan, I.A., Edwards, D.J. and Shah, A. (2004) *In vivo* assessment of botanical supplementation on human cytochrome P450 phenotypes: *Citrus aurantium*, *Echinacea purpurea*, milk thistle, and saw palmetto. *Clin. Pharmacol. Ther.* **76**, 428–440.

Gurley, B.J., Gardner, S.F., Hubbard, M.A., Williams, D.K., Gentry, W.B., Cui, Y. and Ang, C.Y. (2005) Clinical assessment of effects of botanical supplementation on cytochrome P450 phenotypes in the elderly: St. John's wort, garlic oil, panax ginseng and ginkgo biloba. *Drugs Aging* **22**, 525–539.

Gurley, B.J., Gardner, S.F., Hubbard, M.A., Williams, D.K., Gentry, W.B., Khan, I.A. and Shah, A. (2006) *In vivo* effects of goldenseal, kava kava, black cohosh, and valerian on human cytochrome P450 1A2, 2D6, 2E1, and 3A4/5 phenotypes. *Clin. Pharmacol. Ther.* **77**, 415–426.

Helsby, N.A., Chipman, J.K., Gescher, A. and Kerr, D. (1998) Inhibition of mouse and human CYP 1A- and 2E1-dependent substrate metabolism by the isoflavonoids genistein and equol. *Food Chem. Toxicol.* **36**, 375–382.

Hugo, F., Dittmar, T., Treutler, E.K., Zanker, K.S. and Kuehn, J.J. (2005) The *Viscum album* extract Iscador P does not cause an autocrine interleukin-6 loop in B-non-Hodgkin's lymphoma cell lines. *Onkologie* **28**, 415–420.

Humpel, N. and Jones, S.C. (2006) Gaining insight into the what, why and where of complementary and alternative medicine use by cancer patients and survivors. *Eur. J. Cancer Care (Engl.)* **15**, 362–368.

Huntley, A.L. and Ernst, E. (2003) A systematic review of herbal medicinal products for the treatment of menopausal symptoms. *Menopause* **10**, 465–476.

Hsiu, S.L., Hou, Y.C., Wang, Y.H., Tsao, C.W., Su, S.F. and Chao, P.D. (2002) Quercetin significantly decreased cyclosporin oral bioavailability in pigs and rats. *Life Sci.* **72**, 227–235.

Imai, Y., Tsukahara, S., Asada, S. and Sugimoto, Y. (2004) Phytoestrogens/flavonoids reverse breast cancer resistance protein/ABCG2-mediated multi-drug resistance. *Cancer Res.* **64**, 4346–4352.

Jin, J., Shahi, S., Kang, H.K., van Veen, H.W. and Fan, T.P. (2006) Metabolites of ginsenosides as novel BCRP inhibitors. *Biochem. Biophys. Res. Commun.* **345**, 1308–1314.

Jodoin, J., Demeule, M. and Beliveau, R. (2002) Inhibition of the multi-drug resistance P-glycoprotein activity by green tea polyphenols. *Biochim. Biophys. Acta* **1542**, 149–159.

Jurkstiene, V., Kondrotas, A.J. and Kevelaitis, E. (2004) Compensatory reactions of immune system and action of Purple Coneflower (*Echinacea purpurea* (*L.*) *Moench*) preparations. *Medicina* (*Kaunas*) **40**, 657–662.

Kelemen, L.E. (2006) The role of folate receptor alpha in cancer development, progression and treatment: Cause, consequence or innocent bystander? *Int. J. Cancer* **119**, 243–250.

Kelter, G. and Fiebig, H.H. (2006) Absence of tumor growth stimulation in a panel of 26 human tumor cell lines by mistletoe (*Viscum album L.*) extracts Iscador *in vitro. Arzneimittelforschung* **56**, 435–440.

Kemp, D.E. and Franco, K.N. (2002) Possible leukopenia associated with long-term use of echinacea. *J. Am. Board Fam. Pract.* **15**, 417–419.

Kenny, F.S., Pinder, S.E., Ellis, I.O., Gee, J.M., Nicholson, R.I., Bryce, R.P. and Robertson, J.F. (2000) Gamma linolenic acid with tamoxifen as primary therapy in breast cancer. *Int. J. Cancer* **85**, 643–648.

Kenny, F.S., Gee, J.M., Nicholson, R.I., Ellis, I.O., Morris, T.M., Watson, S.A., Bryce, R.P. and Robertson, J.F. (2001) Effect of dietary GLA+/-tamoxifen on the growth, ER expression and fatty acid profile of ER positive human breast cancer xenografts. *Int. J. Cancer* **92**, 342–347.

Kent, U.M., Aviram, M., Rosenblat, M. and Hollenberg, P.F. (2002) The licorice root derived isoflavan glabridin inhibits the activities of human cytochrome P450S 3A4, 2B6, and 2C9. *Drug Metab. Dispos.* **30**, 709–715.

Kim, S.W., Kwon, H.Y., Chi, D.W., Shim, J.H., Park, J.D., Lee, Y.H., Pyo, S. and Rhee, D.K. (2003) Reversal of P-glycoprotein-mediated multi-drug resistance by ginsenoside Rg(3). *Biochem. Pharmacol.* **65**, 75–82.

King, M.L., Adler, S.R. and Murphy, L.L. (2006) Extraction-dependent effects of American ginseng (*Panax quinquefolium*) on human breast cancer cell proliferation and estrogen receptor activation. *Integr. Cancer Ther.* **5**, 236–243.

Kitagawa, S., Nabekura, T. and Kamiyama, S. (2004) Inhibition of P-glycoprotein function by tea catechins in KB-C2 cells. *J. Pharm. Pharmacol.* **56**, 1001–1005.

Labriola, D. and Livingston, R. (1999) Possible interactions between dietary antioxidants and chemotherapy. *Oncology* (*Williston Park*) **13**, 1003–1008.

Lavastre, V., Pelletier, M., Saller, R., Hostanska, K. and Girard, D. (2002) Mechanisms involved in spontaneous and *Viscum album* agglutinin-I-induced human neutrophil apoptosis: *Viscum album* agglutinin-I accelerates the loss of antiapoptotic Mcl-1 expression and the degradation of cytoskeletal paxillin and vimentin proteins via caspases. *J. Immunol.* **168**, 1419–1427.

Lee, Y.J., Jin, Y.R., Lim, W.C., Park, W.K., Cho, J.Y., Jang, S. and Lee, S.K. (2003) Ginsenoside-Rb1 acts as a weak phytoestrogen in MCF-7 human breast cancer cells. *Arch. Pharm. Res.* **26**, 58–63.

Lefebvre, T., Foster, B.C., Drouin, C.E., Krantis, A., Livesey, J.F. and Jordan, S.A. (2004) *In vitro* activity of commercial valerian root extracts against human cytochrome P450 3A4. *J. Pharm. Pharm. Sci.* **7**, 265–273.

Lengacher, C.A., Bennett, M.P., Kip, K.E., Gonzalez, L., Jacobsen, P. and Cox, C.E. (2006) Relief of symptoms, side effects, and psychological distress through use of complementary and alternative medicine in women with breast cancer. *Oncol. Nurs. Forum* **33**, 97–104.

Limtrakul, P., Khantamat, O. and Pintha, K. (2005) Inhibition of P-glycoprotein function and expression by kaempferol and quercetin. *J. Chemother.* **17**, 86–95.

Liu, J., Burdette, J.E., Xu, H., Gu, C., van Breemen, R.B., Bhat, K.P., Booth, N., Constantinou, A.I., Pezzuto, J.M., Fong, H.H., Farnsworth, N.R. and Bolton, J.L. (2001) Evaluation of estrogenic activity of plant extracts for the potential treatment of menopausal symptoms. *J. Agric. Food Chem.* **49**, 2472–2479.

Luettig, B., Steinmuller, C., Gifford, G.E., Wagner, H. and Lohmann-Matthes, M.L. (1989) Macrophage activation by the polysaccharide arabinogalactan isolated from plant cell cultures of *Echinacea purpurea*. *J. Natl. Cancer. Inst.* **81**, 669–675.

Maggiolini, M., Statti, G, Vivacqua, A., Gabriele, S., Rago, V., Loizzo, M., Menichini, F. and Amdo, S. (2002) Estrogenic and anti-proliferative activities of isoliquiritigenin in MCF7 breast cancer cells. *J. Steroid Biochem. Mol. Biol.* **82**, 315–322.

Markowitz, J.S., Devane, C.L., Chavin, K.D., Taylor, R.M., Ruan, Y. and Donovan, J.L. (2003a) Effects of garlic (*Allium sativum L.*) supplementation on cytochrome P450 2D6 and 3A4 activity in healthy volunteers. *Clin. Pharmacol. Ther.* **74**, 170–177.

Markowitz, J.S., Donovan, J.L., Devane, C.L., Taylor, R.M., Ruan, Y., Wang, J.S. and Chavin, K.D. (2003b) Multiple doses of saw palmetto (*Serenoa repens*) did not alter cytochrome P450 2D6 and 3A4 activity in normal volunteers. *Clin. Pharmacol. Ther.* **74**, 536–542.

Markowitz, J.S., Donovan, J.L., Lindsay DeVane, C., Sipkes, L. and Chavin, K. (2003c) Multiple-dose administration of *Ginkgo biloba* did not affect cytochrome P-450 2D6 or 3A4 activity in normal volunteers. *J. Clin. Psychopharmacol.* **23**, 576–581.

Mei, Y., Qian, F., Wei, D. and Liu, J. (2004) Reversal of cancer multi-drug resistance by green tea polyphenols. *J. Pharm. Pharmacol.* **56**, 1307–1314.

Messina, M., McCaskill-Stevens, W. and Lampe, J.W. (2006) Addressing the soy and breast cancer relationship: Review, commentary, and workshop proceedings. *J. Natl. Cancer Inst.* **98**, 1275–1284.

Messmann, R.A. and Allegra, C. (2001) Antifolates. In: *Cancer Chemotherapy and Biotherapy*, 3rd ed. (eds.) Chabner, B.A. and Logo, D. Lippincott, Williams & Wilkins, Philadelphia, PA, USA, p. 138.

Morazzoni, P., Cristoni, A., Di Pierro, F., Avanzini, C., Ravarino, D., Stornello, S., Zucca, M. and Musso, T. (2005) *In vitro* and *in vivo* immune stimulating effects of a new standardized *Echinacea angustifolia* root extract (Polinacea). *Fitoterapia* **76**, 401–411.

Morris, M.E. and Zhang, S. (2006) Flavonoid-drug interactions: Effects of flavonoids on ABC transporters. *Life Sci.* **78**, 2116–2130.

Mu, Y., Zhang, J., Zhang, S., Zhou, H.H., Toma, D., Ren, S., Huang, L., Yaramus, M., Baum, A., Venkataramanan, R. and Xie, W. (2006) Traditional Chinese medicines Wu Wei Zi (*Schisandra chinensis* Baill) and Gan Cao (*Glycyr-rhiza uralensis* Fisch) activate pregnane X receptor and increase warfarin clearance in rats. *J. Pharmacol. Exp. Ther.* **316**, 1369–1377.

Muto, S., Fujita, K., Yamazaki, Y. and Kamataki, T. (2001) Inhibition by green tea catechins of metabolic activation of procarcinogens by human cytochrome P450. *Mutat. Res.* **479**, 197–206.

Natural Medicines Comprehensive Database (2006a) http://www. naturaldatabase.com. Product search: Astragalus.

Natural Medicines Comprehensive Database (2006b) http://www. naturaldatabase.com. Product search: Borage.

Netsch, M.I., Gutmann, H., Luescher, S., Brill, S., Schmidlin, C.B., Kreuter, M.H. and Drewe, J. (2005) Inhibitory activity of a green tea extract and some of its constituents on multi-drug resistance-associated protein 2 functionality. *Planta Med.* **71**, 135–141.

Netsch, M.I., Gutmann, H., Schmidlin, C.B., Aydogan, C. and Drewe, J. (2006) Induction of CYP1A by green tea extract in human intestinal cell lines. *Planta Med.* **72**, 514–520.

Nishikawa, M., Ariyoshi, N., Kotani, A., Ishii, I., Nakamura, H., Nakasa, H., Ida, M., Nakamura, H., Kimura, N., Kimura, M., Hasegawa, A., Kusu, F., Ohmori, S., Nakazawa, K. and Kitada, M. (2004) Effects of continuous ingestion of green tea or grape seed extracts on the pharmacokinetics of midazolam. *Drug Metab. Pharmacokinet.* **19**, 280–289.

Oerter Klein, K., Janfaza, M., Wong, J.A. and Chang, R.J. (2003) Estrogen bioactivity in fo-ti and other herbs used for their estrogen-like effects as determined by a recombinant cell bioassay. *J. Clin. Endocrinol. Metab.* **88**, 4077–4079.

Pal, D. and Mitra, A.K. (2006) MDR- and CYP3A4-mediated drug-herbal interactions. *Life Sci.* **78**, 2131–2145.

Paolini, M., Barillari, J., Broccoli, M., Pozzetti, L., Perocco, P. and Cantelli-Forti, G. (1999) Effect of liquorice and glycyrrhizin on rat liver carcinogen metabolizing enzymes. *Cancer Lett.* **145**, 35–42.

Patel, J., Buddha, B., Dey, S., Pal, D. and Mitra, A.K. (2004) *In vitro* interaction of the HIV protease inhibitor ritonavir with herbal constituents: Changes in P-gp and CYP3A4 activity. *Am. J. Ther.* **11**, 262–277.

Pommier, Y.G., Goldwasser, F. and Strumberg, D. (2001) Topoisomerase II inhibitors: Epipodophyllotoxins, acridines, ellipticines and bisdioxo-piperazines. In: Cancer Chemotherapy and Biotherapy, 3rd ed. (eds.) Chabner, B.A. and Logo, D. Lippincott, Williams & Wilkins, Philadelphia, PA, USA, pp. 539–578.

Prager, N., Bickett, K., French, N. and Marcovici, G. (2002) A randomized, double-blind, placebo-controlled trial to determine the effectiveness of botanically derived inhibitors of 5-alpha-reductase in the treatment of androgenetic alopecia. *J. Altern. Complement. Med.* **8**, 143–152.

Rahden-Staron, I., Czeczot, H. and Szumilo, M. (2001) Induction of rat liver cytochrome P450 isoenzymes CYP 1A and CYP 2B by different fungicides, nitrofurans, and quercetin. *Mutat. Res.* **498**, 57–66.

Ray, S.D., Parikh, H., Hickey, E., Bagchi, M. and Bagchi, D. (2001) Differential effects of IH636 grape seed proanthocyanidin extract and a DNA repair modulator 4-aminobenzamide on liver microsomal cytochrome 4502E1-dependent aniline hydroxylation. *Mol. Cell. Biochem.* **218**, 27–33.

Relling, M.V., Nemec, J., Schuetz, E.G., Schuetz, J.D., Gonzalez, F.J. and Korzekwa, K.R. (1994) O-demethylation of epipodophyllotoxins is catalyzed by human cytochrome P450 3A4. *Mol. Pharmacol.* **45**, 352–358.

Roberts, D.W., Doerge, D.R., Churchwell, M.I., Gamboa da Costa, G., Marques, M.M. and Tolleson, W.H. (2004) Inhibition of extrahepatic human cytochromes P450 1A1 and 1B1 by metabolism of isoflavones found in *Trifolium pratense* (red clover). *J. Agric. Food Chem.* **52**, 6623–6632.

Rowinsky, E.K. and Donehower, R.C. (2001) Antimicrotubule agents. In: *Cancer Chemotherapy and Biotherapy*, 3rd ed. (eds.) Chabner, B.A. and Logo, D. Lippincott, Williams & Wilkins, Philadelphia, PA, USA, pp. 329–372.

Seidlova-Wuttke, D., Hesse, O., Jarry, H., Christoffel, V., Spengler, B., Becker, T. and Wuttke, W. (2003) Evidence for selective estrogen receptor modulator activity in a black cohosh (*Cimicifuga racemosa*) extract: Comparison with estradiol-17beta. *Eur. J. Endocrinol.* **149**, 351–362.

Schroder, H., Clausen, N., Ostergard, E. and Pressler, T. (1986) Folic acid supplements in vitamin tablets: A determinant of hematological drug tolerance in maintenance therapy of childhood acute lymphoblastic leukaemia. *Pediatr. Hematol. Oncol.* **3**, 241–247.

Scripture, C.D., Sparreboom, A. and Figg, W.D. (2005) Modulation of cytochrome P450 activity: Implications for cancer therapy. *Lancet Oncol.* **6**, 780–789.

Sketris, I.S., Farmer, P.S. and Fraser, A. (1984) Effect of vitamin C on the excretion of methotrexate. *Cancer Treat. Rep.* **68**, 446–447.

South, E.H. and Exon, J.H. (2001) Multiple immune functions in rats fed echinacea extracts. *Immunopharmacol. Immunotoxicol.* **23**, 411–421.

Sparreboom, A., Danesi, R., Ando, Y., Chan, J. and Figg, W.D. (2003) Pharmacogenomics of ABC transporters and its role in cancer chemotherapy. *Drug Resist. Update* **6**, 71–84.

Sparreboom, A., Cox, M.C., Acharya, M.R. and Figg, W.D. (2004) Herbal remedies in the United States: Potential adverse interactions with anti-cancer agents. *J. Clin. Oncol.* **22**, 2489–2503.

Sridar, C., Goosen, T.C., Kent, U.M., Williams, J.A. and Hollenberg, P.F. (2004) Silybin inactivates cytochromes P450 3A4 and 2C9 and inhibits major hepatic glucuronosyltransferases. *Drug Metab. Dispos.* **32**, 587–594.

Stimpel, M., Proksch, A., Wagner, H. and Lohmann-Matthes, M.L. (1984) Macrophage activation and induction of macrophage cytotoxicity by purified polysaccharide fractions from the plant *Echinacea purpurea. Infect. Immun.* **46**, 845–849.

Sun, J.L., Hu, Y.L., Wang, D.Y., Zhang, B.K. and Liu, J.G. (2006) Immunologic enhancement of compound Chinese herbal medicinal ingredients and their efficacy comparison with compound Chinese herbal medicines. *Vaccine* **24**, 2343–2348.

Sun, Y., Hersh, E.M., Lee, S.L., McLaughlin, M., Loo, T.L. and Mavligit, G.M. (1983) Preliminary observations on the effects of the Chinese medicinal herbs *Astragalus membranaceus* and *Ligustrum lucidum* on lymphocyte blastogenic responses. *J. Biol. Response Mod.* **2**, 227–237.

Takimoto, C.H. and Arbruck, S. (2001) Topoisomerase I targeting agents: The camptothecins. In: *Cancer Chemotherapy and Biotherapy*, 3rd ed. (eds.) Chabner, B.A. and Logo, D. Lippincott, Williams & Wilkins, Philadelphia, PA, USA, pp. 579–646.

Tascilar, M., de Jong, F.A., Verweij, J. and Mathijssen, R.H. (2006) Complementary and alternative medicine during cancer treatment: Beyond innocence. *Oncologist* **11**, 732–741.

Tian, R., Koyabu, N., Morimoto, S., Shoyama, Y., Ohtani, H. and Sawada, Y. (2005) Functional induction and de-induction of P-glycoprotein by St. John's wort and its ingredients in a human colon adenocarcinoma cell line. *Drug Metab. Dispos.* **33**, 547–554.

Unger, M. and Frank, A. (2004) Simultaneous determination of the inhibitory potency of herbal extracts on the activity of six major cytochrome P450 enzymes using liquid chromatography/mass spectrometry and automated online extraction. *Rapid Commun. Mass Spectrom.* **18**, 2273–2281.

Valko, M., Leibfritz, D., Moncol, J., Cronin, M.T., Mazur, M. and Telser, J. (2007) Free radicals and antioxidants in normal physiological functions and human disease. *Int. J. Biochem. Cell Biol.* **39**, 44–84.

Verhoef, M.J., Balneaves, L.G., Boon, H.S. and Vroegindewey, A. (2005) Reasons for and characteristics associated with complementary and alternative medicine use among adult cancer patients: A systematic review. *Integr. Cancer Ther.* **4**, 274–286.

Wang, W., Zhao, Y., Rayburn, E.R., Hill, D.L., Wang, H. and Zhang, R. (2007) *In vitro* anti-cancer activity and structure-activity relationships of natural products isolated from fruits of Panax ginseng. *Cancer Chemother.* **59**, 589–601.

Wang, Y., Cao, J. and Zeng, S. (2005a) Involvement of P-glycoprotein in regulating cellular levels of Ginkgo flavonols: Quercetin, kaempferol, and isorhamnetin. *J. Pharm. Pharmacol.* **57**, 751–758.

Wang, Y.P., Yan, J., Fu, P.P. and Chou, M.W. (2005b) Human liver microsomal reduction of pyrrolizidine alkaloid N-oxides to form the corresponding carcinogenic parent alkaloid. *Toxicol. Lett.* **155**, 411–420.

Wartenberg, M., Gronczynska, S., Bekhite, M.M., Saric, T., Niedermeier, W., Hescheler, J. and Sauer, H. (2005) Regulation of the multi-drug resistance transporter P-glycoprotein in multicellular prostate tumor spheroids by hyperthermia and reactive oxygen species. *Int. J. Cancer* **113**, 229–240.

Weber, C.C., Kressmann, S., Fricker, G. and Muller, W.E. (2004) Modulation of P-glycoprotein function by St. John's wort extract and its major constituents. *Pharmacopsychiatry* **37**, 292–298.

Werneke, U. and McCready, V.R. (2004) Complementary alternative medicine and nuclear medicine. *Eur. J. Nucl. Med. Mol. Imaging* **31**, 599–603.

Werneke, U., Earl, J., Seydel, C., Horn, O., Crichton, P. and Fannon, D. (2004a) Potential health risks of complementary alternative medicines in cancer patients. *Br. J. Cancer* **90**, 408–413.

Werneke, U., Ladenheim, D. and McCarthy, T. (2004b) Complementary alternative medicine for cancer: A review of effectiveness and safety. *Cancer-Therapy* **2B**, 475–500.

Werneke, U., Turner, T. and Priebe, S. (2006) Complementary alternative medicine in psychiatry: A review of effectiveness and safety. *Br. J. Psych.* **188**, 109–121.

Xia, Q., Chou, M.W., Edgar, J.A., Doerge, D.R. and Fu, P.P. (2006) Formation of DHP-derived DNA adducts from metabolic activation of the prototype heliotridine-type pyrrolizidine alkaloid, lasiocarpine. *Cancer Lett.* **231**, 138–145.

Yale, S.H. and Glurich, I. (2005) Analysis of the inhibitory potential of *Ginkgo biloba*, *Echinacea purpurea*, and *Serenoa repens* on the metabolic activity of cytochrome P450 3A4, 2D6, and 2C9. *J. Altern. Complement. Med.* **11**, 433–439.

Yan, J., Allendorf, D.J. and Brandley, B. (2005) Yeast whole glucan particle (WGP) beta-glucan in conjunction with anti-tumour monoclonal antibodies to treat cancer. *Expert Opin. Biol. Ther.* **5**, 691–702.

Yang, S.P. and Raner, G.M. (2005) Cytochrome P450 expression and activities in human tongue cells and their modulation by green tea extract. *Toxicol. Appl. Pharmacol.* **202**, 140–150.

Zhao, L.Z., Huang, M., Chen, J., Ee, P.L., Chan, E., Duan, W., Guan, Y.Y., Hong, Y.H., Chen, X. and Zhou, S. (2006) Induction of propranolol metabolism by *Ginkgo biloba* extract EGb 761 in rats. *Curr. Drug Metab.* **7**, 577–587.

Zhou-Pan, X.R., Seree, E., Zhou, X.J., Placidi, M., Maurel, P., Barra, Y. and Rahmani, R. (1993) Involvement of human liver cytochrome P450 3A in vinblastine metabolism: Drug interactions. *Cancer Res.* **53**, 5121–5126,.

Zhu, H.J. and Liu, G.Q. (2004) Glutamate up-regulates P-glycoprotein expression in rat brain microvessel endothelial cells by an NMDA receptor-mediated mechanism. *Life Sci.* **75**, 1313–1322.

Zou, L., Harkey, M.R. and Henderson, G.L. (2002) Effects of herbal components on cDNA-expressed cytochrome P450 enzyme catalytic activity. *Life Sci.* **71**, 1579–1589.

List of English and Scientific Names of Plants

English Names	Scientific Names
American ginseng	*Panax quinquefolium*
Astragalus	*Astragalus membranaceus*
Beta-glucans	1-3, 1-6-beta-glucan
Black cohosh	*Actaea racemosa*
Borage/star flower	*Borago officinalis*
Cat's claw	*Uncaria tomentosa*
Chaste berry	*Vitex agnus castus*
Dong quai	*Angelica sinensis*
Echinacea species	*Echinacea*
Evening primrose	*Oenothera biennis*
Grape seed	*Vitis vinifera*
Green tea	*Camellia sinensis*
Hops	*Humulus lupulus*
Kava	*Piper methysticun*
Liquorice	*Glycyrrhiza glabra*
Mistletoe	*Viscum album*
Panax ginseng	*Panax ginseng*
Red clover	*Trifolium pratense*
Saw palmetto	*Serenoa repens*
Soy	*Glycine max*
Tomato	*Lycopersicon esculentum*
Tumeric	*Curcuma longa*
Wild yam	*Dioscorea alata*

Chapter 8

Complementary Therapies for Cancer Patients

Barrie R. Cassileth, Jyothirmai Gubili & K. Simon Yeung

Abstract

Complementary therapies are increasingly sought by cancer patients to control treatment-related symptoms. Unproven methods that do not actually treat cancer are often promoted falsely as cancer cures. These are termed "alternative therapies." Typically expensive and potentially harmful, they can interact with chemotherapy drugs and other medication. Complementary therapies such as music, massage, acupuncture and meditation are non-invasive, gentle techniques applied to control physical and emotional symptoms commonly experienced by cancer patients. These therapies are used as adjuncts to mainstream cancer treatment. Patients and physicians should be aware of the distinction between questionable methods that are not helpful, and complementary therapies that successfully reduce symptoms and enhance quality of life. Easy access to information and misinformation about these therapies via the Internet and print media compounds this problem.

Keywords: Cancer; Symptom Control; Complementary Therapies; Alternative Therapies; Acupuncture.

8.1 Introduction

Since the beginning of civilization, all cultures have developed means of treating illness. Herbs and minerals were used as medicine, and many spiritual and physical practices were also applied to restore health. This knowledge was passed along to subsequent generations, recorded in classical textbooks, and came to form what we know today as Traditional Medical Systems (Table 8.1).

More recently, advances in science have dramatically transformed the study and practice of medicine. Today, physicians visualize the inner organs for abnormalities with sophisticated techniques such as MRI, test blood for genetic defects and prescribe powerful synthetic drugs. While these advances enable cures for many previously incurable illnesses, including cancer, they are not always successful. Chemotherapy and other therapies that are successful against disease cause adverse effects. This has led many cancer patients to seek treatments outside of conventional care for cure and also to relieve distressing symptoms.

The umbrella term, "Complementary and Alternative Medicine (CAM)" today is commonly used in the US. However, the differences between complementary and alternative therapies are important to understand. "Alternative" therapies are not supported by evidence. Most are expensive and potentially harmful as they may worsen the disease state or interact with drugs used in standard treatments. Patients may also delay seeking more effective mainstream treatment in hopes of cure offered by such therapies, which may be falsely claimed to be more natural as well as effective.

Complementary therapies, on the other hand, serve as adjuncts to mainstream care. They can relieve symptoms commonly experienced by cancer patients, and enhance patients' physical, mental and spiritual well-being. As scientific evidence increasingly supports the value of acupuncture and other complementary therapies, these therapies have gradually been incorporated into modern mainstream medical care. They are now offered in many hospitals' cancer programs as therapies for symptom control.

8.2 The Prevalence of Complementary and Alternative Medicine (CAM) Therapies

The rates of CAM usage internationally are higher among cancer patients than in other groups. A systematic review in 1998 (Ernst and Cassileth, 1998) of 26 surveys in cancer patients from 13 countries showed that the average prevalence of CAM use across all studies was 31%. This number has ballooned to 45% in this decade based on ten other similar studies published after 2000. Prevalence rates vary from 30% among prostate cancer patients in Canada (Boon *et al.*, 2003) to as high as 98% among

Table 8.1. World Health Organization fact sheet on traditional medicine.

- In China, traditional herbal preparations account for 30%–50% of the total medicinal consumption.
- In Europe, North America and other industrialized regions, over 50% of the population have used CAM at least once.
- In San Francisco, London and South Africa, 75% of people living with HIV/AIDS use TM/CAM.
- 70% of the population in Canada has used complementary medicine at least once.
- In Germany, 90% of the population has used a natural remedy at some point in their life. Between 1995 and 2000, the number of doctors who underwent special training in natural medicine had almost doubled to 10,800.
- In the United States, 158 million of the adult population use complementary medicines and according to the USA Commission for alternative and complementary medicines, US$17 billion was spent on traditional remedies in 2000.
- In the United Kingdom, annual expenditure on alternative medicine is US$230 million.
- The global market for herbal medicines currently stands at over US$60 billion annually and is growing steadily.

Source: [*WHO*]*http://www.who.int/mediacentre/factsheets/fs134/en*

breast cancer patients in China (Cui *et al.*, 2004). Commonly used therapies include herbs, homeopathy, hypnotherapy, imagery or visualization, meditation, megavitamins, relaxation and spiritual healing (Table 8.2).

8.2.1 *CAM literature*

In the 1970s and early 1980s, unconventional therapies typically were reported in medical journals as quackery. In the last two decades, however, a significant increase in high quality research articles on complementary therapies publications has occurred. A MEDLINE search using "Complementary Therapies" as key words reveals this trend. In the 1980s, the medical literature contained 2800 articles with only 71 (3%) randomized controlled trials (RCTs). In the 1990s, of 3000 articles listed, 255 (8%) were RCTs. The increase is even greater in the 2000s. In the past seven years, more than 4000 articles were Medline indexed and the number of RCT doubled to more than 500 (12%).

Table 8.2. North American classification of complementary therapies.

CAM categories	Modalities derived from TCM
Whole Medical Systems include naturopathic and homeopathic medicine as well as traditional systems derived from non-western cultures.	Traditional Chinese medicine
Mind-Body Medicine involves treatment techniques that connect the mind to body's physical functions and to treat symptoms of disease. Meditation, prayer, as well as art, dance, and music therapies fall into this category.	*Tai Chi*
Biologically Based Practices usually refer to using natural products like herbs, minerals, vitamins, and diet to alter disease outcome. These include many unproved cancer therapies such as shark cartilage and Essiac.	Chinese herbal medicine, green tea, mushroom products
Manipulative and Body-Based Practices are therapies based on moving and/or manipulating body parts or joints. Some examples are massage and chiropractic manipulation.	Acupuncture, moxibustion, *Tui Na*
Energy Medicine involves use of purported energy flow to treat diseases. It can be divided into Biofield therapies such as *Qi Gong* and *Reiki* that use energy emitted from the healer or the patient; and bioelectromagnetic-based therapies that use magnet or other electric current fields as therapy.	*Qi Gong*

8.2.2 *Herbal remedies*

Herbs and dietary supplements are the most popular CAM therapies. Medicinal herbal agents, or phytomedicinals, are made from the whole plant or its leaves, stems, flowers, seeds, and/or roots. Herbal supplements may consist of a single herb or a combination of several, as used in traditional Chinese medicine and Ayurvedic medicine from India. According to the World Health Organization, 80% of the world's population continues to use botanicals as the primary source of medicine today. Many cancer

Table 8.3. Herbal products with potentially serious adverse effects.

Product (responsible constituents if known)	Adverse effects
Aristolochia, *Bragantia* or *Asarum* species (aristolochic acid)	Renal toxicity that can lead to renal failure
Common comfrey, prickley comfrey, and Russian comfrey (pyrrolizidine alkaloids)	Hepatotoxicity, veno-occlusive disease
Ma huang (ephedrine alkaloids)	Sympathomimetic activity, hypertension, tachycardia, increased risks for stroke, heart attack and heart failure
Phytoestrogens	Estrogenic effects
Kava kava	Hepatotoxicity
St. John's Wort	Potent cytochrome P4503A4 inducer, altered metabolism of many drugs

Source: *U.S. Food and Drug Administration.*

patients use herbal supplements for relief from symptoms associated with cancer treatments. However, safety and efficacy of many botanicals are not known.

For example, the herb "*Ma Huang*" traditionally used in China to treat respiratory congestion was marketed as a dietary supplement for weight loss in the US. However, over-dosage led to at least a dozen deaths, heart attacks, and strokes. In Belgium, at least 70 people required renal transplant or dialysis for interstitial fibrosis of the kidney after taking an herbal preparation made from the wrong species of plant as slimming treatment (Table 8.3).

8.3 Complementary Therapies

8.3.1 *Mind-body techniques*

The very existence of placebo effect, in which suggestions and expectancy can induce biological change, demonstrates the connection between mind and body. The potential to influence health with our minds is an appealing concept and an under-utilized opportunity. It affirms the power of the individual. Some mind-body interventions have moved from the category of alternative, unconventional therapies into mainstream complementary or supportive care. For example, the effectiveness of meditation, biofeedback, and yoga in stress reduction and the control of some physiologic reactions have been documented (Deng and Cassileth, 2005). Mind-body therapies in palliative care are geared to decrease distress and promote relaxation in different ways.

Hypnotherapy for pain is well supported (Sellick and Zaza, 1998). This can be integrated into different stages (the Initial Crisis, Transition, Acceptance, and Preparation for Death) of patient's reaction to the lack of curative options (Marcus *et al.*, 2003). Other techniques, including visualization and progressive relaxation, also decrease pain and promote well-being (Walker *et al.*, 1999).

Meditation can help stress reduction. In a randomized wait-list control study of 109 cancer patients, participation in a 7-week Mindfulness-Based Stress Reduction Program was associated with significant improvement in mood disturbance and symptoms of stress (Speca *et al.*, 2000). Another single arm study of breast and prostate cancer patients showed significant improvement in overall quality of life, stress and sleep quality, but symptom improvement was not significantly correlated with program attendance or minutes of home practice (Carlson *et al.*, 2004).

In another study, Tibetan yoga that incorporates controlled breathing and visualization significantly decreased sleep disturbance when compared to wait-list controls (Cohen *et al.*, 2004). Mindfulness-Based Stress Reduction techniques must be practiced regularly to produce beneficial effects (Astin *et al.*, 2003).

8.3.2 *Acupuncture*

Conventional medical regimens may not satisfactorily treat cancer-related pain. The acceptance of complementary medicine as an adjunct to treatments opens a wide array of tactics to treat pain syndromes. Several complementary medicine modalities such as hypnosis, massage, music therapy, mind-body exercises, and dietary supplementation have been shown to reduce anxiety as well as chronic pain.

Acupuncture is perhaps the most extensively studied complementary modality for pain control. A randomized placebo-controlled trial tested auricular acupuncture for patients with pain despite stable medication. Pain intensity decreased by 36% at two months from baseline in the treatment group, a statistically significant difference compared with the two control groups, for whom little pain reduction was seen. Most patients in this study had neuropathic pain, which is often refractory to conventional treatment.

Neurophysiologic studies show that acupuncture-induced analgesic effects appear mediated by endogenous opioids and other neurotransmitters. Functional brain imaging studies suggest that acupuncture also modulates the affective-cognitive aspect of pain perception. Correlations between functional MRI signal intensities and analgesic effects induced by acupuncture have been reported.

Large clinical trials support the efficacy of acupuncture as a treatment for various cancer-related symptoms. Although acupuncture in an integral part of TCM, it is practiced more often than any other modalities of Chinese medicine in non-Asian countries. Among patient groups internationally, however, acupuncture is used by less than 10% of cancer patients. This is true even in countries where acupuncture has been used traditionally. For example, fewer than 5% of cancer patients in China and Japan use acupuncture (Cui *et al.*, 2004; Hyodo *et al.*, 2005). In Europe, 4% of patients had tried acupuncture but only 2% continue to receive treatments after cancer diagnosis (Molassiotis *et al.*, 2005).

Most acupuncture research has been conducted in analgesia models. Acupuncture was shown to be effective for both acute (e.g. post-operative dental pain) and chronic (e.g. headache) pain (Benson *et al.*, 2004; Melchart *et al.*, 1999). A recent randomized controlled trial of 570 patients with osteoarthritis of the knee found that a 26-week course of acupuncture significantly improved pain and dysfunction when compared to sham-acupuncture control (Berman *et al.*, 2004).

In another study, a randomized placebo-controlled trial tested auricular acupuncture for cancer patients with pain despite use of pain medication. Ninety patients were randomized to needles placed at correct acupuncture points (treatment group), versus acupuncture or pressure at non-acupuncture points. Pain intensity decreased by 36% at two months from baseline in the treatment group, a statistically significant difference compared with two control groups, in whom little pain reduction was seen (Alimi *et al.*, 2003).

Acupuncture also helps lessen nausea and vomiting associated with chemotherapy and surgery, as well as with pregnancy and motion sickness (Berman *et al.*, 2004; Ezzo *et al.*, 2006; Chernyak and Sessler, 2005; Jewell and Young, 2003). In one study, 104 breast cancer patients receiving highly emetogenic chemotherapy were randomized to receive electro-acupuncture at the PC6 acupuncture point, minimal needling at non-acupuncture points, or pharmacotherapy alone. Electroacupuncture significantly reduced the number of episodes of total emesis when compared with pharmacotherapy only (Shen *et al.*, 2000).

Acupuncture has been reported to reduce xerostomia (severe dry mouth) caused by salivary gland injury from radiation therapy for head and neck cancer. Acupuncture improved Xerostomia Inventory scores in 18 patients with head and neck cancer and pilocarpine-resistant xerostomia in uncontrolled trials (Johnstone *et al.*, 2001).

Post-chemotherapy fatigue has few reliable treatments in patients without a correctable cause such as anemia. It can be a major contributing factor in lowering the quality of life in palliative care patients. In an uncontrolled trial of fatigue after chemotherapy, acupuncture reduced fatigue 31% after six weeks of treatment. Among those with severe fatigue at baseline, 79% had non-severe fatigue scores at follow-up (Vickers *et al.*, 2004). An uncontrolled study cannot answer the important question of whether the fatigue would have abated on its own during the same time period, however.

Investigation of acupuncture's mechanisms reveal that its effects are due to modulation of the nervous system (Kaptchuk, 2002; Han, 2004).

8.3.3 *Massage therapy*

Numerous approaches involve touch and manipulation techniques, including hands-on massage, very light touch or no touch at all. No-touch therapies such as Reiki or therapeutic touch have been termed "energy medicine," but more recently deemed to be mind-body interventions. A similar method is therapeutic touch (TT), which, despite its name, involves no direct contact. In TT, healers move their hands a few inches above a patient's body and sweep away "blockages" to the patient's energy field, although a study in the *Journal of the American Medical Association* showed that experienced TT practitioners were unable to detect the investigator's "energy field" (Rosa *et al.*, 1998). The clinical effect of the purported bioenergy field, as well as its response to practitioner manipulation, has never been convincingly demonstrated.

Massage involves application of pressure to muscle and connective tissue to reduce tension and pain, improve circulation, and encourage relaxation. Swedish massage, the most common form of massage, is gentle and comprised of five basic strokes (stroking, kneading, friction, percussion and vibration). The movement is rhythmic and free-flowing. Other variations include reflexology, *shiatsu* and *tui na*.

The benefits of massage therapy are documented in palliative care populations (Wilkinson *et al.*, 1999). Massage was shown effective for pain reduction in cancer patients at various stages of illness (Ferrell-Torry and Glick, 1993). Other studies found similar results for patients with post-operative pain. In an analysis of 1290 patient reports of symptom severity pre- and post-massage therapy, pain, fatigue, stress/anxiety, nausea, and depression were reduced by approximately 50%, even for patients reporting high baseline scores. Benefits persisted with no return toward baseline scores throughout 48-hour follow-up (Vickers *et al.*, 2004).

In a randomized trial of 150 post-operative cancer patients, providing massage and acupuncture in addition to standard care resulted in decreased pain and depressive mood (Mehling *et al.*, 2007). Massage has also been demonstrated to be effective in control of nausea in breast cancer patients (Billhult *et al.*, 2007).

8.3.4 *Tai Chi*

Tai Chi has its roots in ancient Chinese martial art and traditional medicine. Simplified and modernized forms are now practiced as exercise programs by people of all ages around the world. Its sequence of precise body movements together with meditation can improve health and well-being. *Tai chi* movements are designed to express a sense of balance and harmony, yet it improves stamina and agility. The practice of synchronized breathing may help reduce stress and improve pulmonary functions.

In a randomized controlled study of 256 elderly patients, *Tai Chi* exercise programs resulted in significantly fewer falls, and fewer injurious falls when compared with the stretching control group (Li *et al.*, 2005). Recent reviews also show that *Tai Chi* can improve quality of life, alleviation of pain, and improved flexibility and strength (Klein and Adams, 2004; Taylor-Piliae and Froelicher, 2004). A clinical study showed that *Tai Chi* exercises slowed bone loss in early post-menopausal women (Chan *et al.*, 2004). Unlike other form of exercise, *Tai Chi* is gentle with minimal stress on the body. It can be modified to suit the physical capability of cancer patients in different stages. In fact, preliminary data showed that regular *Tai Chi* exercise (three times a week for 60 minutes) improved the quality of life and self-esteem of breast cancer survivors (Mustian *et al.*, 2004).

8.3.5 *Music therapy*

Music offers creative, lyrical and symbolic means to address existential and spiritual needs, is aesthetic, beautiful and expressive, brings form, order, comfort and hope, transcends predicaments, space and time, and affirms or re-establishes relationship with self, others and the universe. Formal music therapy programs in palliative medicine exist in many major institutions. Although music therapy extends back to folklore and Greek mythology, it has been studied scientifically only in recent years.

Studies in oncology setting showed that music therapy can benefit cancer patients. In a randomized controlled study of cancer patients undergoing autologous stem cell transplantation, music significantly reduced mood disturbance and psychological distress (Cassileth *et al.*, 2003). Listening to music also reduces anxiety and increase comfort in hospitalized children with cancer (Barrera *et al.*, 2002) and in patients undergoing radiation therapy (Smith *et al.*, 2001). Other data suggest that music may improve the quality of life of terminal stage cancer patients (Smith *et al.*, 2001).

Music therapy was also shown to be effective in reducing both laboratory-induced pain (Beck, 1991) and chronic pain (Zimmerman *et al.*, 1989) in cancer patients.

Table 8.4. Reputable sources of online information on complementary and alternative medicine.

Medline Plus: http://www.nlm.nih.gov/medlineplus/druginformation.html
British Medical Journal: http://www.biomedcentral.com/bmccomplementalternmed/
Memorial Sloan-Kettering Cancer Center: http://www.mskcc.org/aboutherbs
National Center for Complementary and Alternative Medicine (NCCAM): http://nccam.nih.gov
American Cancer Society: http://www.cancer.org/docroot/ETO/ETO_5.asp?sitearea=ETO
NIH Office of Dietary Supplements: http://dietary-supplements.info.nih.gov
US Pharmacopeia: http://www.usp.org/dietarySupplements

8.4 Summary

Medical professionals should be aware that many spurious techniques are falsely promoted as viable treatments for cancer. Table 8.4 lists reliable sources of information about these and also about useful complementary therapies that can help reduce symptoms and improve quality of life. Although many complementary therapies have been practiced over time as components of traditional medical systems, efforts to study them scientifically only started in recent decades. These investigations have produced a body of evidence that supports the use of acupuncture, massage therapy, music and mind-body therapies to reduce physical and emotional symptoms.

Many mainstream medical centers and practices have established Integrative Medicine services to incorporate complementary therapies into multidisciplinary treatment plans. Professional societies such as the Society for Integrative Oncology (www.IntegrativeOnc.com) have also been established to raise awareness and encourage use of evidence-based complementary therapies in palliative and supportive care. These therapies have an important role in the total care of cancer patients, so that symptoms faced by patients can be addressed.

References

Alimi, D., Rubino, C., Pichard-Leandri, E., Fermand-Brule, S., Dubreuil-Lemaire, M.L. and Hill, C. (2003) Analgesic effect of auricular acupuncture for cancer pain: A randomized, blinded, controlled trial. *J. Clin. Oncol.* **21**(22), 4120–4126.

Astin, J.A., Shapiro, S.L., Eisenberg, D.M. and Forys, K.L. (2003) Mind-body medicine: State of the science, implications for practice. *J. Am. Board Fam. Pract.* **16**(2), 131–147.

Barrera, M.E., Rykov, M.H. and Doyle, S.L. (2002) The effects of interactive music therapy on hospitalized children with cancer: A pilot study. *Psycho-Oncology* **11**(5), 379–388.

Beck, S.L. (1991) The therapeutic use of music for cancer-related pain. *Oncol. Nurs. Forum* **18**(8), 1327–1337.

Benson, A.B., 3rd, Ajani, J.A., Catalano, R.B., Engelking, C., Kornblau, S.M., Martenson, J.A., Jr., *et al.* (2004) Recommended guidelines for the treatment of cancer treatment-induced diarrhea. *J. Clin. Oncol.* **22**(14), 2918–2926.

Berman, B.M., Lao, L., Langenberg, P., Lee, W.L., Gilpin, A.M. and Hochberg, M.C. (2004) Effectiveness of acupuncture as adjunctive therapy in osteoarthritis of the knee: A randomized, controlled trial. *Ann. Intern. Med.* **141**(12), 901–910.

Billhult, A., Bergbom, I. and Stener-Victorin, E. (2007) Massage relieves nausea in women with breast cancer who are undergoing chemotherapy. *J. Altern. Complement. Med.* **13**(1), 53–58.

Boon, H., Westlake, K., Stewart, M., Gray, R., Fleshner, N., Gavin, A., *et al.* (2003) Use of complementary/alternative medicine by men diagnosed with prostate cancer: Prevalence and characteristics. *Urology* **62**(5), 849–853.

Carlson, L.E., Speca, M., Patel, K.D. and Goodey, E. (2004) Mindfulness-based stress reduction in relation to quality of life, mood, symptoms of stress and levels of cortisol, dehydroepiandrosterone sulfate (DHEAS) and melatonin in breast and prostate cancer outpatients. *Psychoneuroendocrinology* **29**(4), 448–474.

Cassileth, B.R., Vickers, A.J. and Magill, L.A. (2003) Music therapy for mood disturbance during hospitalization for autologous stem cell transplantation: A randomized controlled trial. *Cancer* **98**(12), 2723–2729.

Chan, K., Qin, L., Lau, M., Woo, J., Au, S., Choy, W., *et al.* (2004) A randomized, prospective study of the effects of Tai Chi Chun exercise on bone mineral density in postmenopausal women. *Arch. Phys. Med. Rehabil.* **85**(5), 717–722.

Chernyak, G.V. and Sessler, D.I. (2005) Perioperative acupuncture and related techniques. *Anesthesiology* **102**(5), 1031–1049.

Cohen, L., Warneke, C., Fouladi, R.T., Rodriguez, M.A. and Chaoul-Reich, A. (2004) Psychological adjustment and sleep quality in a randomized trial of the effects of a Tibetan yoga intervention in patients with lymphoma. *Cancer* **100**(10), 2253–2260.

Cui, Y., Shu, X.O., Gao, Y., Wen, W., Ruan, Z.X. and Jin, F., *et al.* (2004) Use of complementary and alternative medicine by Chinese women with breast cancer. *Breast Cancer Res. Treat.* **85**(3), 263–270.

Deng, G. and Cassileth, B.R. (2005) Integrative oncology: Complementary therapies for pain, anxiety, and mood disturbance. *Cancer J. Clin.* **55**(2), 109–116.

Ernst, E. and Cassileth, B.R. (1998) The prevalence of complementary/alternative medicine in cancer: A systematic review. *Cancer* **83**(4), 777–782.

Ezzo, J., Streitberger, K. and Schneider, A. (2006) Cochrane systematic reviews examine P6 acupuncture-point stimulation for nausea and vomiting. *J. Altern. Complement. Med.* **12**(5), 489–495.

Ferrell-Torry, A.T. and Glick, O.J. (1993) The use of therapeutic massage as a nursing intervention to modify anxiety and the perception of cancer pain. *Cancer Nurs.* **16**(2), 93–101.

Han, J.S. (2004) Acupuncture and endorphins. *Neurosci. Lett.* **361**(1–3), 258–261.

Hyodo, I., Amano, N., Eguchi, K., Narabayashi, M., Imanishi, J., Hirai, M., *et al.* (2005) Nationwide survey on complementary and alternative medicine in cancer patients in Japan. *J. Clin. Oncol.* **23**(12), 2645–2654.

Jewell, D. and Young, G. (2003) Interventions for nausea and vomiting in early pregnancy. *Cochrane Database Syst. Rev.* **4**, CD000145.

Johnstone, P.A., Peng, Y.P., May, B.C., Inouye, W.S. and Niemtzow, R.C. (2001) Acupuncture for pilocarpine-resistant xerostomia following radiotherapy for head and neck malignancies. *Int. J. Radiat. Oncol. Biol. Phys.* **50**(2), 353–357.

Kaptchuk, T.J. (2002) Acupuncture: Theory, efficacy, and practice. *Ann. Intern. Med.* **136**(5), 374–383.

Klein, P.J. and Adams, W.D. (2004) Comprehensive therapeutic benefits of Taiji: A critical review. *Am. J. Phys. Med. Rehabil.* **83**(9), 735–745.

Li, F., Harmer, P., Fisher, K.J., McAuley, E., Chaumeton, N., Eckstrom, E., *et al.* (2005) Tai Chi and fall reductions in older adults: A randomized controlled trial. *J. Gerontol. A. Biol. Sci. Med. Sci.* **60**(2), 187–194.

Marcus, J., Elkins, G. and Mott, F. (2003) The integration of hypnosis into a model of palliative care. *Integr. Cancer Ther.* **2**(4), 365–370.

Mehling, W.E., Jacobs, B., Acree, M., Wilson, L., Bostrom, A., West, J., *et al.* (2007) Symptom management with massage and acupuncture in ostoperative cancer patients: A randomized controlled trial. *J. Pain Symptom Manage.* **33**(3), 258–266.

Melchart, D., Linde, K., Fischer, P., White, A., Allais, G., Vickers, A., *et al.* (1999) Acupuncture for recurrent headaches: A systematic review of randomized controlled trials. *Cephalalgia* **19**(9), 779–786.

Molassiotis, A., Fernadez-Ortega, P., Pud, D., Ozden, G., Scott, J.A., Panteli, V., *et al.* (2005) Use of complementary and alternative medicine in cancer patients: A European survey. *Ann. Oncol.* **16**(4), 655–663.

Mustian, K.M., Katula, J.A., Gill, D.L., Roscoe, J.A., Lang, D. and Murphy, K. (2004) Tai Chi Chuan, health-related quality of life and self-esteem: A randomized trial with breast cancer survivors. *Support Care Cancer* **12**(12), 871–876.

Rosa, L., Rosa, E., Sarner, L. and Barrett, S. (1998) A close look at therapeutic touch. *JAMA* **279**(13), 1005–1010.

Sellick, S.M. and Zaza, C. (1998) Critical review of five non-pharmacologic strategies for managing cancer pain. *Cancer Prev. Control* **2**(1), 7–14.

Shen, J., Wenger, N., Glaspy, J., Hays, R.D., Albert, P.S., Choi, C., *et al.* (2000) Electroacupuncture for control of myeloablative chemotherapy-induced emesis: A randomized controlled trial. *JAMA* **284**(21), 2755–2761.

Smith, M., Casey, L., Johnson, D., Gwede, C. and Riggin, O.Z. (2001) Music as a therapeutic intervention for anxiety in patients receiving radiation therapy. *Oncol. Nurs. Forum* **28**(5), 855–862.

Speca, M., Carlson, L.E., Goodey, E. and Angen, M. (2000) A randomized, wait-list controlled clinical trial: The effect of a mindfulness meditation-based stress reduction program on mood and symptoms of stress in cancer outpatients. *Psychosom. Med.* **62**(5), 613–622.

Taylor-Piliae, R.E. and Froelicher, E.S. (2004) Effectiveness of *Tai Chi* exercise in improving aerobic capacity: A meta-analysis. *J. Cardiovasc. Nurs.* **19**(1), 48–57.

Vickers, A.J., Straus, D.J., Fearon, B. and Cassileth, B.R. (2004) Acupuncture for postchemotherapy fatigue: A phase II study. *J. Clin. Oncol.* **22**(9), 1731–1735.

Walker, L.G., Walker, M.B., Ogston, K., Heys, S.D., Ah-See, A.K., Miller, I.D., *et al.* (1999) Psychological, clinical and pathological effects of relaxation training and guided imagery during primary chemotherapy. *Br. J. Cancer* **80**(1–2), 262–268.

Wilkinson, S., Aldridge, J., Salmon, I., Cain, E. and Wilson, B. (1999) An evaluation of aromatherapy massage in palliative care. *Palliat. Med.* **13**(5), 409–417.

Zimmerman, L., Pozehl, B., Duncan, K. and Schmitz, R. (1989) Effects of music in patients who had chronic cancer pain. *West. J. Nurs. Res.* **11**(3), 298–309.

Chapter 9

Positive Findings about Herbs and Natural Products Action on Cancer

Muriel J. Montbriand

Abstract

Recent findings show that 27 herbs and natural products have potential to decrease cancer growth or to be used as adjuncts with cancer therapy. This discussion provides an update on evidence-based findings from preliminary *in vitro* and *in vivo* studies, and some initial clinical trials. Clearly, the testing for these herbs and products has not advanced to proven efficacy, yet these initial research findings show promising results. This discussion includes scientific and common names, a typical dose of the product where possible, and adverse or dangerous side-effects. Also included are potential interactions with prescriptions, other herbs, laboratory tests, and diseases or conditions. Sources include selections from Natural Medicines Comprehensive Database (2006) plus recent refereed research publications. A table and references are provided to help health care professionals peruse products and herbs that may be beneficial to patients undergoing cancer treatment. Through this information health professionals are encouraged to become better resource persons for their patients.

Keywords: Herbs; Natural Products; Cancer.

9.1 Introduction

Twenty-seven herbs and natural products show potential to benefit individuals with cancer, according to preliminary evidence-based research. These products may be used as adjuvants with conventional cancer therapy, or they may be used as treatment for side-effects of conventional cancer therapy. Some of these products show potential in regression of metastatic tumors. However, caution is advised because the evidence-based research cited here is preliminary and awaiting future research to confirm or reject the value of each product or herb. Yet at the same time, this discussion chapter is designed to show these preliminary and promising results of evidence-based research studies, providing quick references in text and table form. Health professionals are encouraged to understand the possible potential of these products and become better resource persons for their patients.

The use and appeal of herbal and natural products has steadily increased over the past years, with up to 89% reported use (Barnes *et al.*, 2004; Barqawi *et al.*, 2004; Eisenberg *et al.*, 1993 and 1998; Harnack *et al.*, 2001; Kennedy, 2005; Montbriand, 1994, 1995a and b, 1997 and 2000a; Skelly, 1997). A major reason for the increase seems related to consumers' perceptions that these products are environmentally pure and without side-effects. While herbs and natural products enjoy continued popularity with consumers, 60% to 75% of consumers avoid telling their health professionals that they use these products (Montbriand, 1994, 1995a and b, 1997 and 2000a; Eisenberg *et al.*, 2001). Reasons for the non-disclosure include lack of trust in conventional medical professionals, popularity of lay sources, and encouragement by consumers' social-groups (Montbriand, 2000a).

Contrasted to the non-disclosure by patients, health professionals may be inadvertently avoiding the subject of herbal or natural product use because or their own lack of evidence-based knowledge on these products. Findings show that 97% of health care professionals admit to a lack of this information, usually because of time commitments to their own practice knowledge and in some cases cost of obtaining sources (Montbriand, 2000a and b). Yet, according to Montbriand (2000a and b), professionals embraced the idea of being better resource persons for their patients, especially if access to evidence-based information on herbal and natural products could be more accessible, organized and succinct.

Information in this chapter may be useful to health professionals in their efforts to help patients make informed choices when receiving care for cancer. The research cited here shows potential that these products may be useful as adjuvants to cancer treatment or may decrease cancer growth. *The information given in this chapter is not intended as a recommendation for any of these herbs or natural products.* When the words "recommended dosage" are used, the recommendation comes from either US-FDA or Health Canada or are doses used in a quoted research. Previous studies show that individuals tend to self-medicate with higher than recommended doses (Montbriand, 1994, 1995a and b, 1997 and 2000a). Disclosure of self-medication with these products and the dosages used should be encouraged. Findings show that individuals tend to be cautious about use of herbals and natural products if a health professional gives information to ensure patients can make informed choices.

This free exchange of information between health-professionals and patients is critical. While information consumers generally receive is mainly advertisement or anecdotal from their social group (Montbriand, 1994, 1995a and b), a growing body of evidence-based research is showing the interactions of herbs and natural products with prescription drugs, diseases, other herbs, and laboratory tests. Therefore, the importance of helping health care professionals become better resource persons is paramount.

The information in this chapter is an update to previous publications about alternative products and herbals (Montbriand, 1999, 2004a–c and 2005). This chapter specifically is an update on the herbs and natural products that may decrease cancer growth (Montbriand, 2004a). Notice that some of the previously reported information in one of Montbriand's latest articles (2004a) has undergone changes, eliminating 15 herbs and natural products, and introducing 11 new herbs and products, which now show new and promising research. Selections of the herbs and natural products for this discussion are from Natural Medicines Comprehensive Database (2006). Discussion about these herbs and products is based on cited scientific literature. *In vitro* studies (preformed on tissue from living organisms in glass) or *in vivo* studies (preformed on living animal tissue) are reported here, with only a few studies in the preliminary stages of human clinical trials. The clinical trials usually reported are Phases I/II. Phase I trials are now increasingly including persons with specific diseases, although in the past they were designated for healthy individuals to determine dose-related pharmacological toxicities of new drugs. Now Phase I trials are often including persons for whom all conventional therapies have failed (e.g. terminal cancer). These latter trials should properly be designated as mixed Phases I/II or pure Phase II clinical trials, which examine short-term pharmacological toxicity in populations with specific diseases. Pharmaceutical research is conventionally made up of four phases. A few Phase III clinical trials are included in this discussion. When testing advances to Phase III trials, the purpose is to look for pharmacological efficacy of the potential new drug and short term toxicities.

The following herbs will not be included in the discussion because they have already been accepted as cancer treatment drugs. Biomedical chemotherapy agents derived from herbal plants are as follows (Tyler, 1994):

(1) vincristine sulfate (Oncovin® Eli Lilly and Company, Indianapolis, IN) or vinblastine sulfate (Velban® Eli Lilly and Company, Indianapolis, IN) derived from the herb *Catharanthus roseus*, also known as *Vinca rosea*, common names periwinkle, old maid, myrtle, and others;
(2) Etoposide (VePesid® Bristol-Myers Squibb Oncology, Princeton, NJ), Teniposide (Vumon® Bristol-Myers Squibb Oncology) is derived from the herb *Podophyllum peltatum*, common name Mayapple, American mandrake, or American podophyllum; and
(3) Taxol® (Bristol-Myers Squibb Oncology, Princeton, NJ) is derived from the herb *Taxus brevifolia*, common name pacific yew.

All three herbs have very toxic properties. Podophylum is lethal. Additional references for these three herbs are Bisset (1994), Duke (1987), Duke and Vasquez (1994), Facts and Comparisons (2001), and Tyler (1993 and 1994). None of the above herbs appear on the provided table at the end of the comments on herbs and products.

Neither the author nor publisher makes any medical claims for any of the herbs or natural products in this review or tables. This is informational literature. Note some of the herbs described are deadly poisons and some are extremely dangerous.

The information presented here does not pretend to be all-inclusive, but has been selected to include discussion and findings from only recognized professional authors or advisory boards. Common names and scientific names for all herbs and natural products are provided when possible. Herbal scientific names include the Genus (classification of a plant group with common properties) followed by the Species name (each plant group has many species).

Information about the herbs and natural products that follows is in alphabetic order. Included are the scientific name(s), usual reason for self-medication, positive evidence associated with cancer treatment, and possible dose, when possible. An easy-to-use table is provided at the end of the following information. This table contains herb and natural product common-names along with potential interactions with prescriptions, other herbs or products, laboratory tests, diseases or conditions, plus a symbol to remind the reader of possible toxic or adverse effects.

9.2 Comments about Herbs and Natural Products

Astragalus, scientific name *Astragalus membranaceus*, is an herb used with conventional therapies by individuals who have breast, cervical, and lung cancer. Preliminary evidence seems to indicate that astragalus taken with glossy privet, *Ligustrum lucidum* (another herb), adjuvantly with con-ventional cancer treatment may improve survival of breast cancer patients (Upton, 1999). Use of astragalus as an adjuvant with platinum-based chemotherapy seems to be advantageous in treatment of advanced non-small cell lung cancer (Xu *et al.*, 2006). Doses of 1 to 30 grams per day seem to be typical, but Upton (1999) indicates that doses greater than 28 grams might cause immunosuppression.

Beta-glucans, scientific names *1–3, 1–6-beta-glucan, beta-1, 3-D-glucan* and *beta-1–6, 1–3-beta-glucan*, is popular as an immunostimulant by individuals who have conditions such as chronic fatigue syndrome. Beta-glucans is also used by individuals with cancer who are receiving chemotherapy or radiation. Others self-medicate with beta-glucans for help with conditions such as HIV/AIDS cancer, or diabetes (Natural Medicines Comprehensive Database, 2006). Considerable research indicates that lentinan, a beta-glucan, appears to prolong the life of patients with gastric cancer when it is used in combination with chemotherapy (Kimura *et al.*, 2003; Nagahashi *et al.*, 2004; Nakano *et al.*, 1999; Nimura *et al.*, 2006). These multi centered and institutional trials show marked improvement in appetite and sleep quality for cancer patients. Yeast-derived beta-glucans seem well-tolerated orally (Nicolosi *et al.*, 1999). Beta-glucans has been used in oral doses of 7.5 grams twice daily added to juice (Nicolosi *et al.*, 1999).

Cesium, scientific names *Cesium*, *Cs* and *atomic number 55*, is self-medicated to treat cancer and depression. Preliminary research found that if cesium was taken together with minerals, such as magnesium, potassium, and selenium and some vitamins and chelating agents, there appeared to be 50% chance of recovery for patients with primary breast, colon, prostate, pancreas, lung and liver cancer, lymphoma, Ewing sarcoma of the pelvis, and adeno-cancer of the gallbladder (Sartori, 1984). Caution: high exposure to cesium can result in burns and death because cesium is used in radiation therapy (EPA, 2002). A maximum daily dosage of 6 to 9 grams has been given safely (Sartori, 1984). However, Neulieb (1984) reports side-effects of nausea, diarrhea, anorexia, and tingling of the lips, hands, and feet when 6 grams per day are ingested in a self-experiment.

Chrysin, same scientific name, is used to treat various conditions including anxiety, baldness, HIV/AIDS and to prevent cancer. Chrysin is a natural component of passionflower, silver linden, honey, and bee propolis (Galijatovic *et al.*, 1999). A string of research report a 20-fold induction of glucuronidation of bilirubin by chrysin-treated cells, which may reduce the bioavilability of dietary carcinogens (Galijatovic *et al.*, 2000 and 2001; Walle *et al.*, 2000). Similarly, chrysin may reduce estrogen synthesis by acting as an estrogen inhibitor, in a way similar to the action of breast cancer drugs, anastrozole and letrozole (Jeong *et al.*, 1999; Kao *et al.*, 1998). No toxic effects have been recorded. Manufacturers suggest various dosages for chrysin, but none have been tested on humans.

Coenzyme Q-10, same scientific name, is self-medicated for the cardiotoxic side-effect of chemotherapy agent doxorubicin. It is also self-medicated for treatment of breast cancer. Products with coenzyme Q-10 are also used for treatment of other heart conditions, diabetes, inadequate immune system, and migraine headaches. While research is preliminary, coenzyme Q-10 has been shown to facilitate regression of breast cancer when given as an adjuvant with conventional cancer therapy (Lockwood *et al.*, 1994 and 1995). These studies also include adjuvant use of other antioxidants, omega-3, and omega-6 fatty acids with coenzyme Q-10. The following researchers have not found toxic effects associated with ingestion of coenzyme Q-10 (Bresolin *et al.*, 1990; Shults *et al.*, 2002; Huntington, 2001). A daily dose of 100 mg per day or less is recom-mended to minimize adverse effects (Fuke, 2000).

Coriolus mushroom, scientific name of *Coriolus versicolor* synonymous with *Trametes versicolor*, is self-medicated to treat conditions such as chronic fatigue syndrome and inadequate immune system. Some patients with cancer use coriolus mushroom to treat side-effects of chemotherapy or radiation treatments. Some use coriolus mushroom to enhance the effects of chemotherapy. Coriolus mushroom shows anti-tumor and immuno-modulating effects (Dong *et al.*, 1996 and 1997; Harada *et al.*, 1997; Kanoh *et al.*, 1994; Kim *et al.*, 1999; Kobayashi *et al.*, 1995; Maehara *et al.*, 1993; Mizutani and Yoshida, 1991; Ng, 1998; Tsukagoshi *et al.*, 1984; Wang *et al.*, 1996). In Japan, this plant product has been used as a biological response modifier in cancer chemotherapy treatments (Harada *et al.*, 1997; Maehara *et al.*, 1993; Hayakawa *et al.*, 1997; Morimoto *et al.*, 1996; Nakazato *et al.*, 1994; Nio *et al.*, 1992; Sugimachi *et al.*, 1997; Toi *et al.*, 1992). Some authors report few adverse effects from use of coriolus mushroom (Mizutani and Yoshida, 1991; Ng, 1998). However, some patients using this plant adjunctly with chemotherapy experience nausea, leukopenia, and liver function impairment (Nakazato *et al.*, 1994). As an adjuvant, 3 grams has been used daily (Morimoto *et al.*, 1996; Nio *et al.*, 1992; Toi *et al.*, 1992, Yokoe *et al.*, 1997).

Diindolylmethane, scientific name 3,3′-*Diindolylmethane*, is self-medicated to prevent breast and uterine cancers. The American diet contains between 2 to 24 mg of diindolylmethane (Balk, 2000; Riby *et al.*, 2000). Preliminary, *in vivo*, studies established that diidolylmethane has estrogen receptor agonist and antagonistic activities; therefore, this product may be useful in treatment of breast cancer (Riby *et al.*, 2000; Chen *et al.*, 1998; Chen *et al.*; 1996; McDougal *et al.*, 2000). Reports of toxic effects or typical doses are unavailable.

Gamma linolenic acid (GLA), scientific name of (*ZZZ*)-*Octadeca-6,9,12-trienoic acid*, is often self-medicated by individuals with rheumatoid arthritis or pre-menstrual syndrome. Research has found that GLA can hasten the response of tamoxifen (Kenny *et al.*, 2000). GLA is found in two herbs: oil of primrose (*Oenothera biennis*) and borage (*Borago officinalis*). Capsules and tablets of evening of primrose are available according to Facts and Comparisons (2001); however, the stability of tablets is questionable. Further, some capsules on the market may be adulterated, containing only soy or safflower oil. According to Tyler (1994), the American Food and Drug Administration put evening primrose oil on the unapproved food additive list. Tyler (1994) also indicates that some borage contains unsaturated pyrrolizidine alkaloids (UPAs), and when given in even minute amounts this substance can be toxic. Only borage products labeled UPA free are safe to use. However, other scholars warn that even when borage is taken in therapeutic amounts the level of UPA can be toxic (Fetrow and Avila, 1999). An adverse effect of GLA may be prolonged bleeding time (Guivernau *et al.*, 1994). Daily doses of GLA can vary between 1.6 grams and 360 mg, but these are for other conditions, not the use as an adjuvant for cancer treatment (Natural Medicines Comprehensive Database, 2006).

Genistein Combined Polysaccharide, same scientific name, is self-medicated by individuals with prostate and breast cancer. Preliminary research points to genistein having both antioxidant and anti-angiogenic effects on cancer (Barnes *et al.*, 2000). Researchers have found that genistein appears to decrease the expression of aromatase and 5-alpha reductase (Ghafar *et al.*, 2002), possibly giving anti-proliferative effects especially against hormone-dependent cancers such as prostate or breast cancers (Barnes *et al.*, 2000). Using a mouse model, Yuan, *et al.* (2003) found genistein seemed to inhibit breast cancer tumors. However, due to GCP's estrogenic effect, women with estrogen-sensitive cancers should avoid this product (Barnes *et al.*, 2000). Estrogen-sensitive conditions include breast, uterine and ovarian cancers, endometriosis and uterine fibroids. No other adverse effects of GCP are available. Ghafar *et al.* (2002) used a dose of 1.5 grams per day.

Germanium, scientific name *Ge* or *atomic number 32*, is self-medicated for various conditions, including cancer, pain relief, and rheumatoid arthritis. Some evidence indicates that germanium is beneficial in treating breast, colon, prostate, ovary, head and neck, and lung cancers, especially for patients with poor prognosis and approaching palliative care (Budman *et al.*, 1982; Ettinger *et al.*, 1989; Mainwaring *et al.*, 2000; Schein *et al.*, 1980; Vogelzang *et al.*, 1985). Except for one case study showing a patient with complete remission (Mainwaring *et al.*, 2000), all of the above studies found were Phases I or II trials, and all the following studies and case reports suggest germanium is unsafe because of life-threatening adverse effects (Budman *et al.*, 1982; Ettinger *et al.*, 1989; Vogelzang *et al.*,

1985; Krapf *et al.*, 1992; Sanai *et al.*, 1990; Takeuchi *et al.*, 1992). The adverse effects of oral ingestion of germanium are anemia, hepatic steatosis, lactic acidosis, muscle weakness, myopathy, renal degeneration, peripheral neuro-pathy, renal failure, and death (Krapf *et al.*, 1992; Sanai *et al.*, 1990; Takeuchi *et al.*, 1992; Asaka *et al.*, 1995; Hess *et al.*, 1993; Higuchi *et al.*, 1989; Matsusaka *et al.*, 1988; Schauss, 1991; Tao and Bolger, 1997; Yanagisawa *et al.*, 2000). No dosage is available.

Gingkgo, scientific *Gingko biloba*, is an herb with wide popularity in self-medication for memory loss, dementia, and Alzheimer's disease. A combination of ginkgo extract (EGb 761) and 5-fluorouracil, given intravenously, seems to have a positive effect on colorectal cancer (Hauns *et al.*, 2001). The leaf extract of ginkgo seems to be tolerated well in typical doses (Kurz and Van Baelen, 2004). Extracts of ginkgo up to 240 mg were reported by LeBars *et al.* (1997), and Oken *et al.* (1998). Mild adverse reactions to ginkgo leaf extract include gastrointestinal difficulty, headaches, dizziness, palpitations, constipation and skin allergic reactions (Cesarani *et al.*, 1998; Diamond *et al.*, 2000; Kudolo, 2000). However, case reports have indicated concern with severe adverse reactions to ginkgo, such as intracerebral bleeding leading to permanent neurological damage and even death (Meisel *et al.*, 2003; Vale, 1998). Of interest, while individuals speak of ginkgo leaf extract, is the Chinese term *Yin-Kuo*, "silver apricot" (Diamond *et al.*, 2000). *Gingko biloba* trees are reported to live for thousands of years, and fruit and leaves have been used in Chinese pharmacopoeia since 2600 BC.

Gossypol, scientific name *Gossyplum hirsutum* or *Gossypium herbaceum*, is known commonly as cottonseed oil. This oil is used as a male contraceptive and self-medicated for metastatic carcinoma of the endometrium or ovary. Gossypol is also used by individuals who are HIV-positive. Glossypol shows cytotoxic and anti-tumor properties on many cytosolic and mitochondrial enzyme systems, suggested by *in vivo* and *in vitro* research; these enzyme systems are fundamental for tumor cell growth such as melanoma, endometrial, colon, lung, prostate breast, brain, and adrenocortical cancer (Coyle *et al.*, 1994; Gilbert *et al.*, 1995; Liang *et al.*, 1995; Shidaifat *et al.*, 1996; Wu, 1989). Typical doses are unavailable. Gossypol is potentially toxic and considered unsafe for self-medication (Facts and Comparisons, 2001).

Gotu Kola, scientific name *Centella asiatica* synonymous with *Hydrocotyle asiatica*, is self-medicated for conditions such as anxiety, peptic ulcer disease, trauma, shingles, diabetes, and many other conditions. Preliminary studies show that gotu kola seems to exhibit cytotoxic and anti-tumor properties and tends to be selective in toxicity, leaving normal lymphocytes unharmed (Babu *et al.*, 1995). Babu *et al.* (1995) also found gotu kola increased the life of tumor bearing mice. Typical doses, 600 mg of dried leaves, three times a day have been tolerated well (Gruenwald *et al.*, 1998). However, an important adverse effect is gotu kola's photosensitivity properties (Newall *et al.*, 1996). If individuals take gotu kola, indicate the need to wear sunscreen and sun-protective clothing.

Graviola, scientific name *Annona muricata*, is self-medicated for such conditions as cancer and herpes. Graviola is also used as an antibiotic, or as a sedative. The important class of chemicals found in graviola is acetogenins. Researchers have found that acetogenins obstruct the production of adenosine triphosphate, which in turn inhibits the pump that removes cancer drugs from the cell. Thus, the chemotherapy remains in the cell and is more effective against the cancer (Oberlies *et al.*, 1997). Oberlies *et al.* (1997) also speculates that acetogenin may have potential use against multidrug resistant cancers. However, graviola may cause movement disorders similar to Parkinson's disease (Lannuzel *et al.*, 2002). No typical dose is available.

Greater celandine, scientific name *Chelidonium majus*, is self-medicated for conditions such as stomach cancer, gastroenteritis, or liver and gallbladder disorders. Some evidence indicates that a semi-synthetic alkaloid derivative of this plant called Ukrain has some anti-cancer properties (Ernst and Schmidt, 2005; Panzer *et al.*, 2000b). Ernst and Schmidt's (2005) research was a meta-analysis, which also includes their speculation that most of the research they reviewed was of poor methodological quality. Panzer *et al.* (2000b) used a low dose *in vitro* study and found Ukrain to be selectively toxic to malignant cells. This finding was confirmed by other studies (Cordes *et al.*, 2002; Panzer *et al.*, 2000a; Roublevskaia *et al.*, 2000). Caution is advised in use of Greater celandine because these studies are very preliminary. Cases of acute liver injury have been noted with the intake of Greater celandine, but rapid recovery followed withdrawal of Greater celandine from the treatment regimen (Benninger *et al.*, 1999; Stickel *et al.*, 2003). Greater celandine, at a dose of 1 ml three times a day, has been reported by Melzer *et al.* (2004) who conducted a meta-analysis of six randomized-controlled trials. No doses are given specifically for Ukrain.

IP-6, with a scientific name of *Inositol hexaphosphate*, is self-medicated for numerous conditions including cancer, increasing white blood cells counts, preventing heart attacks, or treating kidney stones (Natural Medicines Comprehensive Database, 2006). Preliminary animal research show that IP-6 has anti-cancer potential in breast, colon, liver, prostate and hematological cancers (Challa *et al.*, 1997; Deliliers *et al.*, 2002; Saied and Shamsuddin, 1998; Shamsuddin and Vucenik, 1999; Shamsuddin and Yang, 1995; Thompson and Zhang, 1991; Vucenik *et al.*, 1998 and 2004). A recent *in vitro* study by Tantivejkul *et al.* (2003) found that IP-6 together with adriamycin or tamoxifen seems effective against estrogen receptor alpha-negative cells and adriamycin-resistant cancer cells. No adverse reactions or possible dose are available because all these studies are *in vivo* or *in vitro*. Since none of these studies are conducted on humans, caution is advised.

Lentinan (LNT) is a polysaccharide derived from shitake mushroom, scientific name *Lentinus edodes*, also called *Lenticus edodes*, and *Lentinan edodes*, *Lentinula edodes*, *Tricholomopsis edodes*. This polysaccharide has been given intravenously, intramuscularly, and intraperitoneally as an adjunct treatment for cancer and HIV. According to Kosaka *et al.* (1987) these post-surgery injections showed greater regression of tumor growth after surgery. Not only was there marked atrophy of tumors, there was also intense infiltration of T cells, B cells, and macrophages into the stoma around the tumor. Slow drip parental infusion of lentinan seemed to be tolerated well. Clinical trials used a dose of 1–4 mg per week (Gordon *et al.*, 1995; Wada *et al.*, 1987; Yoshiyuki *et al.*, 1994).

Limonene, with the same scientific name, is self-medicated for prevention of cancer or treatment of bronchitis. An *in vivo* trial by Raphael and Kuttan (2003) shows that limonene appeared to have positive effects on the immune system. Preliminary clinical trials, Phases I and II, were initiated by Vigushin *et al.* (1998) to assess the toxicity and use of D-limonene. They found three patients with colorectal cancer had prolonged stable disease. The dosage they used for breast cancer patients was 8 g/m^2 per day (Vigushin *et al.*, 1998). Finding this dose well tolerated with potential clinical activity, they suggest further evaluation of limonene.

Magnesium, scientific name of *Mg* and *atomic number 12*, is self-medicated to prevent or treat hypomagnesemia, and for treatment of asthma, constipation, heart conditions, leg cramps, or pre-menstrual syndrome. In a clinical study, 12 oncology patients who responded poorly to morphine for their neuropathic pain were given intravenous doses of magnesium sulfate. Two patients received partial relief and one patient reported that the pain was unchanged (Crosby *et al.*, 2000). A single dose of 500 mg to 1 gram was used, and it seemed to relieve neuropathic pain for a period of at least four hours. This finding requires further evaluation. Oral self-medication of magnesium for pain is not advisable because this mineral is fatal in large doses. Magnesium also interacts with numerous drugs, herbs and supplements, and diseases or conditions, making the self-medication of this mineral prohibitive.

Marijuana, scientific name of *Cannabis sativa*, is often used recreationally. Self-medication of marijuana (inhalation, usually three or four "joints" (cigarettes) per day) for cancer and AIDS is reported to decrease pain, relieve nausea and vomiting induced by chemotherapy, and stimulate appetite; however, these claims are not substantiated in bio-medical research. *In vitro* studies shows regression of malignant tumors in Wistar rats (Galve-Roperh *et al.*, 2000). However, two other preliminary studies show conflicting results, suggesting that Delta-9-tetrahydrocannabinol (THC), the main psychoactive component of marijuana, accelerated tumor growth in normal mice (Klein *et al.*, 2000; Zhu *et al.*, 2000). Regular smoking of three to four joints of marijuana per day may cause as much histological damage as smoking 20 to 22 tobacco cigarettes per day (Johnson *et al.*, 2000). The prescription products used in treatment of cancer chemotherapy-induced nausea and vomiting are Delta-9-tetrahydrocannabinol (chemical name) Marinol® (Sanofi-Synthelabo Canada Inc., Markham, ON) and nabilone (a synthetic creation of THC) Cesamet® (ICN Canada Ltd., Montreal, QC). Typical dosage is 5 to 15 mg every two to four hours (Beal *et al.*, 1995).

Melatonin, scientific name of *N-acetyl-5-methoxytryptamine*, is self-medicated for cancer of the breast, brain, lung, prostate, head, neck and gastrointestinal tract, with a most popular use for jet lag or insomnia.

Preliminary research, on metastatic prostate cancer patients in poor clinical condition, indicated that giving melatonin together with injections of triptorelin to these patients, resulted in an achieved one year longer survival (Lissoni *et al.*, 1997). When used concomitantly with interleukin-2 or conventional chemotherapy or hormone therapy, melatonin seems associated with regression of cancer tumors of the breast, gastrointestinal tract, kidney, liver, and lung (Lissoni *et al.*, 1992b, 1994b and c, 1995, 1996a and 1999). For patients with advanced cancer, melatonin has shown promise as an adjunct when given with chemotherapy; it is tolerated well and seems to reduce toxicity of chemotherapy (Lissoni *et al.*, 1997b and 1999). For patients with advanced untreatable cancers, some preliminary studies show that administering melatonin, alone, prolonged the survival time (Lissoni *et al.*, 1991, 1992a, 1994a and 1998).

The adverse effects of melatonin use are headaches, transient depression, daytime fatigue and drowsiness, dizziness, abdominal cramps, irritability (Wagner *et al.*, 1998) and reduced alertness (Dollins *et al.*, 1993). A typical safe dose is not established.

Pomegranate, scientific name *Lythraceae* or *Punicaceae*, has been used in folk medicines by many cultures, ancient and present. In the present day, pomegranate is self-medicated for conditions such as prostate cancer, artherosclerosis, hypertension, HIV disease, and as an astringent for diarrhea and dysentery. Two Phase II studies found significant prolonged doubling time for PSA when patients with prostate cancer drank eight ounces of pomegranate juice daily for two years (Pantuck *et al.*, 2006a and b). All patients with prostate cancer had undergone surgery or radiation before starting the daily regimen of pomegranate juice.

Strontium, scientific name *Sr* and *atomic number 38*, also has the common name strontium chloride noted in dietary supplements. Individuals self-medicate with this product for oesteoporosis, bone pain, sensitive teeth, or seizures. Two preliminary studies conclude that treatment with Sr-89 (strontium) appears to be effective for patients with chemotherapy-refractory prostate cancer (Gunawardana *et al.*, 2004; Oosterhof *et al.*, 2003). However, the Natural Medicines Comprehensive Database (2006) cautions individuals to avoid taking dietary supplements containing strontium chloride because long-term safety has not been established for this substance.

Theanine, scientific name *5-N-ethylglutamine*, is self-medicated by individuals who believe it enhances the effect of chemotherapy. Interest in using theanine as an adjuvant with cancer treatment has been initiated because theanine increases the doxorubicin and adriamycin in tumors, which block cancer drug efflux from tumor cells. This is especially important in drug-sensitive and multi-drug resistant tumors (Sadzuka *et al.*, 1996; 2000; Sugiyama *et al.*, 2001; Sugitama and Sadzuka, 1998). Theanine is a major amino acid found in green tea (Natural Medicines Comprehensive Database, 2006). Green tea seems to have properties that may protect against cancer. Adverse effects and typical doses of theanine are not available.

Tiratricol, scientific name of *3,3′,5-triiodothyroaceic acid*, is self-medicated as a thyroid supplement and also may be used by individuals with thyroid cancer. Research has shown tiratricol to be effective in minimizing serum thyrotrophin concentration in differentiated thyroid cancer (Jaffiol *et al.*, 1995; Mueller-Gaertner and Schneider, 1988). Yet, conclusions from Mechelany *et al.* (1991) determined that there was no justification for using tiratricol as a supplement in treatment of patients with thyroid cancer. The former studies did tests with 127 and 25 patients with differentiated thyroid cancer, and the latter study did tests on 22 patients, respectively. In clinical trials, doses of 10–24 mcg twice daily have been used initially. This dose has then been titrated to less then 0.1 mU/L (Sherman and Ladenson, 1992). The Natural Medicines Comprehensive Database (2006) points to the FDA designating tiratricol as an orphan drug under study for use with levo-thyroxine for patients with well-differentiated thyroid cancer. Patients with differentiated thyroid cancer who are interested in tiratricol should discuss the product with their oncologist. Individuals with normal thyroid function should avoid this product.

Turmeric has a scientific name *Curcuma longa* and is synonymous with *Curcuma domestica* and also *Curcuma aromatica*. Individuals self-medicate with turmeric for gastro-intestinal and respiratory conditions, as well as for fibromyalgia and for cancer. A preliminary study with patients who had advanced colorectal cancer showed that inclusion of turmeric with other cancer treatments resulted in radiologically stable disease in five patients for two to four months of treatment (Sharma *et al.*, 2001). Topical use of turmeric for skin cancer also showed a relief of adverse symptoms

(Kuttan *et al.*, 1987). The dose used in the colorectal cancer study was between 440 and 2200 mg per day, containing 36–180 mg of turmeric.

Whey Protein, no scientific name, is used as a food supplement or as a milk alternative by people with lactose intolerance. Whey protein is also

Table 9.1. Herbs and natural products with potential to use as adjuvant with cancer treatments or with potential to decrease cancer growth.*

Herb or Natural Product *Common Names*	**Interactions with Prescription Drugs (Rx), Herbs and Supplements, Laboratory (Lab) Tests, Disease or Conditions**
ASTRAGALUS (Upton, 1999)* *Other names*: Astragali, *Beg Kei, Bei Qi, Buck Qi, Huang Qi, Huang Qi, Hwanggi*, Membranous Milk Vetch, Milk Vetch, Mongolian Milk, Ogi	*Rx*: Cyclophosphamide (Upton, 1999), Immunosuppresants (Upton, 1999; Sun *et al.*, 1983) *Diseases*: Autoimmune diseases (Upton, 1999; Sun *et al.*, 1983)
BETA GLUCANS *Other names*: Beta-Glycans, Gifolan (GRN), Lentinan, PGG Glucan, Poly-(1–6)-Beta-D-Glucopyranosyl-(1–3)-Beta-D-Glucopyranose, Schizophyllan (SPG), SSG, Yeast-Derived Beta-Glucan	*Rx*: Immunosuppressants (Duvic *et al.*, 1987; Browden *et al.*, 1990) *Lab Tests*: White blood cell counts (Babineau *et al.*, 1995) *Diseases*: Acquired immunodeficiency syndrome (AIDS) or AIDS-related complex (ARC) (Duvic *et al.*, 1987)
CESIUM (Neulib, 1984)* *Other names*: Caesium, Cesium-137, Cesium Chloride, CsCl, High pH Therapy	*Rx*: Potassium-depleting drugs (Sartori, 1984; Neulieb, 1984) *Lab Tests*: Potassium (Sartori, 1984; Neulieb, 1984)
CHRYSIN *Other names*: 5,7-Dihydroxy-flavone, Flavone X, Flavonoid, Galangin Flavanone	*Rx*: Aromatase inhibitors (Jeong *et al.*, 1999; Walle *et al.*, 1999), Cytochrome P450 (CYP1A2) substrates (Lee *et al.*, 1998; Lautraite *et al.*, 2002), Glucuronidated drugs (Galijatovic *et al.*, 2000; 2001) *Herbs and Supplements*: Androstenedione (Kellis and Vickery, 1984; Brown *et al.*, 2000)

*Potential for toxic or adverse effect. Please see text or reference(s).

Table 9.1. (*Continued*)

Herb or Natural Product *Common Names*	**Interactions with Prescription Drugs (Rx), Herbs and Supplements, Laboratory (Lab) Tests, Disease or Conditions**
COENZYME Q-10 *Other names*: Co, Q10	*Rx*: Anti-hypertensive drugs (Langsjoen *et al.*, 1994; Hodgson *et al.*, 2002), Chemotherapy (Kishi *et al.*, 1977; Zhou and Chowbay, 2002; Lund *et al.*, 1998), Warfarin (Spigset, 1994; Heck *et al.*, 2000; Engelsen *et al.*, 2002) *Rx That Affect Coenzyme Q-10 Levels* (Fuke *et al.*, 2000; Hanaki *et al.*, 1993) *Herbs and Supplements*: *L*-Carnitine (Bertelli and Ronca, 1990; Robbers and Tyler, 1999) *Lab Tests*: Glycosylated haemoglobin (haemoglobin A1C, Hg A1C) (Hodgson *et al.*, 2002; Playford, 2003), Liver enzymes (Hodgson *et al.*, 2002), T4/T8 ratio (Folker *et al.*, 1991)
CORIOLUS MUSHROOM (Nakazato *et al.*, 1994)* *Other names*: *Boletus versicolor*, Coriolus, Kawaratake, Krestin, *Polyporus versicolor*, Polysaccharide Peptide, Polysaccharide-K, *Polystictus versicolor*, PSK, PSP, Turkey Tail, *Yun-Zhi* (cloud mushroom)	No known interactions
DIINDOLYLMETHANE *Other names*: DIM	*Rx*: Cytochrome P450 1A2 (CYP1A2) substrates (Lake *et al.*, 1998)
GAMMA LINOLENIC ACID (Tyler, 1994; Fetrow and Avila, 1999; Guivernau *et al.*, 1994)* *Other names*: Gamolenic Acid, GLA	*Rx*: Anti-coagulant/Anti-platelet drugs (Guivernau *et al.*, 1994) *Herbs and Supplements*: Herbs with anti-coagulant/anti-platelet potential (Newall *et al.*, 1996; Brinker, 1996) *Lab Tests*: Bleeding time (Guivernau *et al.*, 1994), Lipid profile (*ibid.*) *Diseases or Conditions*: Bleeding disorders (*ibid.*)

*Potential for toxic or adverse effect. Please see text or reference(s).

Table 9.1. (*Continued*)

Herb or Natural Product *Common Names*	**Interactions with Prescription Drugs (Rx), Herbs and Supplements, Laboratory (Lab) Tests, Disease or Conditions**
GENISTEIN COMBINED POLYSACCHARIDE *Other names*: Basidomycetes Polysaccaride, Fermented Genistein, Fermented Isoflavone, Genistein Polysaccharide, GCP, Isoflavone Combined Polysaccharide, Soy Isoflavone Polysaccharide	*Diseases or Conditions*: Estrogen-sensitive cancers or conditions (Barnes *et al.*, 2000)
GERMANIUM (Budman *et al.*, 1982; Ettinger *et al.*, 1989; Vogelzang *et al.*, 1985; Kraot *et al.*, 1992; Sanai *et al.*, 1990; Takeuchi *et al.*, 1992; Asaka *et al.*, 1995; Hess *et al.*, 1993; Higuichi *et al.*, 1989; Matsusaka *et al.*, 1988; Schauss *et al.*, 1991; Tao and Bolger, 1997; Yanagisawa *et al.*, 2000)* *Other names*: Carboxyethylgermanium Sesquioxide, Ge-132, Ge-Oxy 132, Germanium Sesquioxide, Inorganic Germa-nium, Organic Germanium, Spirogermanium	*Rx*: Furosemide (Lasix) (Becker, 1996)

*Potential for toxic or adverse effect. Please see text or reference(s).

Table 9.1. (*Continued*)

Herb or Natural Product *Common Names*	**Interactions with Prescription Drugs (Rx), Herbs and Supplements, Laboratory (Lab) Tests, Disease or Conditions**
GINKGO (Cesarani *et al.*, 1998; Diamond *et al.*, 2000; Kudolo, 2000; Meisel *et al.*, 2003; Vale, 1998)* *Other names*: Adiantifolia, *Bai Guo Ye*, *Baiguo*, Fossil Tree, Ginkgo Folium, Japanese Silver Apricot, Kew Tree, Maidenhair Tree, *Salisburia Adiantifolia*, *Yinhsing*	*Rx*: Alprazolam (Xanax) (Markowitz *et al.*, 2003), Anti-coagulant/anti-platelet drugs (Heck *et al.*, 2000; Kudolo, 2002), Anti-convulsants (Miwa *et al.*, 2001), Anti-diabetes drugs (Matthews, 1998; Kudolo, 2006), Buspirone (BuSpar) (Spinella and Eaton, 2002), Cytochrome P450 1A2 (CYP1A2) substrates (Gurley *et al.*, 2000 and 2002; Budzinski *et al.*, 2000), Cytochrome P450 2C19 (CYP2C19) substrates (Yin *et al.*, 2004), Cytochrome P450 2C9 (CYP2C9) substrates (Yale and Glurich, 2005; Gaudineau *et al.*, 2004), Cytochrome P450 2D6 (CYP2D6) substrates (Gurley *et al.*, 2000 and 2002; Markowitz *et al.*, 2003; Yasui-Furukori *et al.*, 2004), Cytochrome P450 3A4 (CYP3A4) substrates (Gurley *et al.*, 2000 and 2002; Markowitz *et al.*, 2003; Yasui-Furukori *et al.*, 2004), Fluoxetine (Prozac) (Spinella and Eaton, 2002), Ibuprofen (Meisel *et al.*, 2003), Omeprazole (Prilosec) (Yin *et al.*, 2004), Seizure threshold lowering drugs (Miwa *et al.*, 2001; Gregory, 2001; Granger, 2001), Trazodne (Desyrel) (Galluzzi *et al.*, 2000), Warfarin (Coumadin) (Matthews, 1998; Gaudineau *et al.*, 2004; Jiang *et al.*, 2005) *Herbs and Supplements*: Anti-coagulant/anti-platelet herbs and supplements (Kudolo, 2000), Seizure threshold lowering herbs and supplements (Spinella and Eaton, 2002; Gregory, 2001; Granger, 2001) *Diseases or Conditions*: Bleeding disorders (Heck *et al.*, 2000), Diabetes (Kudolo, 2000 and 2006), Epilepsy (Miwa *et al.*, 2001; Gregory, 2001), Infertility Ondrizek *et al.*, 1999a and b) Surgery (Fessenden *et al.*, 2001; Yagmur *et al.*, 2005)

*Potential for toxic or adverse effect. Please see text or reference(s).

Table 9.1. (*Continued*)

Herb or Natural Product *Common Names*	**Interactions with Prescription Drugs (Rx), Herbs and Supplements, Laboratory (Lab) Tests, Disease or Conditions**
GOSSYPOL (Facts and Comparisons, 2001)* *Other names*: Cottonseed Oil	*Rx*: Digoxin (Lanoxin) (Facts and Comparisons, 2001), Diuretic drugs (Facts and Comparisons, 2001), Nonsteroidal anti-inflammatory drugs (NSAIDs) (Miller, 1998), Stimulant laxatives (Brinker, 1998), Theophylline (Cowart *et al.*, 1994) *Herbs and Supplements*: Cardiac glycoside-containing herbs (Brinker, 1998), licorice/horsetail (*ibid.*), stimulant laxative herbs (*ibid.*) *Diseases or Conditions*: Hypokalemia (Guo and Reidenberg, 1998), Urogenital irritation or sensitivity (McGuffin *et al.*, 1997)
GOTU KOLA (Newall *et al.*, 1996)* *Other names*: Brahma-Buti, Centella, Gotu Cola, Hydrocotyle, Idrocotyle, Indian Pennywort, Indian Water Navelwort, Marsh Penny, Talepetraka, Tsubo-Kusa, White Rot	*Rx*: Cholesterol-reducing drugs (Newall *et al.*, 1996), Diabetes drugs (*ibid.*), Drugs with sedative properties (*ibid.*) *Herbs and Supplements*: Herbs with sedative properties (Newall *et al.*, 1996; Brinker, 1998) *Diseases or Conditions*: Diabetes (Newall *et al.*, 1996)
GRAVIOLA (Lannuzel *et al.*, 2002)* *Other names*: Brazillian Cherimoya, Brazillian Paw Paw, Corossolier, Durian Benggal, Guanavana, Soursop	No known interactions
GREATER CELANDINE (Benninger *et al.*, 1999; Stickel *et al.*, 2003)*	*Rx*: Hepatotoxic drugs (Stickel *et al.*, 2003) *Herbs and Supplements*: Hepatotoxic herbs and supplements (Stickel *et al.*, 2003) *Lab Tests*: Liver function tests (Stickel *et al.*, 2003)

*Potential for toxic or adverse effect. Please see text or reference(s).

Table 9.1. (*Continued*)

Herb or Natural Product *Common Names*	**Interactions with Prescription Drugs (Rx), Herbs and Supplements, Laboratory (Lab) Tests, Disease or Conditions**
IP-6 *Other names*: Fytic Acid, Insitol Hexaphosphate, Phytic Acid	*Rx*: Anti-coagulant/Anti-platelet drugs (Vucenik *et al.*, 1999) *Herbs and Supplements*: Calcium, Iron, Zinc (Zhou and Erdman, 1995), Herbs with anti-coagulant/anti-platelet potential (Vucenik *et al.*, 1999) *Lab Tests*: Cholesterol/triglycerides (Jariwalla, 1999) *Diseases or Conditions*: Clotting disorders (Vucenik *et al.*, 1999), Iron-deficiency anemia (Jariwalla, 1999), Osteoporosis/osteopenia (Paget's Disease) (Zhou and Erdman, 1995)
LENTINAN *Other names*: None	*Lab Tests*: CD4 Counts (Gordon *et al.*, 1995) *Diseases or Conditions*: Malnutrition (Nishihira *et al.*, 1988)
LIMONENE *Other names*: Alpha-Limonene, Dipentene, D-Limonene, L-Limonene, r-Limonene, S-Limonene	*Rx*: Cytochrome P450 2C19 (CYP2C19) inducers (Crowell, 1999; Miyazawa *et al.*, 2002), Cytochrome P450 2C19 (CYP2C19) inhibitors (*ibid.*), Cytochrome P450 2C9 (CYP2C9) inducers (*ibid.*), Cytochrome P450 2C9 (CYP2C9) inhibitors (*ibid.*), Cytochrome P450 2C9 (CYP2C9) substrates (*ibid.*)
MAGNESIUM (Martindale, 1999; Birrer *et al.*, 2002) *Other names*: Magnesium Sulfate, Magnesium Aspartate, Magnesium Carbonate, Magnesium Citrate, Magnesium Gluconate, Magnesium Hydroxide	*Rx*: Aminoglycoside antibiotics (L'Hommedieu *et al.*, 1983), Bisphosphonates (Dunn and Goa, 2001), Calcium channel blockers (Hansten and Horn, 1997), Potassium-sparing diuretics (Ryan, 1987; Hollifield, 1987; Heidenreich, 1990), Quinolone antibiotics (Hansten, and Horn, 1997), Skeletal muscle relaxants (*ibid.*), Tetracycline antibiotics (Sompolinsky and Samra, 1972)

Table 9.1. (*Continued*)

Herb or Natural Product *Common Names*	**Interactions with Prescription Drugs (Rx), Herbs and Supplements, Laboratory (Lab) Tests, Disease or Conditions**
MAGNESIUM (Martindale, 1999; Birrer *et al.*, 2002) *Other names*: Magnesium Sulfate, Magnesium Aspartate, Magnesium Carbonate, Magnesium Citrate, Magnesium Gluconate, Magnesium Hydroxide	*Rx Influences on Nutrient Levels and Depletion*: Aldesleukin (interleukin-2, IL-2, proleukin) (Kozeny *et al.*, 1988), Amifostine (Ethyol, WR-2721) (Hirschel-Scholz *et al.*, 1988), Aminoglycosides (L'Hommedieu *et al.*, 1983), Amphotericin-B (Abelcet, Amphotec, AmBisome, Amphocin, Fungizone) (Sabra and Branch, 1990), Beta-2 agonists (Tveskov *et al.*, 1994; Whyte *et al.*, 1987; Khilnani *et al.*, 1992; Bos *et al.*, 1988; Gastafson *et al.*, 1996; Rolla *et al.*, 1990), Carboplatin (Paraplatin), Cisplatin (Platinol-AQ) (Martin *et al.*, 1992), Cholestyramine (Questran) (Watkins *et al.*, 1985; Runeberg *et al.*, 1972), Corticosteroids (glucocorticoids) (Quamme, 1986; Kleeman *et al.*, 1975; Rickers *et al.*, 1984), Cyclosporine (Neoral, Sandimmune) (Rahman and Ing, 1989; Thomson *et al.*, 1984; Allen *et al.*, 1985), Digoxin (Lanoxin, Lanoxicaps) (Ryan, 1987; Gottlieb, 1989), Diuretics (Ryan, 1987; Hollifield, 1987), Estrogens and estrogen-containing oral contraceptives (Seelig, 1993; Stanton and Lowenstein, 1987), Fluoroquinolones (Hansten and Horn, 1997), Foscarnet (Foscavir) (Gearhart and Sort, 1993), Insulin (De Leeuw *et al.*, 2004), Penicillamine (Cuprimine) (Cantilena and Klaassen, 1982; Seelig, 1982), Pentamidine (NebuPent, Pentacarinat, Pentam 300) (Shah *et al.*, 1990; Burnett and Reents, 1990; Gradon *et al.*, 1991), Sodium phosphates (monobasic sodium phosphate and dibasic sodium phosphate, fleet phospho-soda) (Schwarz and Zagala-Navarez, 2002), Tacrolimus (FK506, Prograf) (Lote *et al.*, 2000), Tetracyclines (Murry and Healy, 1991)

Table 9.1. (*Continued*)

Herb or Natural Product *Common Names*	**Interactions with Prescription Drugs (Rx), Herbs and Supplements, Laboratory (Lab) Tests, Disease or Conditions**
MAGNESIUM (Martindale, 1999; Birrer *et al.*, 2002) *Other names*: Magnesium Sulfate, Magnesium Aspartate, Magnesium Carbonate, Magnesium Citrate, Magnesium Gluconate, Magnesium Hydroxide	*Herbs and Supplements*: Boron (Meacham *et al.*, 1995; Nielsen *et al.*, 1987), Calcium (Spencer *et al.*, 1994; Sojka *et al.*, 1997), Vitamin D (Hardwick *et al.*, 1991; Charles *et al.*, 1987), Zinc (Nielsen and Milne, 2004) *Lab Tests*: Alkaline phosphatase (ALK PHOS) (Young, 1995), Angiotensin-converting enzyme (ACE) (*ibid.*), Blood pressure (Sanjuliani *et al.*, 1996), Calcium (Young, 1995), Diagnex blue (*ibid.*), Electrocardigram (ECG) (Lasserre *et al.*, 1994; Brodsky *et al.*, 1994), Parathyroid hormone (Vetter and Lohse, 2002), Testosterone (Young, 1995) *Diseases or Conditions*: Alcoholism (Rude, 1998), Diabetes (*ibid.*), Elderly (Durlach *et al.*, 1998), Heart block (Santoro *et al.*, 2000), Malabsorption syndromes (Galland, 1988; Geerling *et al.*, 1998), Renal disease (Rude, 1998), Restless leg syndrome (Frankel *et al.*, 1974; Popoviciu *et al.*, 1993)
MARIJUANA (Johnson *et al.*, 2000)* *Other names*: Cannabis, Grass, Hash, Hashish, Hemp, Kif, Mariguana, Marihuana, Pot, Weed	*Rx*: Barbiturates (Hebel, 1998), CNS depressants (*ibid.*), Disulfiram (Antabuse) (*ibid.*), Fluoxetine (Prozac) (*ibid.*), Theophylline (*ibid.*), Alcohol (*ibid.*) *Herbs and Supplements*: Supplements with sedative properties (*ibid.*) *Lab Tests*: Intraocular pressure (Merritt *et al.*, 1980) *Diseases or Conditions*: Cardiovascular diseases (Facts and Comparisons, 2001), Compromised immune function (Klein *et al.*, 2000; Zhu *et al.*, 2000), Respiratory Diseases (Facts and Comparisons, 2001; Johnson *et al.*, 2000), Seizure disorders (Facts and Comparisons, 2001)

*Potential for toxic or adverse effect. Please see text or reference(s).

Table 9.1. (*Continued*)

Herb or Natural Product *Common Names*	**Interactions with Prescription Drugs (Rx), Herbs and Supplements, Laboratory (Lab) Tests, Disease or Conditions**
MELATONIN (Wagner *et al.*, 1998; Dollins *et al.*, 1993)* *Other names*: MEL, MLT, Pineal Hormone	*Rx*: Anti-coagulant/anti-platelet Drugs (Herxheimer and Petrie, 2002), Anti-diabetes drugs (Cagnacci *et al.*, 2001), Benzodiazepines (Djeridane and Touitou, 2001), Caffeine (Wright, 2000), Contraceptive drugs (*ibid.*), Flumazenil (Romazicon) (Golombek *et al.*, 1992), Fluvoxamine (Luvox) (Hartter *et al.*, 2000; Grozinger *et al.*, 2000; von Bahr *et al.*, 2000), Immunosuppressants (Lissoni *et al.*, 1999), Nifedipine Gits (Procardia XL) (Lusardi *et al.*, 2000), Verapamil (Calan, Covera, Isoptin, Verelan) (Wikner *et al.*, 1997) *Herbs and Supplements*: Herbs with anti-coagulant/anti-platelet potential (Herxheimer and Petrie, 2002), Herbs/supplements with sedative properties (Avery *et al.*, 1998) *Lab Tests*: Blood pressure (Lusardi *et al.*, 2000), Heart rate (*ibid.*), Human growth hormone (Valcavi *et al.*, 1993), Luteinizing hormone (Nordlund and Lerner, 1977), Oxytocin (Forsling *et al.*, 1999), Vasopressin (*ibid.*) *Diseases or Conditions*: Cancer (Lissoni *et al.*, 1996b), Depression (Carman *et al.*, 1976), Diabetes (Cagnacci *et al.*, 2001), Hypertension (Lusardi *et al.*, 2000), Seizure disorders (Bazil *et al.*, 2000)
POMEGRANATE (Gaig *et al.*, 1999)* *Other names*: Dadima, Fruit of the Dead, Granada, Grenade, Grenadier, Roma, *Shi Liu Gen Pi*, *Shi Liu Pi*	*Rx*: Ace Inhibitors (ACEIs) (Aviram and Dornfeld, 2001), Anti-hypertensive drugs (*ibid.*), Cytochrome P450 2D6 (CYP2D6) substrates (Kim *et al.*, 2002), Cytochrome P450 3A4 (CYP3A4) substrates (Hidaka *et al.*, 2005), Rosuvastatin (Crestor) (Sorokin *et al.*, 2006) *Herbs and Supplements*: Herbs and supplements with hypotensive effects (Aviram and Dornfeld, 2001) *Diseases or Conditions*: Plant allergies (Gaig *et al.*, 1999)

*Potential for toxic or adverse effect. Please see text or reference(s).

Table 9.1. (*Continued*)

Herb or Natural Product *Common Names*	**Interactions with Prescription Drugs (Rx), Herbs and Supplements, Laboratory (Lab) Tests, Disease or Conditions**
STRONTIUM (Natural Medicines Comprehensive Database, 2006)* *Other names*: Stable Strontium, Strontium Chloride, Strontium-89 Chloride, Strontium Citrate, Strontium Ranelate	*Rx that can Affect Strontium Levels*: Androgens (Eisenberg, 1996), Corticosteriuds (*ibid.*), Estrogens (*ibid.*) *Lab Tests*: Blood cell counts (Metastron Prescribing Information, 1998) Creatine phosphokinase (Meunier *et al.*, 2002 and 2004) *Diseases or Conditions*: Bone disease (Gutteridge *et al.*, 1968), Renal insufficiency (Verberckmoes *et al.*, 2003)
THEANINE *Other names*: Gamma-Glutamylethylamide, L-Theanine	*Rx*: Anti-hypertensive drugs (Yokogoshi and Kobayashi, 1998), Stimulant drugs (Kimura and Murata, 1986)
TIRATRICOL (Natural Medicines Comprehensive Database, 2006; McKevoy, 1998; FDA, 2000)* *Other names*: Triac, Triodothyroacetic Acid	*Rx*: Anti-coagulant/anti-platelet drugs (McKevoy, 1998), Anti-diabetes drugs (*ibid.*), Cholestyramine (Questran) (*ibid.*), Stimulant drugs (*ibid.*), Thyroid hormone (Mueller-Gaertner and Schneider, 1988) *Herbs and Supplements*: Herbs and supplements with sympathomimetic activity (McKevoy, 1998), Herbs with thyroid activity (*ibid.*), Vitamin K (*ibid.*) *Lab Tests*: Prothrombin Time (PT), International Normalization Ratio (INR) (*ibid.*), Thyroid function tests (FDA, 2007), Thyroid Stimulating Hormone (TSH) (Menegay *et al.*, 1989), Thyrotrpin-Releasing Hormone (TRH) stimulation (Mueller-Gaertner and Schneider, 1988; Sherman and Ladenson, 1992) *Diseases or Conditions*: Adrenal insufficiency, Diabetes, Hypopituitarism (McKevoy, 1998), Angina, Cardiovascular disease, Hypertension (*ibid.*), Diabetes (*ibid.*), Liver disease (Jean-Pastor *et al.*, 1986), Myxedema (McKevoy, 1998), Prolonged clotting time (*ibid.*)

*Potential for toxic or adverse effect. Please see text or reference(s).

Table 9.1. (*Continued*)

Herb or Natural Product *Common Names*	**Interactions with Prescription Drugs (Rx), Herbs and Supplements, Laboratory (Lab) Tests, Disease or Conditions**
TURMERIC *Other names*: *Curcumae longae rhizoma*, Curcumin, Halada, Haldi, Haridra, Indian Saffron, *Nisha*, *Radix curcumae*, *Rajani*, *Rhizoma cucurmae longae*	*Rx*: Anti-coagulant/anti-platelet drugs (Shah *et al.*, 1999) *Herbs and Supplements*: Herbs with anti-coagulant/anti-platelet potential (*ibid.*) *Diseases or Conditions*: Bile duct obstruction and gallstones (Rasyid *et al.*, 2002)
WHEY PROTEIN (Laoprasert *et al.*, 1998)* *Other names*: Bovine Whey Protein Concentrate, Whey Peptides	*Rx*: Alendronate (Fosamax) (Martindale, 1999), Levodopa (Semia *et al.*, 1998), Quinoline antibiotics (Martindale, 1999), Tetracycline antibiotics (*ibid.*) *Lab Tests*: Blood Urea Nitrogen (BUN) (Wong and Watson, 1995) *Diseases or Conditions*: Milk allergy (Laoprasert *et al.*, 1998)

*Potential for toxic or adverse effect. Please see text or reference(s).

self-medicated to treat metastatic carcinoma and colon cancer. Researchers have become aware that a high concentration of glutathione (GSH) is present in most tumor cells and seems to be a factor in resistance to chemotherapy (Kennedy *et al.*, 1995). A Phases I/II clinical study on patients, with various cancers, showed that by administering an oral dose of 30 grams of whey protein daily for six months, these patients showed a sustained drop in lymphocyte GSH levels. This finding suggests that whey protein may deplete GSH in tumor cells and may make these cells more vulnerable to chemotherapy. More research is needed to confirm this finding. Kennedy *et al.* (1995) used a dose of 30 grams per day in their research. Individuals allergic to milk products should avoid whey protein, according to Laoprasert *et al.* (1998) who report an anaphylactic reaction to a product containing whey protein.

As indicated above, Table 9.1 follows with information about the potential interactions of each of the above herb or natural products with prescriptions, other herbs, laboratory tests, or diseases. Scientific and common names are also included.

Conclusion and Implications

This review chapter provides information to help health care professionals become better resource persons for their patients. Through awareness of significant clinical roles as resource persons. All professionals are encouraged to improve liaisons between themselves and with patients to discuss the possible benefits or dangers in use of these herbs and natural products. All herbs and natural products presented show promise in treatment of cancer.

An update to a recent publication (Montbriand, 2004a), this review specifically presents the latest evidence based research on 27 herbs and natural products with potential to decrease growth of cancers or to use as adjuncts with cancer treatments. All of the research presented is from *in vivo*, *in vitro*, and early Phases I/II trials; therefore, the results are at best preliminary, but all the same encouraging. Since the last review (Montbriand, 2004a), several new herbs and natural products have come to the forefront through new and promising research. Other products that showed promise only a few years ago, are now showing less promise and have been eliminated from this review. Until products and herbs are proven beneficial in clinical trials, health care professionals must stay constantly alert to new findings. This constant vigilance can only be a benefit to the health profession and especially to patients with cancer.

The scientific and common names of natural products and herbs have been included in this review. Pay careful attention to the spelling of these names on all products of interest. Manufacturers who are careful about the spelling of their products may be more attentive to the quality of the product they sell, according to Tyler (1996). Manufacturers may also provide doses for their products, but these doses should be noted with caution. The typical doses provided in this review, while not recommended doses, are doses used by the researchers cited in their clinical trial or case study. The references for these studies can be found in the reference list. These doses have at least some preliminary testing and seem more prudent than doses found on manufacturers' publication.

In most cases, herbs come in capsules or tablets, usually powder or crushed forms of a whole plant. In some cases, the whole plant is available. Keep in mind that the whole plant is a conglomerate of many chemical components, some medicinal, some benign, and some possibly poisonous. One example is the elderberry. The inner bark has been used by the North American natives as a medicinal tea, yet the stems and berries of the elderberry contain cyanide (Facts and Comparisons, 2001). Encourage patients who have grown herbs on their own, or who use scavenged herbs from the wild for personal concoctions to talk about their experimentation to health professionals. Some plants, such as mushrooms found in the wild, are difficult to identify. Some plants are poisonous, and an inexperienced individual may make mistakes in identification of wild plants, with tragic results.

Even when a plant is correctly identified, one cannot be assured of the quality or quantity of any medicinal components in that herb. The growing conditions of that herb can vary considerably with the quality of the soil, seed, bulb, or plant. This caution also applies to herbals or products. Therefore, one should always be aware that when using an herb or natural product, the amount of the medicinal component is not constant and may not even be present.

On the other hand, all prescriptions and some herbal or natural products have DIN (drug identification numbers) guaranteeing that the specified medicinal components will be present. For example, Tanacet 125® (Ashbury Biologicals/Herbal Laboratories) contains the medicinal component (tanacet) of the herb feverfew, scientific name, *Tanacetum partheniu* that has been used for headaches. When a product such as Tanacet 125® has a DIN number, this means that it is quality controlled. The product will contain an exact amount of the medicinal component, and in the example of the above case, tanacet is found in the exact amount specified. Conversely, when the consumer buys an herbal product, such as feverfew, the amount of the medicinal component is unknown, in the above case tanacet.

This review also contains information to help identify situations where herbs or natural products may interact with prescription medications, other herbs or products, lab tests, or with diseases or conditions. Notations are also given to ensure identification of possible dangers in using these herbs or products. These notations have been provided on a table to ensure quick reference. Keep in mind that these cautions are preliminary and may change.

While this review may seem overlain with cautions, health care professionals and patients may be encouraged to see the progress made by the research community in discovering possible potentially useful herbs and natural products that interact positively with cancer. However, this encouragement should be taken responsibly. Patients with cancer often are desperate to find a potential cure; therefore, health care professionals have the unique opportunity in helping these patients make informed choices. Health care professionals, should be aware that while this information is available in the evidence-based research from biomedicine, the alternative system targets individuals with cancer, encouraging them to try products that have not been subject to the rigorous testing required in conventional health care. Often the alternative system insists that their products have undergone rigorous testing; yet, these rigorous tests cannot be found in published refereed medical, pharmacy, nursing, or other health-science journals. My experience has been that patients appreciate and want current evidence-based information from health professionals. Even if the information seems overlain with technical terms, patients have often informed me that they do not want just the vernacular version. Patients want to be part of the whole discussion and want to be allowed to make informed choices in their care. Being current with the latest evidence-based information on potential cancer developments is a unique opportunity for health care professionals and patients with cancer.

Acknowledgments

I acknowledge with thanks the continuing support of Dr. Carl D'Arcy, Director, Applied Research/Psychiatry, University of Saskatchewan. During this work, I was a recipient of two Health Services Utilization and Research Commission, Socio-Health Grants. Saskatchewan, Canada.

References

Allen, R.D., Hunnisett, A.G. and Morris, P.J. (1985) Cyclosporine and magnesium. *Lancet* **1**, 1283–1284.

Asaka, T., Nitta, E., Makifuchi, T., Shibazaki, Y., Kitamura, Y., Ohara, H., *et al.* (1995) Germanium intoxication with sensory ataxia. *J. Neurol. Sci.* **130**, 220–223.

Avery, D., Lenz, M. and Landis, C. (1998) Guidelines for prescribing melatonin. *Ann. Med.* **30**, 122–130.

Aviram, M. and Dornfeld, L. (2001) Pomegranate juice consumption inhibits serum angiotensin converting enzyme activity and reduces systolic blood pressure. *Atherosclerosis* **158**, 195–198.

Babineau, T.J., Hackford, A., Kenler, A., Bistrian, B., Forse, R.A., Fairchild, P.G., *et al.* (1995) A phase II multicenter, double-blind, randomized, placebo-controlled study of three dosages of an immunomodulator (PGG-glucan) in high-risk surgery patients. *Ann. Surg.* **222**, 689–690.

Babu, T.D., Kuttan, G. and Padikkala, J. (1995) Cytotoxic and anti-tumour properties of certain taxa of *Umbelliferae* with special reference to *Centella asiatica* (*L.*) *Urban*. *J. Ethnopharmacol.* **48**, 53–57.

Balk, J.L. (2000) Indole-3-carbinol for cancer prevention. *Altern. Med. Alert.* **3**, 105–107.

Barnes, P.M., Powell-Griner, E., McFann, K. and Nahin, R.L. (2004) Complementary and alternative medicine use among adults: United States, 2002. *Adv. Data* **343**, 1–9.

Barnes, S., Kim, H., Darley-Usmar, V., Patel, R., Xu, J., Boersma, B., *et al.* (2000) Beyond ERalpha and Erbeta: Estrogen receptor binding is only part of the isoflavone story. *J. Nutr.* **130**, 656S–657S.

Barqawi, A., Gamito, E., O'Donnell, C. and Crawford, E.D. (2004) Herbal and vitamin supplement use in a prostate cancer screening population. *Urology* **63**, 288–292.

Bazil, C.W., Short, D., Crispin, D. and Zheng, W. (2000) Patients with intractable epilepsy have low melatonin, which increases following seizures. *Neurology* **55**, 1746–1748.

Beal, J.E., Olson, R., Laubenstein, L., Morales, J.O., Bellman, P. and Yangco, B. (1995) Dronabinol as a treatment for anorexia associated with weight loss in patients with AIDS. *J. Pain Symptom. Manage.* **10**, 89–97.

Becker, B.N. (1996) Ginseng-induced diuretic resistance. *JAMA* **276**, 606–607.

Benninger, J., Schneider, H.T., Schuppan, D., Kirchner, T. and Hahn, E.G. (1999) Acute hepatitis induced by greater celandine (*Chelidonium majus*). *Gastroenterology* **117**, 1234–1237.

Bertelli, A. and Ronca, G. (1990) Carnitine and coenzyme Q10: Biochemical properties and functions, synergism and complementary actions. *Int. J. Tissue React.* **12**, 183–186.

Birrer, R.B., Shallash, A.J. and Totten, V. (2002) Hypermagnesemia-induced fatality following epsom salt gargles. *J. Emerg. Med.* **22**, 185–188.

Bisset, N.G. (ed.) (1994) *Max Wichtl Herbal Drugs and Phytopharmaceuticals. A Handbook for Practice on a Scientific Basis*. Medpharm Scientific Publishers, Stuttgart, London.

Bos, W.J., Postma, D.S. and van Doormaal, J.J. (1988) Magnesiuric and calciuric effect of terbutaline in man. *Clin. Sci.* **74**, 595–597.

Bresolin, N., Doriguzzi, C., Ponzetto, C., Angelini, C., Moroni, I., Castelli, E., *et al.* (1990) Ubidecarenone in the treatment of mitochondrial myopathies: A multicenter double-blind trial. *J. Neurol. Sci.* **100**, 70–78.

Brinker, F. (1996) *Herb Contraindications and Drug Interactions*. The Pharmaceutical Press, London, UK.

Brinker, F. (1998) *Herb Contraindications and Drug Interactions*, 2nd ed. Eclectic Medical Publications, Sandy, OR.

Brodsky, M.A., Orlov, M.V., Capparelli, E.V., Allen, B.J., Iseri, L.T., Ginkel, M., *et al.* (1994) Magnesium therapy in new-onset atrial fibrillation. *Am. J. Cardiol.* **73**, 1227–1229.

Browden, W., Williams, D., Pretus, H., Olivero, G., Enrichens, F., Mao, P., *et al.* (1990) Beneficial effect of enhanced macrophage function in the trauma patient. *Ann. Surg.* **211**, 605–612.

Brown, G.A., Vukovich, M.D., Reifenrath, T.A., Uhl, N.L., Parsons, K.A., Sharp, R.L., *et al.* (2000) Effects of anabolic precursors on serum testosterone concentrations and adaptations to resistance training in young men. *Int. J. Sport. Nutr. Exerc. Metab.* **10**, 340–359.

Budman, D.R., Schulman, P., Vinciguerra, V. and Degnan, T.J. (1982) Phase I trial of spirogermanium given by infusion in a multiple-dose schedule. *Cancer Treat. Rep.* **66**, 173–175.

Budzinski, J.W., Foster, B.C., Vanderhoek, S. and Arnason, J.T. (2000) An *in vitro* evaluation of human cytochrome P450 3A4 inhibition by selected commercial herbal extracts and tinctures. *Phytomedicine* **7**, 273–282.

Burnett, R.J. and Reents, S.B. (1990) Severe hypomagnesemia induced by pentamidine. *Ann. Pharmacother.* **24**, 239–240.

Cagnacci, A., Arangino, S., Renzi, A., Paoletti, A.M., Melis, G.B., Cagnacci, P., *et al.* (2001) Influence of melatonin administration on glucose tolerance and insulin sensitivity of postmenopausal women. *Clin. Endocrinol.* **54**, 339–346.

Cantilena, L.R. and Klaassen, C.D. (1982) The effect of chelating agents on the excretion of endogenous metals. *Toxicol. Appl. Pharmacol.* **63**, 344–350.

Carman, J.S., Post, R.M., Buswell, R. and Goodwin, F.K. (1976) Negative effects of melatonin on depression. *Am. J. Psychiatry* **133**, 1181–1186.

Cesarani, A., Meloni, F., Alpini, D., Barozzi, S., Verderio, L. and Boscani, P.F. (1998) *Gingko biloba* (EGb 761) in the treatment of equilibrium. *Adv. Ther.* **15**, 291–304.

Challa, A., Rao, D.R. and Reddy, B.S. (1997) Interactive suppression of aberrant crypt foci induced by azoxymethane in rat colon by phytic acid and green tea. *Carcinogenesis* **18**, 2023–2036.

Charles, P., Mosekilde, L., Sondergard, K. and Jensen, F.T. (1987) Treatment with high-dose oral vitamin D2 in patients with jejunoileal bypass for morbid obesity. Effects on calcium and magnesium metabolism, vitamin D metabolites and faecal lag time. *Scand. J. Gastroenterol.* **19**, 1031–1038.

Chen, I., Safe, S. and Bjeldanes, L. (1996) Indole-3-carinol and diindolylmethane as aryl hydrocarbon (Ah) receptor agonists and antagonists in T47D human breast cancer cells. *Biochem. Phamacol.* **51**, 1069–1076.

Chen, I., McDougal, A., Wang, F. and Safe, S. (1998) Aryl hydrocarbon receptor-mediated antiestrogenic and antitumorigenic activity of diindolylmethane. *Cancinogenesis* **19**, 1631–1639.

Cordes, N., Plasswilm, L., Bamberg, M. and Rodemann, H.P. (2002) Ukrain, an alkaloid thiophosphoric acid derivative of *Chelidonium majus L.* protects human fibroblasts but not human tumour cells *in vitro* against ionizing radiation. *Int. J. Radiat. Biol.* **78**, 17–27.

Cowart, C.L., London, S.N., Vernon, M.W. and Pedigo, N.G. (1994) The effect of cyclic adenosine monophosphate, forskolin, and theophylline on motility parameters in gossypol-treated human sperm. *Fertil. Steril.* **61**, 929–934.

Coyle, T., Levante, S., Shetler, M. and Winfield, J. (1994) *In vitro* and *in vivo* cytotoxicity of gossypol against central nervous system tumor cell lines. *J. Neurooncol.* **19**, 25–35.

Crosby, V., Wilcock, A. and Corcoran, R. (2000) The safety and efficacy of a single dose (500 mg or 1 g) of intravenous magnesium sulfate in nuropathic pain poorly responsive to strong opioid analgesics in patients with cancer. *J. Pain. Symptom Manage.* **20**, 1–2.

Crowell, P.L. (1999) Prevention and therapy of cancer by dietary monoterpenes. *J. Nutr.* **129**, 775S–778S.

De Leeuw, I., Engelen, W., De Block, C. and Van Gaal, L. (2004) Long term magnesium supplementation influences favourably the natural evolution of neuropathy in Mg-depleted type 1 diabetic patients (T1dm). *Magnes. Res.* **17**, 109–114.

Deliliers, G.L., Servida, F., Fracchiolla, N.S., Ricci, C., Borsotti, C., Colombo, G., *et al.* (2002) Effect of inositol hexaphosphate (IP(6)) on human normal and leukaemic haematopoietic cells. *Br. J. Haematol.* **117**, 577–587.

Diamond, B.J., Shiflett, S.C., Feiwel, N., Matheis, R.J., Noskin, O., Richards, J.A., *et al.* (2000) *Gingko biloba* extract: Mechanisms and clinical indications. *Arch. Phys. Med. Rehabil.* **81**, 668–678.

Djeridane, Y. and Touitou, Y. (2001) Chronic diazepam administration differentially affects melatonin synthesis in rat pineal and Harderian glands. *Psychopharmacology* **154**, 403–407.

Dollins, A.B., Lynch, H.J., Wurtman, R.J., Deng, M.H., Kischka, K.U., Gleason, R.E., *et al.* (1993) Effect of pharmacological daytime doses of melatonin on human mood and performance. *Psychopharmacology* **112**, 490–496.

Dong, Y., Kwan, C.Y., Chen, Z.N. and Yang, M.M. (1996) Anti-tumor effects of a refined polysaccharide peptide fraction isolated from *Coriolus versicolor*: *In vitro* and *in vivo* studies. *Res. Comm. Mol. Pathol. Pharmacol.* **92**, 140–148.

Dong, Y., Yang, M.M. and Kwan, C.Y. (1997) *In vitro* inhibition of proliferation of HL-60 cells by tetrandrine and *Coriolus versicolor* peptide derived from Chinese medical herbs. *Life Sci.* **60**, PL135–140.

Duke, J.A. (1987) *CRC Handbook of Medicinal Herbs*. CRC Press, Boca Raton, FL.

Duke, J.A. and Vasquez, R. (1994) *Amazonian Ethnobotanical Dictionary*. CRC Press, Boca Raton, FL.

Dunn, C.J. and Goa, K.L. (2001) Risedronate: A review of its pharmacological properties and clinical use in resorptive bone disease. *Drug* **61**, 685–712.

Durlach, J., Bac, P., Durlach, V., Rayssiguier, Y., Bara, M. and Guiet-Bara, A. (1998) Magnesium status and ageing: An update. *Magnes. Res.* **11**, 25–42.

Duvic, M., Reisman, M., Finley, V., Rapini, R., DiLuzio, N.R. and Mansell, P.W. (1987) Glucan-induced keratoderma in acquired immunodeficiency syndrome. *Arch. Dermatol.* **123**, 751–756.

Eisenberg, D.M., Kessler, R.C., Foster, C., Norlock, F.E., Calkins, D.R. and Delbanco, T.L. (1993) Unconventional medicine in the United States: Prevalence, cost and patterns of use. *N. Engl. Med.* **328**, 246–252.

Eisenberg, D.M., Davis, R.B., Ettner, S.L., Appel, S., Wilkey, S., Van Rompay, M. and Kessler, R.C. (1998) Trends in alternative medicine in the United States, 1990–1997. *JAMA* **280**, 1569–1575.

Eisenberg, D.M., Kessler, R.C., Van Rompay, M.I., Kaptchuk, T.J., Wilkey, S.A., Appel, S. and Davis, R.B. (2001) Perceptions about complementary therapies relative to conventional therapies among adults who use both: Results from a national survey. *Ann. Intern. Med.* **135**, 344–351.

Eisenberg, E. (1966) Effects of androgens, estrogens and corticoids on strontium kinetics in man. *J. Clin. Endocrinol. Metab.* **26**, 566–582.

Engelsen, J., Nielsen, J.D. and Winther, K. (2002) Effect of coenzyme Q10 and *Gingko biloba* on warfarin dosage in stable, long-term warfarin treated outpatients. A randomized, double bind, placebo-crossover trial. *Thromb. Haemost.* **87**, 1075–1076.

Environmental Protection Agency (2002). *Radiation Information*: *Cesium*. Retrieved September 12, 2002 from http://www.epa.gov/radiation/radionuclides/cesium.htm

Ernst, E. and Schmidt, K. (2005) Ukrain — a new cancer cure? A systematic review of randomized clinical trials. *BMC Cancer* **5**, 69.

Ettinger, D.S., Finkelstein, D.M., Donehower, R.C., Chang, A.Y., Green, M., Blum, R., *et al.* (1989) Phase II study of N-methylformamide, spirogermanium, and 4-demethoxydaunorubicin in treatment of non-small cell lung cancer (EST 3583): An Eastern Cooperative Oncology Group study. *Med. Pediatr. Oncol.* **17**, 197–201.

Facts and Comparisons. (2001) *The Lawrence Review of Natural Products® Monograph System*. Walter Kluwer Company, St. Louis.

FDA. (2000) FDA warns against consuming dietary supplements containing tiratricol. Retrieved November 22, 2000 from www.fda.gov/bbs/topics/ANSWERS/ANS01057.html.

FDA. (2007) List of orphan designations and approvals. Office of Orphan Products Development. www.fda.gov/orphan/designat/list.htm.

Fessenden, J.M., Wittenborn, W. and Clarke, L. (2001) *Gingko biloba*: A case report of herbal medicine and bleeding postoperatively from a laparoscopic cholecystectomy. *Am. Surg.* **67**, 33–35.

Fetrow, C.W. and Avila, J.R. (1999) *Professional's Handbook of Complementary and Alternative Medicines*. Springhouse, Springhouse PA, USA.

Folkers, K., Hanioka, T., Xia, L.J., McRee, J.T. Jr. and Langsjoen, P. (1991) Coenzyme Q10 increases T4/T8 ratios of lymphocytes in ordinary subjects and relevance to patients having the AIDS related complex. *Biochem. Biophys. Res. Comm.* **176**, 786–791.

Forsling, M.L., Wheeler, M.J. and Williams, A.J. (1999) The effect of melatonin administration on pituitary hormone secretion in man. *Clin. Endocrinol.* **51**, 637–642.

Frankel, B.L., Patten, B.M. and Gillin, J.C. (1974) Restless leg syndrome. Sleep-electroencephalographic and neurologic findings. *JAMA* **230**, 1302–1303.

Fuke, C., Krikorian, S.A. and Couris, R.R. (2000) Coenzyme Q10: A review of essential functions and clinical trials. *US Pharm.*, pp. 28–41.

Gaig, P., Bartolome, B., Lleonart, R., Garcia-Ortega, P., Palacios, R. and Richard, C. (1999) Allergy to pomegranate (*Punica granatum*). *Allergy* **54**, 287–288.

Galijatovic, A., Otake, Y., Walle, U.K. and Walle, T. (1999) Extensive metabolism of the flavonoid chrysin by human Caca-2 and Hep G2 cell. *Xenobiotica* **29**, 1241–1256.

Galijatovic, A., Walle, U.K. and Walle, T. (2000) Induction of UDP-glucuronosyltransferase by the flavonoids chrysin and guercetin in caco-2 cells. *Pharmacol. Res.* **17**, 21–26.

Galijatovic, A., Otake, Y., Walle, U.K. and Walle, T. (2001) Induction of UDP-glucuronosyltransferase UGT1A1 by the flavonoid chrysin in Caco-2 — potential role in carcinogen bioinactivation. *Pharmacol. Res.* **18**, 374–379.

Galland, L. (1988) Magnesium and inflammatory bowel disease. *Magnesium* **7**, 78–83.

Galluzzi, S., Zanetti, O., Binetti, G., Trabucchi, M. and Frisoni, G.B. (2000) Coma in a patient with Alzheimer's disease taking low dose trazodone and *Gingko biloba. J. Neurol. Neurosurg. Psychiatry* **68**, 679–680.

Galve-Roperh, I., Sanchez, C., Cortes, M.L., del Pulgar, T.G., Izquierdo, M. and Guzman, M. (2000) Anti-tumoral action of cannabinoids: Involvement of sustained ceramide accumulation and extracellular signal-regulated kinase activation. *Nat. Med.* **6**, 313–319.

Gaudineau, C., Beckerman, R., Welbourn, S. and Auclair, K. (2004) Inhibition of human P450 enzymes by multiple constituents of the *Gingko biloba* extract. *Biochem. Biophys. Res. Comm.* **318**, 1072–1078.

Gearhart, M.O. and Sorg, T.B. (1993) Foscarnet-induced severe hypomagnesemia and other electrolyte disturbances. *Ann. Pharmacother.* **27**, 285–289.

Geerling, B.J., Badart-Smook, A., Stockbrugger, R.W. and Brummer, R.J. (1998) Comprehensive nutritional status in patients with long-standing Crohn disease currently in remission. *Am. J. Clin. Nutr.* **67**, 919–926.

Ghafar, M.A., Golliday, E., Bingham, J., Mansukhani, M.M., Anastasiadis, A.G., and Katz, A.E. (2002) Regression of prostate cancer following administration of Genistein Combined Polysaccharide (GCP), a nutritional supplement: A case report. *J. Altern. Complement. Med.* **8**, 493–497.

Gilbert, N.E., O'Reilly, J.E., Chang, C.J., Lin, Y.C. and Brueggemeier, R.W. (1995) Antiproliferative activity of gossypol and gossypolone on human breast cancer cells. *Life Sci.* **57**, 61–67.

Golombek, D.A, Escolar, E., Burin, L.J., De Brito Sanchez, M.G., Fernandez Duque, D. and Cardinali, D.P. (1992) Chronopharmacology of melatonin: Inhibition by benzodiazepine antagonism. *Chronobiol. Int.* **9**, 124–131.

Gordon, M., Guralnik, M., Kaneko, Y., Mimura, T., Goodgame, J., DeMarzo, C., *et al.* (1995) A Phase II controlled study of a combination of the immune modulator, lentinan, with didanosine (ddI) in HIV patients with CD4 cells of 200–500/mm^3. *J. Med.* **26**, 193–207.

Gottlieb, S.S. (1989) Importance of magnesium in congestive heart failure. *Am. J. Cardiol.* **63**, 39G–42G.

Gradon, J.D., Fricchione, L. and Sepkowitz, D. (1991) Severe hypomagnesemia associated with pentamidine therapy. *Rev. Infect. Dis.* **13**, 511–512.

Granger, A.S. (2001) *Gingko biloba* precipitating epileptic seizures. *Age Aging* **30**, 523–525.

Gregory, P.J. (2001) Seizure associated with *Gingko biloba*? *Ann. Intern. Med.* **134**, 344.

Grozinger, M., Hartter, S., Wang, X., Roschke, J., Hiemke, C. and Rose, D.M. (2000) Fluvoxamine strongly inhibits melatonin metabolism in a patient with low-amplitude melatonin profile. *Arch. Gen. Psychiatry* **57**, 812–813.

Gruenwald, J., Brendler, T. and Jaenicke, C. (eds.) (1998) *PDR for Herbal Medicines*. Medical Economics, Montvale, NJ.

Guivernau, M., Meza, N., Barja, P. and Roman, O. (1994) Clinical and experimental study on the long-term effect of dietary gamma-linolenic acid on plasma lipids, platelet aggregation, thromboxane formation, and prostacyclin production. *Prostaglandin Leukot. Essent. Fatty Acids* **51**, 311–316.

Gunawardana, D.H., Lichtenstein, M., Better, N. and Rosenthal, M. (2004) Results of strontium-89 therapy in patients with prostate cancer resistant to chemotherapy. *Clin. Nucl. Med.* **29**, 81–85.

Guo, J. and Reidenberg, M.M. (1998) Inhibition of 11-beta-hydroxysteroid dehydrogenase by bioflavonoids and their interaction with furosemide and gossypol. *J. Lab. Clin. Med.* **132**, 32–38.

Gurley, B.J., Gardner, S.F. and Hubbard, M.A. (2000) Clinical assessment of potential cytochrome P450-medicated herb-drug interactions. In: *AAPS Ann. Mtg. Expo., Indianapolis, IN.*, October 29–November 2, presentation #3460.

Gurley, B.J., Gardner, S.F., Hubbard, M.A., Williams, D.K., Gentry, W.B., Cui, Y., *et al.* (2002) Cytochrome P450 phenotypic ratio for predicting herb-drug interactions in humans. *Clin. Pharmacol. Ther.* **72**, 276–287.

Gustafson, T., Boman, K., Rosenhall, I., Sandstrom, T. and Wester, P.O. (1996) Skeletal muscle magnesium and potassium in asthmatics treated with oral beta 2-agonists. *Eur. Respir. J.* **9**, 237–240.

Gutteridge, D.H., Robinson, C.J. and Joplin, G.F. (1968) Delayed strontium absorption in post-menopausal osteoporosis and osteomalacia. *Clin. Sci.* **34**, 351–363.

Hanaki, Y., Sugiyama, S., Ozawa, T. and Ohno, M. (1993) Coenzyme Q10 and coronary artery disease. *Clin. Invest.* **71**(8 Suppl), S112–115.

Hansten, P.D. and Horn, J.R. (1997) *Drug Interactions Analysis and Management*. Applied Therapeutics Inc, Vancouver, WA.

Harada, M., Matsunaga, K., Oguchi, Y., Iijima, H., Tamada, K., Abe, K., *et al.* (1997) Oral administration of PSK can improve the impaired anti-tumor CD4+ T-cell response in gut-associated lymphoid tissue (GALT) of specific-pathogen-free mice. *Int. J. Cancer* **70**, 362–372.

Hardwick, L.L., Jones, M.R., Brautbar, N. and Lee, D.B. (1991) Magnesium absorption: Mechanisms and the influence of vitamin D, calcium and phosphate. *J. Nutr.* **121,** 13–23.

Harnack, L.J., Rydell, S.A. and Stang, J. (2001) Prevalence of use of herbal products by adults in the Minneapolis/St. Paul, Minn, metropolitan area. *Mayo Clin. Proc.* **76**, 688–694.

Hartter, S., Grozinger, M., Weigmann, H., Roschke, J. and Hiemke, C. (2000) Increased bioavailability of oral melatonin after fluvoxamine coadministration. *Clin. Pharmacol. Ther.* **67**, 1–6.

Hauns, B., Haring, B., Kohler, S., Mross, K. and Unger, C. (2001) Phase II study of combined 5-fluorouracil/*Gingko biloba* extract (GBE 761 ONC) therapy in 5-fluorouracil pretreated patients with advanced colorectal cancer. *Phytother. Res.* **15**, 34–38.

Hayakawa, K., Mitsuhashi, N., Saito, Y., Nakayama, Y., Furuta, M., Nakamoto, S., *et al.* (1997) Effect of Krestin as adjuvant treatment following radical radiotherapy in non-small cell lung cancer patients. *Cancer Detect. Prev.* **21**, 71–77.

Hebel, S.K. (ed.) (1998) *Drug Facts and Comparisons*, 52nd ed. St. Louis, MO.

Heck, A.M., De Witt, B.A. and Lukes, A.L. (2000) Potential interactions between alternative therapies and warfarin. *Am. J. Health Syst. Pharm.* **57**, 1221–1227.

Heidenreich O. (1990) Mode of action of conventional and potassium-sparing diuretics — aspects with relevance to Mg-sparing effects. *Magnesium* **3**, 248–256.

Herxheimer, A. and Petrie, K.J. (2002) Melatonin for the prevention and treatment of jet lag. *Cochrane Database Syst. Rev.* **2**, CD001520.

Hess, B., Raisin, J., Zimmermann, A., Horber, F., Bajo, S., Wyttenbach, A., *et al.* (1993) Tubulointerstitial nephropathy persisting 20 months after discontinuation of chronic intake of germanium lactate citrate. *Am. J. Kidney Dis.* **21**, 548–552.

Hidaka, M., Okumura, M., Fujita, K., Ogikubo, T., Yamasaki, K., Iwakiri, T., *et al.* (2005) Effects of pomegranate juice on human cytochrome p450 3A (CYP3A) and carbamazepine pharmacokinetics in rats. *Drug Metab. Dispos.* **33**, 644–648.

Higuchi, I., Izumo, S., Kuriyama, M., Suehara, M., Nakagawa, M., Fukunaga, H., *et al.* (1989) Germanium myopathy: Clinical and experimental pathological studies. *Acta. Neuropathol.* (*Berl*). **79**, 300–304.

Hirschel-Scholz, S., Pauier, L. and Bonjour, J.P. (1988) Interference of WR-2721 with magnesium metabolism: Mechanism of action. *Miner. Electrolyte Metab.* **14**, 114–120.

Hodgson, J.M., Watts, G.F., Playford, D.A., Burke, V. and Croft, K.D. (2002) Coenzyme Q10 improves blood pressure and glycaemic control: A controlled trial in subjects with type 2 diabetes. *Eur. J. Clin. Nutr.* **56**, 1137–1142.

Hollifield, J.W. (1987) Magnesium depletion, diuretics, and arrhythmias. *Am. J. Med.* **82**, 30–37.

Huntington Study Group. (2001) A randomized, placebo-controlled trial of coenzyme Q10 and remacemide in Huntington's disease. *Neurology* **57**, 397–404.

Jaffiol, C., Daures, J.P., Nsakala, N., Guerenova, J., Baldet, L., Pujol, P., *et al.* (1995) Long term follow up of medical treatment of differentiated thyroid cancer. *Ann. Endocrinol. (Paris)* **56**, 119–129 (article in French).

Jariwalla, R.J. (1999) Inositol hexaphosphate (IP6) as an anti-neoplastic and lipid-lowering agent. *Anti-cancer Res.* **19**, 3699–3702.

Jean-Pastor, M.J., Jean, P., Biour, M., Castot, A., Chichmanian, F., Danan, G., *et al.* (1986) Hepatopathies from treatment with a specialty drug combination of tiratricol-cyclovalon-retinol. *J. Toxicol. Clin. Exp.* **6**, 115–121 (article in French).

Jeong, H.J., Shin, Y.G., Kim, I.H. and Pezzuto, J.M. (1999) Inhibition of aromatose activity by flavonoids. *Arch. Pharm. Res.* **22**, 309–312.

Jiang, X., Williams, K.M., Liauw, W.S., Ammit, A.J., Roufogalis, B.D., Duke, C.C., *et al.* (2005) Effect of ginkgo and ginger on pharmacokinetics and pharmacodynamics of warfarin in healthy subjects. *Br. J. Clin. Pharmacol.* **59**, 425–432.

Johnson, M.K., Smith, R.P., Morrison, D., Laszlo, G. and White, R.J. (2000) Large lung bullae in marijuana smokers. *Thorax* **55**, 340–342.

Kanoh, T., Saito, K., Matsunaga, K., Oguchi, Y., Taniguchi, N., Endoh, H., *et al.* (1994) Enhancement of the anti-tumor effect by the concurrent use of a monoclonal anti-body and the protein-bound polysaccharide PSK in mice bearing a human cancer cell line. *In Vivo* **8**, 242–245.

Kao, Y.C., Zhou, C., Sherman, M., Laughton, C.A. and Chen, S. (1998) Molecular basis of thc inhibition of human aromatase (estrogen syntheses) by flavone and isoflavone phytoestrogens: A site-directed mutagenesis study. *Environ. Health Perspect.* **106**, 85–92.

Kellis, J.T. Jr. and Vickery, L.E. (1984) Inhibition of human estrogen synthetase (aromatase) by flavones. *Science* **225**, 1032–1034.

Kennedy, J. (2005) Herb and supplement use in the US adult population. *Clin. Ther.* **27**, 1832–1833.

Kennedy, R.S., Konok, G.P., Bounous, G., Baruchel, S. and Lee, T.D. (1995) The use of a whey protein concentration in the treatment of patients with metastatic carcinoma: A phase I–II clinical study. *Anti-cancer Res.* **15**(6B), 2643–2649.

Kenny, F.S., Pinder, S.E., Ellis, I.O., Gee, J.M., Nicholson, R.I., Bryce, R.P., *et al.* (2000) Gamma linolenic acid with tamoxifen as primary therapy in breast cancer. *Int. J. Cancer* **85**, 643–648.

Khilnani, G., Parchani, H. and Toshniwal, G. (1992) Hypomagnesemia due to beta 2-agonist use in bronchial asthma. *J. Assoc. Physician India* **40**, 346.

Kim, H.S., Kacew, S. and Lee, B.M. (1999) *In vitro* chemopreventive effects of plant polysaccharides (*Aloe barbadensis Miller*, *Lentinus edodes*, *Ganoderma lucidum* and *Coriolus versicolor*). *Carcinogenesis* **20**, 1637–1640.

Kim, N.D., Mehta, R., Yu, W., Neeman, I., Livney, T., Amichay, A., *et al.* (2002) Chemopreventive and adjuvant therapeutic potential of pomegranate (*Punica granatum*) for human breast cancer. *Breast Cancer Res. Treat.* **71**, 203–217.

Kimura, R. and Murata, T. (1986) Effect of theanine on norepinephrine and serotonin levels in rat brain. *Chem. Pharm. Bull.* **34**, 3053–3057.

Kimura, Y., Iijima, S., Kato, T., Tsujie, M., Naoi, Y., Hayashi, T., *et al.* (2003) Usefulness of TS-1 and lentinan combination immunochemotherapy in advanced or recurrent gastric cancer — pilot study aimed at a randomized trial. *Gan To Kagaku Ryoho* **30**, 1125–1130.

Kishi, T., Watanabe, T. and Folkers, K. (1977) Bioenergetics in clinical medicine XV. Inhibition of coenzyme Q10-enzymes by clinically used adrenergic blockers of beta-receptors. *Res. Comm. Chem. Pathol. Pharmacol.* **17**, 157–164.

Kleeman, C.R., Levi, J. and Better, O. (1975) Kidney and adrenocortical hormones. *Nephron* **15**, 261–278.

Klein, T.W., Newton, C.A., Nakachi, N. and Friedman, H. (2000) Delta 9-tetrahydrocannaboinal treatment suppresses immunity and early IFN-gamma, IL-12, and IL-12 receptor beta 2 responses to *Legionella pneumophila* infection. *J. Immunol.* **164**, 6461–6466.

Kobayashi, H., Matsunaga, K. and Oguchi, Y. (1995) Anti-metastatic effects of PSK (Krestin), a protein-bound polysaccharide obtained from *basidiomycetes*: An overview. *Cancer Epidemiol. Biomarkers Prev.* **4**, 275–281.

Kosaka, A., Kuzuoka, M., Yamafuji, K., Imaizumi, A., Hattori, Y. and Yamashita, A. (1987) Synergistic action of lentinan (LNT) with endocrine therapy of breast cancer in rats and humans. *Gan To Kagaku Ryoho* **14**, 516–522 (article in Japanese).

Kozeny, G.A., Nicolas, J.D., Creekmore, S., Sticklin, L., Hano, J.E. and Fisher, R.I. (1988) Effects of interleukin-2 immunotherapy on renal function. *J. Clin. Oncol.* **6**, 1170–1176.

Krapf, R., Schaffner, T. and Iten, P.X. (1992) Abuse of germanium associated with fatal lactic acidosis. *Nephron* **62**, 351–356.

Kudolo, G.B. (2000) The effect of 3-month ingestion of *Gingko biloba* extract on pancreatic beta-cell function in response to glucose loading in normal glucose tolerant individuals. *J. Clin. Pharmacol.* **40**, 647–654.

Kudolo, G.B. (2006) The effect of 3-month ingestion of *Gingko biloba* extract (EGb 761) on pancreatic beta-cell function in response to glucose loading in individuals with non-insulin-dependent diabetes mellitus. *J. Clin. Pharmacol.* **46**, 628–634.

Kudolo, G.B., Dorsey, S. and Blodgett, J. (2002) Effect of the ingestion of *Gingko biloba* extract on platelet aggregation and urinary prostanoid excretion in healthy and type 2 diabetic subjects. *Thromb. Res.* **108**, 151–160.

Kurz, A. and Van Baelen, B. (2004) *Gingko biloba* compared with cholinesterase inhibitors in the treatment of dementia: A review based on meta-analyses by the cochran collaboration. *Dement. Geriatr. Cogn. Disord.* **18**, 217–226.

Kuttan, R., Sudheeran, P.C. and Josph, C.D. (1987) Turmeric and curcumin as topical agents in cancer therapy. *Tumori.* **73**, 29–31.

Lake, B.G., Tredger, J.M., Renwick, A.B., Barton, P.T. and Price, R.J. (1998) 3,3″-Diindolylmethane induces CYP1A2 in cultured precision-cut human liver slices. *Xenobiotica* **28**, 803–811.

Langsjoen, P., Langsjoen, P., Willis, R. and Folkers, K. (1994) Treatment of essential hypertension with coenzyme Q10. *Mol. Aspects Med.* **15**(Suppl), S265–272.

Lannuzel, A., Michel, P.P., Caparros-Lefebvre, D., Abaul, J., Hocquemiller, R. and Ruberg, M. (2002) Toxicity of Annonaceae for dopaminergic neurons: Potential role in atypical Parkinsonism in Guadeloupe. *Mov. Disord.* **17**, 84–90.

Laoprasert, N., Wallen, N.D., Jones, R.T., Hefle, S.L., Taylor, S.L. and Yunginger, J.W. (1998) Anaphylaxis in a milk-allergic child following ingestion of lemon sorbet containing trace quantities of milk. *J. Food Prot.* **61**, 1522–1524.

Lasserre, B., Spoerri, M., Moullet, V. and Theubet, M.P. (1994) Should magnesium therapy be considered for the treatment of coronary heart disease? II. Epidemiological evidence in outpatients with and without coronary heart disease. *Magnes. Res.* **7**, 145–153.

Lautraite, S., Musonda, A.C., Doehmer, J., Edwards, G.O. and Chipman, J.K. (2002) Flavonoids inhibit genetic toxicity produced by carcinogens in cells expressing CYP1A2 and CYP1A1. *Mutagenesis* **17**, 45–53.

LeBars, P.L., Katz, M.M., Berman, N., Itil, T.M., Freedman, A.M. and Schatzberg, A.F. (1997) A placebo-controlled, double-blind, randomized trial of an extract of *Gingko biloba* for dementia. North American EGb Study Group. *JAMA* **278**, 1327–1332.

Lee, H., Yeom, H., Kim, Y.G., Yoon, C.N., Jin, C., Choi, J.S., *et al.* (1998) Structure-related inhibition of human hepatic caffeine N3-demethylation by naturally occurring flavonoids. *Biochem. Pharmacol.* **55**, 1369–1375.

L'Hommedieu, C.S., Nicholas, D., Armes, D.A., Jones, P., Nelson, T. and Pickering, L.K. (1983) Potentiation of magnesium sulfate — induced neuromuscular weakness by gentamicin, tobramycin, and amikacin. *J. Pediatr.* **102**, 629–631.

Liang, X.S., Rogers, A.J., Webber, C.L., Ormsby, T.J., Tiritan, M.E., Matlin, S.A., *et al.* (1995) Developing gossypol derivatives with enhanced anti-tumor activity. *Invest. New Drugs* **13**, 181–186.

Lissoni, P., Barni, S., Cattaneo, G., Tancini, G., Esposti, G., Esposti, D. and Fraschini, F. (1991) Clinical results with the pineal hormone melatonin in advanced cancer resistant to standard anti-tumor therapies. *Oncology* **48**, 448–450.

Lissoni, P., Barni, S., Ardizzoia, A., Paolorossi, F., Crispino, S. and Tancini, G. (1992a) Randomized study with the pineal hormone melatonin versus care alone in advanced nonsmall cell lung cancer resistant to a first-line chemotherapy containing cisplatin. *Oncology* **49**, 336–339.

Lissoni, P., Tisi, E., Barni, S., Ardizzoia, A., Rovelli, F., Rescaldani, R., *et al.* (1992b) Biological and clinical results of a neuroimmunotherapy with interleukin-2 and the pineal hormone melatonin as a first line treatment in advanced non-small cell lung cancer. *Br. J. Cancer* **66**, 155–158.

Lissoni, P., Barni, S., Ardizzoia, A., Tancini, G., Conti, A. and Maestroni, G. (1994a) A randomized study with the pineal hormone melatonin versus supportive care alone in patients with brain metastases due to solid neoplasms. *Cancer* **73**, 699–701.

Lissoni, P., Barni, S., Cazzaniga, M., Ardizzoni, A., Rovelli, F., Brivio, F., *et al.* (1994b) Efficacy of the concomitant administration of the pineal hormone melatonin in cancer immunotherapy with low-dose IL-2 in patients with advanced solid tumors who had progressed on IL-2 alone. *Oncology* **51**, 344–347.

Lissoni, P., Barni, S., Tancini, G., Ardizzoia, A., Ricci, G., Aldeghi, R., *et al.* (1994c) A randomized study with subcutaneous low-dose interleukin 2 alone versus interleukin 2 plus the pineal neurohormone melatonin in advanced solid neoplasma other than renal cancer and melanoma. *Br. J. Cancer* **69**, 196–199.

Lissoni, P., Barni, S., Meregalli, S., Fossati, V., Cazzaniga, M., Esposti, D., *et al.* (1995) Modulation of cancer endocrine therapy by melatonin: A Phase II study of tamoxifen plus melatonin in metastatic breast cancer patients progressing under tamoxifen alone. *Br. J. Cancer* **71**, 854–856.

Lissoni, P., Paolorossi, F., Tancini, G., Ardizzoia, A., Barni, S., Brivio, F., *et al.* (1996a) A Phase II study of tamoxifen plus melatonin in metastatic solid tumour patients. *Br. J. Cancer* **74**, 1466–1468.

Lissoni, P., Pittalis, S., Ardizzoia, A., Brivio, F., Barni, S., Tancini, G., *et al.* (1996b) Prevention of cytokine-induced hypotension in cancer patients by the pineal hormone melatonin. *Support Care Cancer* **4**, 313–316.

Lissoni, P., Cazzaniga, M., Tancini, G., Scardino, E., Musci, R., Barni, S., *et al.* (1997a) Reversal of clinical resistance to LHRH analogue in metastatic prostate cancer by the pinel hormone melatonin: Efficacy of LHRH analogue plus melatonin in patients progressing on LHRH analogue alone. *Eur. Urol.* **31**, 178–181.

Lissoni, P., Paolorossi, F., Ardizzoia, A., Barni, S., Chilelli, M., Mancuso, M., *et al.* (1997b) A randomized study of chemotherapy with cisplatin plus etoposide versus chemoendocrine therapy with cisplatin, etoposide and the pineal hormone melatonin as a first-line treatment of advanced non-small cell lung cancer patients in a poor clinical state. *J. Pineal Res.* **23**, 15–19.

Lissoni, P., Giani, L., Zerbini, S., Trabottoni, P. and Rovelli, F. (1998) Biotherapy with the pineal immunomodulating hormone melatonin versus melatonin plus aloe vera in untreatable advanced solid neoplasms. *Nat. Immun.* **16**, 27–33.

Lissoni, P., Barni, S., Mandala, M., Ardizzoia, A., Paolorossi, F., Vaghi, M., *et al.* (1999) Decreased toxicity and increased efficacy of cancer chemothrapy using the pineal hormone melatonin in metastatic solid tumour patients with poor clinical status. *Eur. J. Cancer* **35**, 1688–1692.

Lockwood, K., Moesgaard, S. and Folkers, K. (1994) Partial and complete regression of breast cancer in patients in relation to dosage of coenzyme Q-10. *Biochem. Biophys. Res. Comm.* **199**, 1504–1508.

Lockwood, K., Moesgaard, S., Yamamoto, T. and Folkers, K. (1995) Progress on therapy of breast cancer with vitamin Q10 and the regression of metastases. *Biochem. Biophys. Res. Comm.* **212**, 172–177.

Lote, C.J., Thewles, A., Wood, J.A. and Zafar, T. (2000) The hypomagnesaemic action of FK506: Urinary excretion of magnesium and calcium and the role of parathyroid hormone. *Clin. Sci.* **99**, 285–292.

Lund, E.L., Quistorff, B., Spang-Thomsen, M. and Kristjansen, P.E. (1998) Effect of radiation therapy on small-cell lung cancer is reduced by ubiquinone intake. *Folia Microbiol.* (*Praha*) **43**, 505–506.

Lusardi, P., Piazza, E. and Fogari, R. (2000) Cardiovascular effects of melatonin in hypertensive patients well controlled by nifedipine: A 24-hour study. *Br. J. Clin. Pharmacol.* **49**, 423–427.

Maehara, Y., Inutsuka, S., Takeuchi, H., Baba, H., Kusumoto, H. and Sugimachi, K. (1993) Postoperative PSK and OK-432 immunochemotherapy for patients with gastric cancer. *Cancer Chemother. Pharmacol.* **33**, 171–175.

Mainwaring, M.G., Poor, C., Zander, D.S. and Harman, E. (2000) Complete remission of pulmonary spindle cell carcinoma after treatment with oral germanium sesquioxide. *Chest.* **117**, 591–593.

Markowitz, J.S., Donovan, J.L., Lindsay DeVane, C., Sipkes, L. and Chavin, K.D. (2003) Multiple-dose administration of *Gingko biloba* did not affect cytochrome P-450 2D6 or 3A4 activity in normal volunteers. *J. Clin. Psychopharmacol.* **23**, 576–581.

Martin, M., Diaz-Rubio, E., Casado, A., Lopez Vega, J.M., Sastre, J. and Almenarez, J. (1992) Intravenous and oral magnesium supplementations in the prophylaxis of cisplatin-induced hypomagnesemia. Results of a controlled trial. *Am. J. Clin. Oncol.* **15**, 348–351.

Martindale, W. (1999) *Martindale the Extra Pharmacopoeia*. Pharmaceutical Press, London, UK.

Matsusaka, T., Fujii, M., Nakano, T., Terai, T., Kurata, A., Imaizumi, M., *et al.* (1988) Germanium-induced nephropathy: Report of two cases and review of the literature. *Clin. Nephrol.* **30**, 341–345.

Matthews, M.K. (1998) Association of *Gingko biloba* with intracerebral hemorrhage. *Neurology* **50,** 1934.

McDougal, A., Sethi Gupta, M., Rammamoorthy, K., Sun, G. and Safe, S.H. (2000) Inhibition of carcinogen-induced rat mammary tumor growth and other estrogen-dependent responses by symmetrical dihalo-substituted analogs of diindolylmethane. *Cancer Lett.* **151**, 168–179.

McGuffin, M., Hobbs, C., Upton, R. and Goldberg, A. (eds.) (1997) *American Herbal Products Association's Botanical Safety Handbook*. CRC Press, LLC, Boca Raton, FL.

McKevoy, G.K. (ed.) (1998) *AHFS Drug Information*. American Society of Health-System Pharmacists, Bethesda, MD.

Meacham, S.L., Taper, L.J. and Volpe, S.L. (1995) Effect of boron supplementation on blood and urinary calcium, magnesium, and phosphorus, and urinary boron in athletic and sedentary women. *Am. J. Clin. Nutr.* **61**, 341–345.

Mechelany, C., Schlumberger, M., Challeton, C., Comoy, E. and Parmentier, C. (1991) TRIAC (3,5,3′-triiodothyroacetic acid) has parallel effects at the pituritary and peripheral tissue levels in thyroid cancer patients treated with L-thyroxine. *Clin. Endocrinol.* **35**, 123–128.

Meisel, C., Johne, A. and Roots, I. (2003) Fatal intracerebral mass bleeding associated with *Gingko biloba* and ibuprofen. *Atherosclerosis* **167**, 367.

Melzer, J., Rosch, W., Reichling, J., Brignoli, R. and Saller, R. (2004) Meta-analysis: Phytotherapy of functional dyspepsia with the herbal drug preparation STW 5 (Iberogast). *Aliment. Pharmacol. Ther.* **20**, 1279–1287.

Menegay, C., Juge, C. and Burger, A.G. (1989) Pharmacokinetics of 3,5,3′-triiodothyroacetic acid and its effect on serum TSH levels. *Acta Endocrinol.* **121**, 651–658.

Merritt, J.C., Crawford, W.J., Alexander, P.C., Anduze, A.L. and Gelbart, S.S. (1980) Effect of marijuana on intraocular and blood pressure in glaucoma. *Ophthalmology* **87**, 222–228.

Metastron Prescribing Information. (1998) Med-Physics, Inc. Amersham Healthcare, Arlington Heights, IL.

Meunier, P.J., Slosman, D.O., Delmas, P.D., Sebert, J.L., Brandi, M.L., Albanese, C., *et al.* (2002) Strontium ranelate: Dose-dependent effects in established postmenopausal vertebral osteoporosis — a 2-year randomized placebo controlled trial. *J. Clin. Endocrinol. Metab.* **87**, 2060–2066.

Meunier, P.J., Roux, C., Seeman, E., Ortolani, S., Badurski, J.E., Spector, T.D., *et al.* (2004) The effects of strontium ranelate on the risk of vertebral fracture in women with postmenopausal osteoporosis. *N. Engl. J. Med.* **350**, 504–506.

Miller, L.G. (1998) Herbal medicinals: Selected clinical considerations focusing on known or potential drug-herb interactions. *Arch. Int. Med.* **158**, 2200–2211.

Miwa, H., Iijima, M., Tanaka, S. and Mizuno, Y. (2001) Generalized convulsions after consuming a large amount of gingko nuts. *Epilepsia* **42**, 280–281, 2001.

Miyazawa, M., Shindo, M. and Shimada, T. (2002) Metabolism of (+)-abd (−)-limonenes to respective carveols and perillyl alcohols by CYP2C9 and CYP2C19 in human liver microsomes. *Drug Metab. Dispos.* **30**, 602–607.

Mizutani, Y. and Yoshida, O. (1991) Activation by the protein-bound polysaccharide PSK (krestin) of cytotoxic lymphocytes that act on fresh autologous tumor cells and T24 human urinary bladder transitional carcinoma cell line in patients with urinary bladder cancer. *J. Urol.* **145**, 1082–1087.

Montbriand, M.J. (1994) *Decision Heuristics of Patients with Cancer: Alternate and Biomedical Choices*. Unpublished doctoral dissertation, College of Medicine, University of Saskatchewan, SK, Canada.

Montbriand, M.J. (1995a) Decision tree model describing alternate health care choices made by oncology patients. *Cancer Nurs.* **18**, 104–117.

Montbriand, M.J. (1995b) Alternative therapies as control behaviors used by cancer patients. *J. Adv. Nurs.* **22**, 646–654.

Montbriand, M.J. (1997) Empowerment of seniors through improved communication about medication. In: *Proceedings of the Sixth Science in Health-Social Services for the Elderly and the Disabled*, Heumann, L.F. (ed.) University of Illinois of Urbana-Champaign, Chicago, IL, pp. 258–264.

Montbriand, M.J. (1999) Past and present herbs used to treat cancer: Medicine, magic, or poison? *Oncol. Nurs. Forum* **26**, 49–60.

Montbriand, M.J. (2000a) Senior and health-professionals' mismatched perceptions and communication about prescription and non-prescription medication. *Can. J. Aging* **19**, 35–56.

Montbriand, M.J. (2000b) Health professionals' attitudes about alternative therapies. *Can. Nurs.* **96**, 22–26.

Montbriand, M.J. (2004a). Herbs or natural that may decrease cancer growth: Part one. *Oncol. Nurs. Forum* **31**, E75–E90. Retrieved November 28, 2006, from www.ons.org/Publications/journals/ONF/Volume31/issue4/pdf/75.pdf

Montbriand, M.J. (2004b) Herbs or natural products that increase cancer growth or reoccurrence: Part two. *Oncol. Nurs. Forum* **31**, E99–E115. Retrieved November 28, 2006, from www.ons.org/publications/journals/ONF/volume31/issue5/3105898.asp

Montbriand, M.J. (2004c) Herbs or natural products that protect against cancer growth: Part three. *Oncol. Nurs. Forum* **31**, E127–E146. Retrieved November 28, 2006, from www.ons.org/publications/journals/ONF/volume31/issue6/3106127.asp

Montbriand, M.J. (2005) Herbs or natural that may cause cancer and harm: Part four. *Oncol. Nurs. Forum* **32**, E20–E29. Retrieved November, 28. 2006, from www.ons.org/publications/journals/ONF/volume32/issue1/320132.asp

Morimoto, T., Ogawa, M., Orita, K., Sugimachi, K., Toge, T., Dohi, K., *et al.* (1996) Postoperative adjuvant randomized trial comparing chemoendocrine therapy chemotherapy and immunotherapy for patients with stage II breast cancer: 5-year results from the Nishinihon Cooperative Study Group of Adjuvant Chemoendocrine Therapy for Breast Cancer (ACETBC) of Japan. *Eur. J. Cancer* **32A**, 235–342.

Mueller-Gaertner, H.W. and Schneider, C. (1988) 3,5,3′-Triiodothyroacetic acid minimizes the pituitary thyrotrophin secretion in patients on levo-thyroxin therapy after ablative therapy for differentiated thyroid carcinoma. *Clin. Endocrinol.* **28**, 345–351.

Murry, J.J. and Healy, M.D. (1991) Drug-mineral interactions: A new responsibility for the hospital dietician. *J. Am. Diet. Assoc.* **91**, 66–73.

Nagahashi, S., Suzuki, H., Nishiwaki, M., Okuda, K., Kurosawa, Y., Terada, S., *et al.* (2004) TS-1/CDDP/Lentinan combination chemotherapy for inoperable advanced gastric cancer. *Gan To Kagaku Ryoho* **31**, 1999–2003.

Nakano, H., Namatame, K., Nemoto, H., Motohashi, H., Nishiyama, K. and Kumada, K. (1999) A multi-institutional prospective study of lentinan in advanced gastric cancer patients with unresectable and recurrent diseases: Effect on prolongation of survival and improvement of quality of life. Kanagawa Lentinan Research Group. *Hepatogastroenterology* **46**, 2662–2668.

Nakazato, H., Koike, A., Saji, S., Ogawa, N. and Sakamoto, J. (1994) Efficacy of immunochemotherapy as adjuvant treatment after curative resection of gastric cancer. Study Group of Immunochemotherapy with PSK for Gastric Cancer. *Lancet* **344**, 1122–1126.

Natural Medicines Comprehensive Database (2006) Retrieved from the Therapeutic Research Faculty National Database, 3120 West March Lane, Stockton, CA 95208, http://www.naturaldatabase.com

Neulieb, R. (1984) Effect of oral intake of cesium chloride: A single case report. *Pharmacol. Biochem. Behav.* **21**, 15–16.

Newall, C.A., Anderson, L.A. and Philpson, J.D. (1996) *Herbal Medicine: A Guide for Health Care Professionals.* The Pharmaceutical Press, London, UK.

Ng, T.B. (1998) A review of research on the protein-bound polysaccharide (polysaccharopeptide, PSP) from the mushroom *Coriolus versicolor* (*Basidiomycetes*: *Polyporaceae*). *Gen. Pharmacol.* **30**, 1–4.

Nicolosi, R., Bell, S.J., Bistrian, B.R., Greenberg, I., Forse, R.A. and Blackburn, G.L. (1999) Plasma lipid changes after supplementation with beta-glucan fiber from yeast. *Am. J. Clin. Nutr.* **70**, 208–212.

Nielsen, F.H. and Milne, D.B. (2004) A moderately high intake compared to a low intake of zinc depresses magnesium balance and alters indices of bone turnover in postmenopausal women. *Eur. J. Clin. Nutr.* **58**, 703–710.

Nielsen, F.H., Hunt, C.D., Mullen, L.M. and Hunt, J.R. (1987) Effect of dietary boron on mineral, estrogen, and testosterone metabolism in postmenopausal women. *FASEB J.* **1**, 394–397.

Nimura, H., Mitsumori, N., Takahashi, N., Kashimura, H., Takayama, S., Kashiwagi, H., *et al.* (2006) S-1 combined with lentinan in patients with unresectable or recurrent gastric cancer. *Gan To Kagaku Ryoho* **33**(1), 106–109.

Nio, Y., Tsubone, M., Tseng, C.C., Morimoto, H., Kawabata, K., Masai, Y., *et al.* (1992) Immunomodulation by orally administered protein-bound polysaccharide PSK in patients with gastrointestinal cancer. *Biotherapy* **4**, 117–128.

Nishihira, T., Akimoto, M. and Mori, S. (1988) Anti-cancer effects of BRMs associated with nutrition in cancer patients. *Gan To Kagaku Ryoho* **15**, 1615–1620 (article in Japanese).

Nordlund, J.J. and Lerner, A.B. (1977) The effects of oral melatonin on skin color and on the release of pituitary hormones. *J. Clin. Endocrinol. Metab.* **45**, 768–774.

Oberlies, N.H., Chang, C.J. and McLaughlin, J.L. (1997) Structure-activity relationships of diverse Annonaceous acetogenins against multidrug resistant human mammary adenocarcinoma (MCF-7/Adr) cells. *J. Med. Chem.* **17**, 84–90.

Oken, B.S., Storzbach, D.M. and Kaye, J.A. (1998) The efficacy of *Gingko biloba* on cognitive function in Alzheimer disease. *Arch. Neurol.* **55**, 1409–1415.

Ondrizek, R.R., Chan, P.J., Patton, W.C. and King, A. (1999a) Inhibition of human sperm motility by specific herbs used in alternative medicine. *J. Assist. Reprod. Genet.* **16**, 87–91.

Ondrizek, R.R., Chan, P.J., Patton, W.C. and King, A. (1999b) An alternative medicine study of herbal effects on the penetration of zona-free hamster oocytes and the integrity of sperm deoxyribonucleic acid. *Fertil. Steril.* **71**, 517–522.

Oosterhof, G.O., Roberts, J.T., de Reijke, T.M., Engelholm, S.A., Horenblas, S., von der Maase, H., *et al.* (2003) Strontium(89) chloride versus palliative local field radiotherapy in patients with hormonal escaped prostate cancer: A Phase III study of the European Organisation for Research and Treatment of Cancer, Genitourinary Group. *Eur. Urol.* **44**, 519–526.

Pantuck, A.J., Leppert, J.T., Zomorodian, N., Aronson, W., Hong, J., Barnard, R.J., *et al.* (2006a) Phase II study of pomegranate juice for men with rising prostate-specific antigen following surgery or radiation for prostate cancer. *Clin. Cancer Res.* **12**, 4018–4026.

Pantuck, A.J., Zomorodian, N. and Belldegrun, A.S. (2006b) Phase II study of pomegranate juice for men with prostate cancer and increasing PSA. *Curr. Urol. Rep.* **7**, 7.

Panzer, A., Hamel, E., Joubert, A.M., Bianchi, P.C. and Seegers, J.C. (2000a) Ukrain(TM), a semisynthetic *Chelidonium majus* alkaloid derivative, acts by inhibition of tubulin polymerization in normal and malignant cell lines. *Cancer Lett.* **28**, 149–157.

Panzer, A., Joubert, A.M., Bianchi, P.C. and Seegers, J.C. (2000b) The antimitotic effects of Ukrain, a *Chelidonium majus* alkaloid derivative, are reversible *in vitro*. *Cancer Lett.* **150**, 85–92.

Playford, D.A., Watts, G.F., Croft, K.D. and Burke, V. (2003) Combined effect of coenzyme Q10 and fenofibrate on forearm microcirculatory function in type 2 diabetes. *Artherosclerosis* **168**, 169–179.

Popoviciu, L., Asgian, B., Delast-Popoviciu, D., Alexandrescu, A., Petrutiu, S. and Bagathal, I. (1993) Clinical, EEG, electromyographic and polysomnographic studies in restless legs syndrome caused by magnesium deficiency. *Rom. J. Neurol. Psychiatry* **31**, 55–61.

Quamme, G.A. (1986) Renal handling of magnesium: Drug and hormone interactions. *Magnesium* **5**, 248–272.

Rahman, M.A. and Ing, T.S. (1989) Cyclosporine and magnesium metabolism. *J. Lab. Clin. Med.* **114**, 213–214.

Raphael, T.J. and Kuttan, G. (2003) Immunomodulatory activity of natural occurring monoterpenes carvone, limonene, and perillic acid. *Immunopharmacol. Immunotoxicol.* **25**, 285–294.

Rasyid, A., Rahman, A.R., Jaalam, K. and Lelo, A. (2002) Effect of different curcumin dosages on human gall bladder. *Asia Pac. J. Clin. Nutr.* **11**, 314–318.

Riby, J.E., Chang, G.H., Firestone, G.L. and Bjeldanes, L.F. (2000) Ligand-independent activation of estrogen receptor function by 3,3″-diindolylmethane in human breast cancer cells. *Biochem. Pharmacol.* **60**, 167–177.

Rickers, H., Deding, A., Christiansen, C. and Rodbro, P. (1984) Mineral loss in cortical and trabecular bone during high-dose prednisone treatment. *Calcif. Tissue Int.* **36**, 269–273.

Robbers, J.E. and Tyler, V.E. (1999) *Tyler's Herbs of Choice: The Therapeutic Use of Phytomedicinals*. The Haworth Herbal Press, New York, NY, 1999.

Rolla, G., Bucca, C., Bugiani, M., Oliva, A. and Branciforte, L. (1990) Hypomagnesemia in chronic obstructive lung disease: Effect of therapy. *Magnes. Trace Elem.* **9**, 132–136.

Roublevskaia, I.N., Polevoda, B.V., Ludlow, J.W. and Haake, A.R. (2000) Induced G2/M arrest and apoptosis in human epidermoid carcinoma cell lines by semisynthetic drug Ukrain. *Anti-cancer Res.* **20**, 3163–3167.

Rude, R.K. (1998) Magnesium deficiency: A cause of heterogeneous disease in humans. *J. Bone. Miner. Res.* **13**, 749–758.

Runeberg, L., Miettinen, T.A. and Nikkila, E.A. (1972) Effect of cholestyramine on mineral excretion in man. *Acta Med. Scand.* **192**, 71–76.

Ryan, M.P. (1987) Diuretics and potassium/magnesium depletion: Directions for treatment. *Am. J. Med.* **82**, 38–47.

Sabra, R. and Branch, R.A. (1990) Amphotericin B nephrotoxicity. *Drug Saf.* **5**, 94–108.

Sadzuka, Y., Sugiyama, T., Miyagishima, A., Nozawa, Y. and Hirota, S. (1996) The effects of theanine, as a novel biochemical modulator, on the anti-tumor activity of adriamycin. *Cancer Lett.* **105**, 203–209.

Sadzuka, Y., Sugiyama, T. and Sonobe, T. (2000) Improvement of idarubicin induced antitumor activity and bone marrow suppression by theanine, component of tea. *Cancer Lett.* **158**, 119–124.

Saied, I.T. and Shamsuddin, A.M. (1998) Up-regulation of the tumor suppressor gene p53 and WAF1 gene expression by IP6 in HT-29 human colon carcinoma cell line. *Anti-cancer Res.* **18**, 1479–1484.

Sanai, T., Okuda, S., Onoyama, K., Oochi, N., Oh, Y., Kobayashi, K., *et al.* (1990) Germanium dioxide-induced nephropathy: A new type of renal disease. *Nephron* **54**, 53–60.

Sanjuliani, F., de Abreu Fagundes, V.G. and Francischetti, E.A. (1996) Effects of magnesium on blood pressure and intracellular ion levels of Brazilian hypertensive patients. *Int. J. Cardiol.* **56**, 177–183.

Santoro, G.M., Antoniucci, D., Bolognese, L., Valenti, R., Buonamici, P., Trapani, M., *et al.* (2000) A randomized study of intravenous magnesium in acute myocardial infarction treated with direct coronary angioplasty. *M. Heart J.* **140**, 891–897.

Sartori, H.E. (1984) Cesium therapy in cancer patients. *Pharmacol. Biochem. Behav.* **21**(1), 11–13.

Schauss, A.G. (1991) Nephrotoxicity and neurotoxicity in humans from organogermanium compounds and germanium dioxide. *Biol. Trace Elem. Res.* **29**, 267–280.

Schein, P.S., Slavik, M., Smythe, T., Hoth, Smith, F., Macdonald, J.S., *et al.* (1980) Phase I clinical trial of spirogermanium. *Cancer Treat. Rep.* **64**, 1051–1056.

Schwarz, R.E. and Zagala-Nevarez, K. (2002) Significant hypomagnesemia after celiotomy: Implications of preoperative bowel cleansing with sodium phosphate purgative. *Surgery* **131**, 236.

Seelig, M.S. (1982) Auto-immune complications of D-penicillamine — A possible result of zinc and magnesium depletion and of pyridoxine inacti-vation. *J. Am. Coll. Nutr.* **1**, 207–214.

Seelig, M.S. (1993) Interrelationship of magnesium and estrogen in cardiovascular and bone disorders, eclampsia, migraine, and premenstrual syndrome. *J. Am. Coll. Nutr.* **12**, 442–458.

Semia, T.P., Beizer, J.L. and Higbee, M.D. (1998) *Geriatric Dosage Handbook*, 4th ed. Lexicomp, Hudson, OH.

Shah, B.H., Nawaz, Z. and Pertani, S.A. (1999) Inhibitory effect of curcumin, a food spice from turmeric, on platelet-activating factor and arachidonic acid-mediated platelet aggregation through inhibition of thromboxane formation and Ca^{2+} signaling. *Biochem. Pharmacol.* **58**, 1167–1172.

Shah, G.M., Avarado, P. and Kirschenbaum, M.A. (1990) Symptomatic hypocalcemia and hypomagnesemia with renal magnesium wasting associated with pentamidine therapy in a patient with AIDS. *Am. J. Med.* **89**, 380–382.

Shamsuddin, A.M. and Vucenik, I. (1999) Mammary tumor inhibition by IP6: A review. *Anti-cancer Res.* **19**, 3671–3674.

Shamsuddin, A.M. and Yang, G.Y. (1995) Inositol hexaphosphate inhibits growth and induces differentiation of PC-3 human prostate cancer cells. *Carcinogenesis* **16**, 1975–1979.

Sharma, R.A., McLelland, H.R., Hill, K.A., Ireson, R., Euden, S.A. and Manson, M.M. (2001) Pharmacodynamic and pharmacokinetic study of oral Curcuma extract in patients with colorectal cancer. *Clin. Cancer Res.* **7**, 1894–1900.

Sherman, S.I. and Ladenson, P.W. (1992) Organ-specific effects of tiratricol: A thyroid hormone analog with hepatic, not pituitary, superagonist effect. *J. Clin. Endocrinol. Metab.* **75**, 901–905.

Shidaifat, F., Canatan, H., Kulp, S.K., Sugimoto, Y., Chang, W.Y., Zhang, Y., *et al.* (1996) Inhibition of human prostate cancer cells growth by gossypol is associated with stimulation of transforming growth factor-beta. *Cancer Lett.* **107**, 37–44.

Shults, C.W., Oakes, D., Kieburtz, K., Beal, M.F., Haas, R., Plumb, S., *et al.* (2002) Effects of coenzyme Q10 in Parkinson disease: Evidence of slowing of the functional decline. *Arch. Neurol.* **59**, 1541–1550.

Skelly, A. (1997) Alternative medicine tried as a second resort. *Med. Post.* **33**, 27.

Sojka, J., Wastney, M., Abrams, S., Lewis, S.F., Martin, B., Weaver, C., *et al.* (1997) Magnesium kinetics in adolescent girls determined using stable isotopes: Effects of high and low calcium intake. *Am. J. Physiol.* **273**, R710–R715.

Sompolinsky, D. and Samra, Z. (1972) Influence of magnesium and manganese on some biological and physical properties of tetracycline. *J. Bacteriol.* **110**, 468–476.

Sorokin, A.V., Duncan, B., Panetta, R. and Thompson, P.D. (2006) Rhabdomyolysis associated with pomegranate juice consumption. *Am. J. Cardiol.* **98**, 705–706.

Spencer, H., Fuller, H., Norris, C. and Williams, D. (1994) Effect of magnesium on the intestinal absorption of calcium in man. *J. Am. Coll. Nutr.* **15**, 485–492.

Spigset, O. (1994) Reduced effect of warfarin caused by ubidecarenone. *Lancet* **334**, 1372–1373.

Spinella, M., Eaton, L.A. (2002) Hypomania induced by herbal and pharma-ceutical psychotropic medicines following mild traumatic brain injury. *Brain Inj.* **16**, 359–367.

Stanton, M.F. and Lowenstein, F.W. (1987) Serum magnesium in women during pregnancy, while taking contraceptives, and after menopause. *J. Am. Coll. Nutr.* **6**, 313–319.

Stickel, F., Poschl, G., Seitz, H.K., Waldherr, R., Hahn, E.G. and Schuppan, D. (2003) Acute hepatitis induced by Greater Celandine (*Chelidonium majus*). *Scand. J. Gastroenterol.* **38**, 565–568.

Sugimachi, K., Maehara, Y., Ogawa, M., Kakegawa, T. and Tomita, M. (1997) Dose intensity of uracil and tegafur in postoperative chemotherapy for patients with poorly differentiated gastric cancer. *Cancer Chemother. Pharmacol.* **40**, 233–238.

Sugiyama, T. and Sadzuka, Y. (1998) Enhancing effects of green tea components on the anti-tumor activity of adriamycin against M5076 ovarian sarcoma. *Cancer Lett.* **133**, 19–26.

Sugiyama, T., Sadzuka, Y., Tanaka, K. and Sonobe, T. (2001) Inhibition of glutamate transporter by theanine enhances the therapeutic efficacy of doxorubicin. *Toxicol. Lett.* **121**, 89–96.

Sun, Y., Hersh, E.M., Lee, S.L., McLaughlin, M., Loo, T.L. and Mavligit, G.M. (1983) Preliminary observations on the effects of the Chinese medicinal herbs *Astragalus membranaceus* and *Ligustrum lucidum* on lymphocyte blastogenic responses. *J. Biol. Response Mod.* **2**, 227–237.

Takeuchi, A., Yoshizawa, N., Oshima, S., Kubota, T., Oshikawa, Y., Akashi, Y., *et al.* (1992) Nephrotoxicity of germanium compounds: Report of a case and review of the literature. *Nephron* **60**, 436–442.

Tantivejkul, K., Vucenik, I., Eiseman, J. and Shamsuddin, A.M. (2003) Inositol hexaphosphate (IP6) enhances the anti-proliferative effects of adriamycin and tamoxifen in breast cancer. *Breast Cancer Res. Treat.* **79**, 301–312.

Tao, S.H. and Bolger, P.M. (1997) Hazard assessment of germanium supplements. *Regul. Toxicol. Pharmacol.* **25**, 211–219.

Thompson, C.B., Sullivan, K.M., June, C.H. and Thomas, E.D. (1984) Association between cyclosporine neurotoxicity and hypomagnesemia. *Lancet* **2**, 1116–1120.

Thompson, L.U. and Zhang, L. (1991) Phytic acid and minerals: Effect on early markers of risk for mammary and colon carcinogenesis. *Carcinogenesis* **12**, 2041–2045.

Toi, M., Hattori, T., Akagi, M., Inokuchi, K., Orita, K., Sugimachi, K., *et al.* (1992) Randomized adjuvant trial to evaluate the addition of tamoxifen and PSK to chemotherapy in patients with primary breast cancer, 5-Year results from the Nishi-Nippon Group of the Adjuvant Chemoendocrine Therapy for Breast Cancer Organization. *Cancer* **70**, 2475–2483.

Tsukagoshi, S., Hashimoto, Y., Fujii, G., Kobayashi, H., Nomoto, K. and Orita, K. (1984) Krestin (PSK). *Cancer Treat. Rev.* **11**, 131–155.

Tveskov, C., Djurhuus, M.S., Klitgaard, N.A.H. and Egstrup, K. (1994) Potassium and magnesium distribution, ECG changes, and ventricular ectopic beats during beta-2-adrenergic stimulation with terbutaline in healthy subjects. *Chest* **106**, 1654–1659.

Tyler, V.E. (1993) *The Honest Herbal*, 3rd ed. Pharmaceutical Products Press, Binghamton, NY.

Tyler, V.E. (1994) *Herbs of Choice: The Therapeutic Use of Phytomedicinals*. Pharmaceutical Products Press, Binghamton, NY.

Tyler, V.E. (1996) What pharmacists should know about herbal remedies. *J. Am. Pharm. Assoc.* **NS36**, 29–37.

Upton, R. (ed.) (1999) *Astragalus Root: Analytical, Quality Control, and Therapeutic Monograph*. American Herbal Pharmacopoeia, Santa Cruz, CA.

Valcavi, R., Zini, M., Maestroni, G.J., Conti, A. and Portioli, I. (1993) Melatonin stimulates growth hormone secretion through pathways other than the growth hormone-releasing hormone. *Clin. Endocrinol.* **39**, 193–199.

Vale, S. (1998) Subarachnoid haemorrhage associated with *Gingko biloba*. *Lancet* **352**, 36.

Verberckmoes, S.C., De Broe, M.E. and D'Haese, P.C. (2003) Dose-dependent effect of strontium on osteoblast function and mineralization. *Kidney Int.* **64**, 534–543.

Vetter, T. and Lohse, M.J. (2002) Magnesium and the parathyroid. *Curr. Opin. Nephrol. Hypertens.* **11**, 403–410.

Vigushin, D.M., Poon, G.K., Boody, A., English, J., Halbert, G.W. and Pagonis, C. (1998) Phase I and pharmacokinetic study of D-limonene in patients with advanced cancer. Cancer Research Campaign Phase I/II Clinical Trials Committee. *Cancer Chemother. Pharmacol.* **42**, 111–117.

Vogelzang, N.J., Gesme, D.H. and Kennedy, B.J. (1985) A phase II study of spirogermanium in advanced human malignancy. *Am. J. Clin. Oncol.* **8**, 341–344.

von Bahr, C., Ursing, C., Yasui, N., Tybring, G., Bertilsson, L. and Rojdmark, S. (2000) Fluvoxamine but not citalopram increases serum melatonin in healthy subjects — an indication that cytochrome P450 CYP1A2 and CYP2C19 hydroxylate melatonin. *Eur. J. Clin. Pharmacol.* **56**, 123–127.

Vucenik, I., Zhang, Z.S. and Shamsuddin, A.M. (1998) IP6 in treatment of liver cancer. II. Intra-tumoral injection of IP6 regresses pre-existing human liver cancer xenotransplanted in nude mice. *Anti-cancer Res.* **18**, 4091–4096.

Vucenik, I., Podczasy, J.J. and Shamsuddin, A.M. (1999) Antiplatelet activity of inositol hexaphosphate. *Anti-cancer Res.* **19**, 3689–3693.

Vucenik, I., Passaniti, A., Vitolo, M.I., Tantivejkul, K., Eggleton, P. and Shamsuddin, A.M. (2004) Anti-angiogenic activity of inostol hexaphosphate (IP6). *Carcinogenesis* **25**, 2115–2123.

Wada, T., Nishide, T., Hatayama, K., Chang, S.W., Tatsuta, M. and Yasutomi, M. (1987) A comparative clinical trial with tegafur plus lentinan treatment at two different doses in advanced cancer. *Gan To Kagaku Ryoho* **14**, 2509–2512 (article in Japanese).

Wagner, J., Wagner, M.L. and Hening, W.A. (1998) Beyond benzodiazepines: Alternative pharmacologic agents for the treatment of insomnia. *Ann. Pharmacother.* **32**, 680–691.

Walle, T.R., Otake, Y., Galijatovic, A., Ritter, J.K. and Walle, U.K. (2000) Induction of UDP-glucuronosyltransferase UGT1A1 by the flavonoid chrysin in the human hepatoma cell line hep G2. *Drug Metab. Dispos.* **28**, 1077–1082.

Walle, U.K., Galijatovic, A. and Walle, T. (1999) Transport of the flavonoid chysin and its conjugated metabolites by the human intestinal cell line Caco-2. *Biochem. Pharmacol.* **58**, 431–438.

Wang, H.X., Ng, T.B., Liu, W.K., Ooi, V.E. and Chang, S.T. (1996) Polysaccharide-peptide complexes from the cultured mycelia of the mushroom *Coriolus versicolor* and their culture medium activate mouse lymphocytes and macrophages. *Int. J. Biochem. Cell. Biol.* **28**, 601–607.

Watkins, D.W., Khalafi, R., Cassidy, M.M. and Vahouny, G.V. (1985) Alterations in calcium magnesium, iron, and zinc metabolism by dietary cholestyramine. *Dig. Dis. Sci.* **30**, 477–482.

Whyte, K.F., Addis, G.J., Whitesmith, R. and Reid, J.L. (1987) Adrenergic control of plasma magnesium in man. *Clin. Sci.* **72**, 135–138.

Wikner, J., Wetterberg, L. and Rojdmark, S. (1997) Does hypercalcaemia or calcium antagonism affect human melatonin secretion or renal excretion? *Eur. J. Clin. Invest.* **27**, 374–379.

Wong, C.W. and Watson, D.L. (1995) Immunomodulatory effects of dietary whey proteins in mice. *J. Dairy Res.* **62**, 359–368.

Wright, K.P. Jr., Myers, B.L., Plenzler, S.C., Drake, C.L. and Badia, P. (2000) Acute effects of bright light and caffeine on nighttime melatonin and temperature levels in women taking and not taking oral contracepives. *Brain Res.* **873**, 310–317.

Wu, D. (1989) An overview of the clinical pharmacology and therapeutic potential of gossypol as a make contraceptive agent and in gynecological disease. *Drug* **38**, 333–341.

Xu, F., Zhang, Y., Xiao, S., Lu, X., Yang, D., Yang, X., *et al.* (2006) Absorption and metabolism of *Astragali radix* decoction: *In silico*, *in vitro*, and a case study *in vivo*. *Drug Metab. Dispos.* **34**, 913–924.

Yagmur, E., Piatkowski, A., Groger, A., Pallua, N., Gressner, A.M. and Kiefer, P. (2005) Bleeding complication under *Gingko biloba* medication. *Am. J. Hematol.* **79**, 343–344.

Yale, S.H. and Glurich, I. (2005) Analysis of the inhibitory potential of *Gingko biloba*, *Echinacea purpurea*, and *Serenoa repens* on the metabolic activity of cytochrome P450 3A4, 2D6, and 2C9. *J. Altern. Complement. Med.* **11**, 433–439.

Yanagisawa, H., Yamazaki, N., Sato, G. and Wada, O. (2000) L-Arginine treatment may prevent tubulointerstitial nephropathy caused by germanium dioxide. *Kidney Int.* **57**, 2275–2284.

Yasui-Furukori, N., Furukori, H., Kaneda, A., Kaneko, S. and Tateishi, T. (2004) The effect of *Gingko biloba* extracts on the pharmacokinetics and pharmacodynamics of donepezil. *J. Clin. Pharmacol.* **44**, 538–542.

Yin, O.Q., Tomlinson, B., Waye, M.M., Chow, A.H. and Chow, M.S. (2004) Pharmacogenetics and herb-drug interactions: Experience with *Gingko biloba* and omeprazole. *Pharmacogenetics* **14**, 841–850.

Yokoe, T., Iino, Y., Takei, H., Horiguchi, J., Koibuchi, Y., Maemura, M., *et al.* (1997) HLA antigen as predictive index for the outcome of breast cancer patients with adjuvant immunochemotherapy with PSK. *Anti-cancer Res.* **17**, 2815–2818.

Yokogoshi, H. and Kobayashi, M. (1998) Hypotensive effect of gamma-glutamylethylamide in spontaneously hypertensive rats. *Life Sci.* **62**, 1065–1068.

Yoshiyuki, T., Onda, M., Tokunaga, A., Teramoto, T., Oguri, T., Fujita, I., *et al.* (1994) Treatment for peritoneal dissemination of gastric cancer by intraperitoneal administration of CDDP through Infuse-a-Port. *Gan To Kagaku Ryoho* **21**, 2323–2325 (article in Japanese).

Young, D.S. (1995) *Effects of Drugs on Clinical Laboratory Tests*, 4th ed. AACC Press, Washington, DC.

Yuan, L., Wagatsuma, C., Yoshida, M., Miura, T., Mukoda, T., Fujii, H., *et al.* (2003) Inhibition of human breast cancer growth by GCP (genistein combined polysaccharide) in xenogeneic athymic mice: Involvement of genistein biotransformation by beta-glucuronidase from tumor tissues. *Mutat. Res.* **523–524**, 55–62.

Zhou, J.R. and Erdman, J.W. Jr. (1995) Phytic acid in health and disease. *Crit. Rev. Food Sci. Nutr.* **35**, 495–508.

Zhou, Q. and Chowbay, B. (2002) Effect of coenzyme Q10 on the disposition of doxorubicin in rats. *Eur. J. Drug Metab. Pharmacokinet.* **27**, 185–192.

Zhu, L.X., Sharma, S., Stolina, M., Gardner, B., Roth, M.D., Tashkin, D.P., *et al.* (2000) Delta-9-tetrahydrocannabinol inhibits anti-tumor immunity by a CB2 receptor-mediated, cytokin-dependent pathway. *J. Immunol.* **165**, 373–380.

Chapter 10

Mechanistic Studies on Combination of Phytochemicals and Synthetic Drugs as Anti-Cancer Agents

Shanmugam HemaIswarya & Mukesh Doble

Abstract

Environmental, endogenous DNA damaging agents and genetic factors cause aberrant changes in the normally functioning genes leading to tumor. The treatment strategies of cancer are varied and mostly they are administered in combination. The application of complementary and alternative medicine, which includes phytochemicals and herbal extracts, leads to chances of herb-drug interactions. The interaction could be adverse or advantageous and it is due to a number of factors which are not fully understood. Changes in cell signaling pathways, pharmacokinetic interactions, reversal of multi-drug resistance, and increase in immunity are a few mechanisms where the phytochemicals can act in synergy with anti-cancer drugs.

Keywords: Phytochemicals; Anti-Cancer Agents; Complementary or Alternative Medicine (CAM); Synergistic Effect.

10.1 Introduction

Cancer is the one of the top two causes of death in most of the industrialized and developing countries. It is estimated that 80% to 90% of all cancers are caused by environmental risk factors including chemicals, radiations and viruses. The different treatment methodologies include chemotherapy, hormonal supplements, surgery, radiation therapy, or complementary or alternative medicine (CAM). With advances in the understanding of the cellular and molecular levels of carcinogenesis, chemoprevention has grown into a promising strategy for treating cancer. Of course this is associated with some limitations and drawbacks such as:

(1) most common tumors are resistant to available anti-neoplastic drug;
(2) limited anti-solid tumor activity;
(3) little impact on survival rates;
(4) when used at high doses, there is increased level of toxicity; and
(5) other side-effects (Surh, 1999).

All these problems can be addressed by the application of combination therapy.

Approximately 16% of the population use herbal remedies with prescription medicines, which increases the risk of adverse herb-drug interactions. The herbs may affect the ADME (absorption, distribution, metabolism and excretion) of the anti-cancer drugs. More than 5000 individual phytochemicals have been identified in fruits, vegetables and grains, which are known to possess curative effects. They broadly fall under the following major classifications, which includes carotenoids, phenolics, alkaloids, nitrogen-containing compounds and organosulfur compounds. Most of the phytochemicals have complementary or similar mechanisms of action (Fig. 10.1). Also it is seen that a purified compound may have a lesser bioactivity than the natural combination of phytochemicals in the whole foods (Liu, 2004).

For instance, Crambene and indole-3-carbinol (I3C), the bioactive phytochemicals present in the cruciferous vegetables, like Brussels sprouts or broccoli were found to synergistically enhance the detoxification enzyme activity against aflatoxin B1 (AFB1). At low concentrations present in the crucifers, the synergy was not observed but on the contrary at high concentrations, crambene and I3C groups demonstrated synergistic protections from AFB1 (Wallig *et al.*, 1993). In addition to these two compounds, cruciferous vegetables also contain sulforaphane, phenyl ethyl isothiocyanate (PEITC), goitrin, 1,2–dithiol-2-thiones and various polyphenols (Guo *et al.*, 1992; Kelley and Bjeldanes, 1995; Kensler *et al.*, 1992; Chu *et al.*, 2002). When rats are fed with crambene, I3C, iberion and PEITC as individual components or as a mixture, the groups that received the mixture showed more activity (induction of Phase II detoxification enzymes) than the sum of individual treatments (Nho and Jeffrey, 2001).

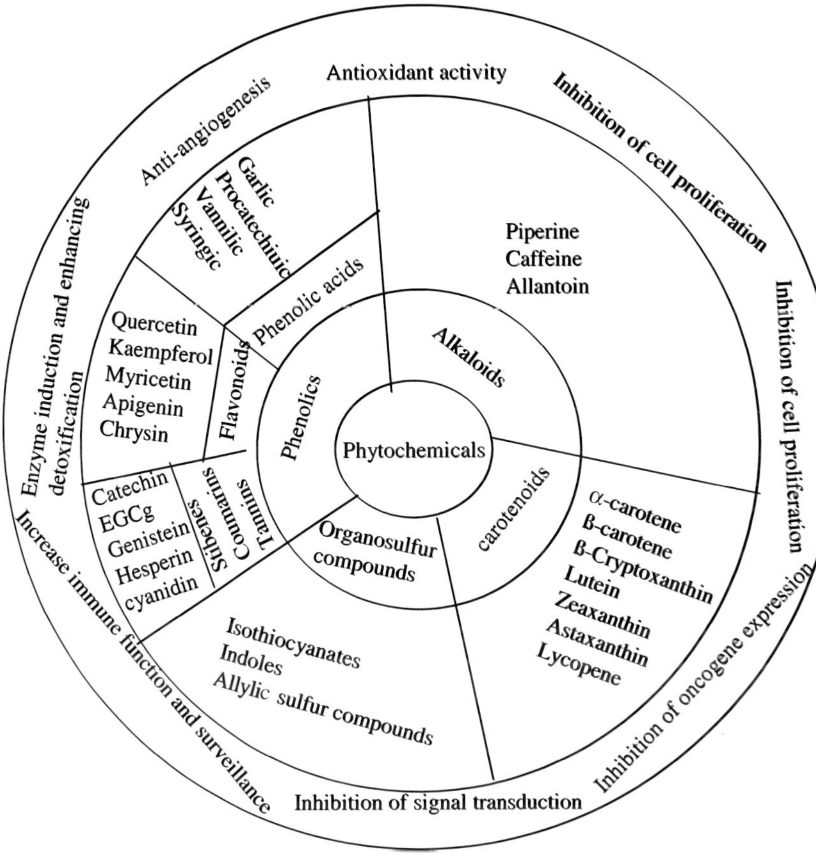

Fig. 10.1. Phytochemicals and mechanism of action.

Selenium, which is readily taken up by the cruciferous vegetables (Banuelos, 2002), was found to act in synergy with retinoids and vitamin E, to inhibit carcinogenesis (Horvath and Ip, 1983; Curphey *et al.*, 1988). The same selenium was found to reduce the sulforaphone and polyphenol content in broccoli, thereby decreasing the chemoprotection activity of these compounds (Finley *et al.*, 2005). But it worked in synergy with crambene to kill MCF-3 canine mammary cells (Wallig, 1993).

The interaction between herbal extracts or phytochemicals and synthetic drugs can be understood by the following example. PC-SPES is a herbal product used for cancer treatment. It is strongly cytotoxic and pro-apoptotic

Table 10.1. Interactions of various drugs with natural products.

No.	Natural products	Synthetic drugs	Target	System studied	References
1.	Quercetin	Carboxytriazole	—	Human breast carcinoma cells	Yeh *et al.* (1995)
2.		Triazofurin	—	Human ovarian carcinoma cells	Shen *et al.* (1999)
3.		*cis*-diamminedichloroplatinum (II)			
4.		Cytosine arabinoside (Ara-C)	—	HL-60 cells Human leukemic cells	Teofili *et al.* (1992)
5.		Reseveratol	Significant alterations in the cell cycle kinetics and induce apoptosis	Human pancreatic carcinoma cells	Mouria *et al.* (2002)
6.				Squamous carcinoma cells	Elatter and Virji (1999)
7.				Human leukemia cells	Mertens-Talcott and Percival (2005)
8.	Tea catechins	Sulindac	Induce apoptosis	Human lung carcinoma cells	Suganuma *et al.* (1999)
9.	Epigallocatechin gallate (EGCg)		Inhibition of intestinal tumors	Min mice	Fugiki *et al.* (2003)

Table 10.1. *(Continued)*

No.	Natural products	Synthetic drugs	Target	System studied	References
10.			—	Levels of gene expression in human lung carcinoma cells	Fugiki *et al.* (2003)
11.		(−)-epicatechin	Induction of apoptosis, growth inhibition	Human lung carcinoma cells	Suganuma *et al.* (1999)
12.			Inhibition of TNF-α release	BALB/c-3T3 cells	
	Tea catechins				
13.	Ep-gallocatechin gallate	Tamoxifen	Induce apoptosis	Human lung carcinoma cells	Suganuma *et al.* (1999)
14.			Inhibition of intestinal tumors	Min mice	Fugiki *et al.* (2003)
15.		Epigallocatechin Epicatechin gallate Epicatechin	Inhibition of induced expression of human CYP1A1 and CYP1A2 (Cyt450 1A)	HepG2 cells	Williams *et al.* (2003)

Table 10.1. (*Continued*)

No.	Natural products	Synthetic drugs	Target	System studied	References
16.	Thearubigins	Genistein	Blocking cell cycle	Human prostrate tumor cell	Sakamoto (2000)
17.	Catechin	NS398	—	Bladder and prostrate cancer cells	Farivar-Mohenseni *et al.* (2004)
18.		Eicosapentanoic acid	Modulation of DNA synthesis through the alteration of glucose oxidation	Human breast carcinoma cells	Nakagawa *et al.* (2000)
19.	Genistein	Tamoxifen	Anti-proliferative effect	Dysplastic and cancerous breast cells	Tanos *et al.* (2002)
20.		5-Fluorouracil	Modulation of AMPK and COX-2 signaling pathways	Colon cancer cells	Hwang *et al.* (2005)

Table 10.1. (*Continued*)

No.	Natural products	Synthetic drugs	Target	System studied	References
21.		Doxorubicin	Inhibition of NF-kB activation	Hepatocellular carcinoma cells	Notarbartolo *et al.* (2005)
22.	Curcumin	Cisplatin	—	Ovarian carcinoma cells	Chan *et al.* (2003)
23.		Genistein	Inhibition of protein kinases	Breast cancer cells	Wolff *et al.* (1993)

towards prostrate carcinoma cells, which was thought to be due to the presence of contaminants. Batches of PC-SPES were removed from the market due to the presence of traces of synthetic drugs like diethyl stiesterol, indomethacin and warfarin as contaminants. Studies concluded that the traces of synthetic drugs found were not responsible for the cytotoxic and pro-apoptotic activities of this herb on small cell lung carcinoma cells, but that the herbal mixture itself was responsible for the observed behavior (Sadava and Winesburg, 2005).

Interactions of various drugs with natural phytochemicals reported in the literature are tabulated in Table 10.1. The mechanism and their targets are not fully known. Experimental techniques to determine the action of combination drugs and to design effective mixtures have not been completely standardized. It is still being practiced as an art using trial and error methods. This review deals with the effect of combination of phytomedicines and drugs acting in synergy at single or multiple target sites and the associated cell signaling network.

10.2 AP1 and NF-κB Pathway

NF-κB (nuclear factor-κB) and the AP-1 (activator protein-1) are a set of transcription factors for genes that promote the cell survival and the proliferation mechanisms. Both induce the transcription of target genes that include cyclin D1, Bcl-2 (B-cell lymphoma-2), BCl-X_2, VEGF (vascular endothelial growth factor), MMP (matrix metalloproteinase), and urokinase-type plasminogen activator, which are involved in cell differentiation, proliferation and angiogenesis (Dorai and Aggarwal, 2004). Several phytochemicals individually or in combination are known to block these initial transmission signals.

For instance, curcumin has more than one defined mechanism of action. It is found to act in synergy with cisplatin and doxorubicin on the hepatocellular carcinoma cell lines. There is down-regulation of NF-κB target genes such as cyclooxygenase-2 (COX-2), Bcl-X_L and c-myc when it is combined with cisplatin (Chan *et al.*, 2003). Pre-treatment with curcumin enhances the anti-proliferative and apoptotic effect of vinorelbine by down-regulating anti-apoptotic Bcl-2 and Bcl-X_L genes, up-regulating pro-apoptotic Bcl-xs and Bax genes and activating caspase-9 and -3 genes. The suppression of NF-κB and AP-1 by both curcumin and vinorelibine may possibly explain the observed anti-proliferative and apoptotic effects (Sen *et al.*, 2005). Curcumin has also been found to act in synergy with other standard cytotoxic drugs through different mechanisms of action as shown in Table 10.1.

10.3 Receptor Tyrosine Kinase (RTK) Related Pathways of Signal Transduction

Various growth factors such as epidermal growth factor (EGF)-receptor and VEGF-receptors promote the cell proliferation signals. They also suppress apoptotic signals, anchorage independence and growth of blood vessels. Many chemopreventive phytochemicals including curcumin, genistein, resveratrol and catechins are known to be potent inhibitors of these growth factor receptors (Korutla *et al.*, 1995). RTKs stimulate the phosphorylation of protein kinases such as the mitogen activated protein kinase (MAPK), thereby activating a cascade of intracellular signals. This includes MEK1/2 (MAPK or ERK kinase), ERK1/2 (extracellular signal regulated kinase), JNK1/2/3 (Jun N-terminal kinase) and p38α/β/γ genes that are involved in signal transduction (Chang and Karin, 2001).

Protein kinases have now emerged as one of the most important groups of drug targets, accounting for 20% to 30% of the drug discoveries of many pharmaceutical companies (Sodhi *et al.*, 2003). RTK inhibitor GW282974A (an analog of GW2016; Lapatinib) is effective in chemo-sensitization of drug resistant EGFR over-expressing cells. This gives rise to a synergistic effect when used in combination with either cisplatin or paclitaxel in chemo-sensitivity assays (Coley *et al.*, 2006). Phytochemicals like curcumin, EGCg are known to inhibit RTK and downstream signaling pathways. Also EGCg can directly inhibit the binding of EGF, platelet derived growth factor (PDGF), and fibroblast growth factor (FGF) to their respective receptors (Korutla *et al.*, 1995; Liang *et al.*, 1997; Sachinidis *et al.*, 2000). Therefore, RTK inhibition by phytochemicals in combination with synthetic drugs is an effective alternative to circumvent tumor cell drug resistance, which occurs in conjunction with the over-expression of EGFR.

10.4 COX-2 and Cancer

COX-2 isozyme is involved in the neoplastic growth and its development. It is highly over-expressed in pre-malignant and malignant tumors. A correlation is also observed between COX-2 expression and increased tumor cell density. COX-2 is related to cancer through direct and indirect mechanisms. Prostaglandins generated by COX enzymes may directly stimulate mitogenesis through a direct effect on fibroblasts, osteoblasts, and mammary cells. COX-2 indirectly affects mutagenesis, angiogenesis, and increased cell migration and apoptosis, so inhibitors of COX-2 expression in tumor have a therapeutic potential (Subbaramaiah and Dannenberg, 2003).

Sulindac, a non-steroidal anti-inflammatory drug (NSAID), which is used as a cancer preventive agent, is also associated with adverse side-effects that include gastrointestinal bleeding. Combining sulindac and tamoxifen (an anti-cancer drug) with EGCg was found to work in synergy on lung cancer PC-9 cells (Suganuma *et al.*, 2001). Also, EGCg in combination with NSAIDs is found to reduce the incidence of tumor in mice with multiple intestinal neoplasia and apoptosis induced against colon carcinogenesis of rats. This is due to the fact that EGCg (blocks COX-2) and NSAIDs (blocks COX-1); both act in tandem as dual inhibitors (Ohishi *et al.*, 2002).

10.5 Regulation of Cell Cycle

Cell cycle machinery controls cell proliferation, and cancer is a disease arising due to inappropriate cell proliferation. The completion of a cell division cycle requires the spatial and temporal coordination of a wide diversity of processes that relies on the activity of a family of protein kinases, namely the Cdks (cyclin-dependent kinases). Normal cells halt their cell cycle progression at the G1/S and G2/M borders. This gives them enough time to repair their damaged DNA in case of exposure to genotoxic stresses. The inactivation of genes involved in these cell cycle checkpoints would allow for the propagation of cells carrying DNA lesions and hence give rise to tumors. Cancer is precisely the imperfections at the cell cycle checkpoints, which prevents the cycle from stopping in the face of adverse conditions, making them vulnerable.

Drugs that block different phases of cell cycle can act in synergy, e.g. quercetin and triazofurin. Quercetin cause cell cycle arrest in the G_0/G_1 phase (Yoshida *et al.*, 1990), the G_2/M phase (Choi *et al.*, 2001), at the G_1 and S phase boundary (Yoshida *et al.*, 1990) and induce caspase-3 activity and apoptosis (Wang *et al.*, 1999). It is found to act in synergy with triazofurin in human carcinoma cells (Shen *et al.*, 1999). Triazofurin reduces the cellular GTP pool and decreases inositol-1,4,5-triphosphate concentration (Weber *et al.*, 1997). The latter is brought about by the blocking of S phase of the cell cycle (Jayaram *et al.*, 1982). Also significant alterations in the cell cycle kinetics induced by the single compounds such as ellagic acid, quercetin, resveratrol and their combinations is observed against human leukemia cells. This interaction synergistically induced the apoptosis and reduced the cell growth (Mertens-Talcott and Percival, 2005).

10.6 Modulation of Multi-Drug Resistance (MDR)

Prolonged cancer chemotherapy may lead to the selective proliferation of MDR cells. Development of MDR is due to:

(1) the up-regulation or activation of transporter proteins;
(2) modification of the detoxification systems;
(3) changes in the target repair mechanisms; and
(4) deregulation of the cell death pathways (Coley, 2003).

One of the best multi-drug resistance mechanisms known is the over-expression of membrane transport proteins including the 170 kDa P-glycoprotein (Pgp). It is an ATP-dependent membrane transporter that extrudes a variety of hydrophobic anti-tumor drugs. Therefore, Pgp inhibitors may resensitize the MDR cells. Examples of such inhibitors are verapamil, reserpine, cephalosporin, gramicidin, cyclosporin A (Castaing *et al.*, 2000). These drugs are associated with severe side-effects (Coley, 2003). They also share common physical and structural characteristics such as cycli-city, lipophilicity and a positive or neutral charge at physiological pH (Anuchapreeda *et al.*, 2002).

The other approach is through the modulation of the MDR1 gene. These types of modulators may either block the induction of MDR1 gene expression or inhibit its promoter and down-regulate Pgp expression (Hu *et al.*, 1996). There are many problems associated with these modulators:

(1) they also become transported by Pgp (Krishna and Mayer, 2000);
(2) since inhibitory effect is through competition, the dose concentration has to be extremely high, which leads to side-effects and toxicity (Fisher *et al.*, 1994; Ozols *et al.*, 1987); and
(3) when these agents are co-administered with former, they influence the pharmacokinetics and biodistribution properties of the anti-cancer agents (Lum and Gosland, 1995).

Due to the limitations of the synthetic modulators, phytochemicals can be tried out in combination with the former. Herbs are known to interact with the ATP binding cassette transporters such as Pgp, MRP1, MRP2, and BCRP and play an important role in the transport of the anti-cancer drugs (Sparreboon and Nooter, 2000; Suzuki *et al.*, 2001; Ejendal and Hrycyna, 2002). The extract of rhizomes from *Alisma orientalis* (Sam) Juzep., which is commonly found in Southern China, show a synergistic inhibitor effect with cancer drugs including actinomycin D, puromycin, paciltaxel, vinblastine and doxorubicin against $HEPG_2$-DR and K562-DR, the two MDR cancer cells expressing Pgp (Fong *et al.*, 2007).

Curcumin down-regulates Pgp expression and reduces Pgp mediated efflux in drug resistant human cervical carcinoma cells by directly interacting with it. It modulates both the expression and function of MDR1 (Anuchapreeda *et al.*, 2002). Commercial curcuminoids contain 77% curcumin (I), 17% demethoxycurcumin (II) and 3% bisdemethoxycurcumin (III). These individual components were compared for their ability to modulate the human MDR1 expression in KB-V1 (Chearwae *et al.*, 2004). Preliminary experiments showed that the compound III was the most active modulator of the three (Limtrakul *et al.*, 2004). But later studies revealed that it was compound I. These compounds in addition also inhibited verapamil stimulated ATPase activity at high concentrations (Chearwae *et al.*, 2004).

Flavonols such as quercetin, Kaempferol and galangin were reported to increase adriamycin efflux from HCT-15 colon cancer cells whereas a hydrophobic quercetin derivative inhibited rhodamine 123 efflux from MCF-7 breast cancer cells and abolish their MDR phenotype (Scambia *et al.*,

1994). Quercetin was also found to prevent the binding of transported drugs such as colchicines (Shapiro and Ling, 1997a) or Hoechst 33342 and also inhibit the MRP1 transporters (Shapiro and Ling, 1997b). Various other flavonols, particularly genistein, inhibited drug efflux from cells over-expressing Pgp (Chieli *et al.*, 1995; Castro and Altenberg, 1997). Modifying flavonoids by prenylation was found to increase the binding affinity and strongly inhibit drug interaction and nucleotide hydrolysis. This approach constitutes a promising potential modulators for MDR (Di Pietro *et al.*, 2002).

10.7 Alteration of Pharmacokinetics

The design of chemotherapy schedules for treatment of malignancies is based on the selection of optimal drug doses with tolerable adverse effects. Inter-individual variation in the ADME may exist for a given dose, which depends upon both the physiological and pathological functions. These factors are important for the outcome of the treatment in terms of efficacy as well as toxicity. As chemotherapy uses combination of drugs, pharmacological interactions may be expected. Many anti-cancer drugs need specific enzymes for their metabolism and phytochemicals given in combination can alter the ADME of the drugs. This is due to the altered expression and functioning of cytochrome P450(CYP) isozymes. CYP450 are a very important drug metabolizing family of isozymes and CYP3A4 is responsible for the metabolism of several classes of currently used anti-cancer drugs. This isoenzyme can be easily induced or inhibited by other drugs or herbs. Interactions combining the drugs that modify the action of detoxification enzymes and the inhibitors of Pgp may result in enhanced adverse effects to patients. Elevated CYP activity decreases the bio-availability of the drug and loss of therapeutic activity whereas an increase in plasma concentrations due to the inhibition of CYP activity will lead to toxicity (Sparreboon *et al.*, 2004). Phytochemicals are known to induce and suppress the different classes of CYP family (Table 10.2). The bioactive agents that up-regulate the detoxification enzymes are divided into two groups, namely: monofunctional inducers that up-regulate a number of Phase II enzymes (quinine reductase and glutathione S-transferases), and bifunctional inducers that up-regulate some of the Phase II and a few

Table 10.2. Induction and suppression of Phase I detoxification enzymes by phytochemicals (Meijerman *et al.*, 2006).

No.	Cytochrome P450	Metabolize the chemotherapeutic drug	Action	Phytochemicals
1.	CYP2C9*1	Cyclophosphamide	Decrease	Fresh garlic Fresh garlic oil Freeze dried garlic
2.	CYP2C19	Teniposide	Decrease	Fresh garlic Fresh garlic oil Freeze dried garlic
			Increase	Ginkgo
3.	CYP2E1	Dacarbazine	Decrease	Diallylsulfide
	CYP2E1	Dacarbazine	Increase	Diallyldisulfide
			Increase	Allylmethyl sulfide Allyl mercaptan Diallyl sulfone Genistein
	CYP3A4	Etoposide Paciltaxel Vinorelbine Vinblastine Tamoxifen	Increase	When the above are administered for long term (> 6 weeks) and at high concentrations
4.	CYP3A4	Etoposide Paciltaxel Vinorelbine Vinblastine Tamoxifen	Decrease	Fresh garlic Fresh garlic oil Freeze dried garlic Extract of Echinacea Quercetin
			Increase	Ginkgo
5.	CYP3A5	Etoposide	Decrease	Fresh garlic Fresh garlic oil Freeze dried garlic Genistein
6.	CYP1A1	Dacarbazine	Increase	Quercetin Kaempferol

Phase I enzymes (CYP1A1). Glucosinolates (I3C and crambene) are a group of secondary metabolites from cruciferous vegetables, which interact to produce synergistic induction of Phase II detoxification enzymes (Nho and Jeffery, 2001). The pharmaceutical behavior of a particular drug can be identified only through preclinical and early clinical evaluation. Changes in drug dose, sequence, or infusion duration, increase of time-interval between drugs, etc. are the measures required to provide an optimal therapeutic dose of combination chemotherapy for the patient with cancer.

10.8 Enhancement of Immune Function

Immune dysfunction has been found to be associated with cancer. Cancer immunotherapy relies on the ability of the immune system to identify and destroy tumor cells and to elicit a long-lasting memory of this interaction. Under ordinary circumstances, however, the ability of tumor cells to trigger an effective immune response is limited. The nominal poor immunogenicity of tumor cells results in part from their weak expression of immune cells. Immunomodulation through natural and synthetic substances may be considered as an alternative for the prevention and cure of neoplastic diseases. *Withania somnifera* is observed to restore the number, and function of immunocompetent cells, immune complexes and immunoglobulins to counteract the side-effects of synthetic anti-cancer drugs, thereby enhancing their efficacy (Senthilnathan *et al.*, 2006).

10.9 Conclusion

The use of dietary supplements, phytochemicals, nutraceuticals in combination with synthetic drugs for the treatment of cancer is increasing day by day, but the risk of their toxicity and side-effects determine the efficacy and safety of the combination therapy. The additive and synergistic effects of the phytochemicals in combination are responsible for the potent antioxidant and anti-proliferative activities. A single antioxidant can never replace a combination of natural phytochemicals due to the synergy of various constituents. The use of phytochemicals in combination with the anti-cancer drugs can be recommended once the entire molecular and physiological interaction mechanisms are fully understood.

References

Anuchapreeda, S., Leechanachai, P., Smith, M.M., Ambudkar, S.V. and Limtraku, P. (2002) Modulation of P-glycoprotein expression and function by curcumin in mulitdrug-resistant human KB cells. *Biochem. Pharmacol.* **64**, 573–582.

Banuelos, G.S. (2002) Irrigation of broccoli and canola with boron- and selenium-laden effluent. *J. Environ. Qual.* **31**, 1802–1818.

Castaing, M., Brouant, P., Loiseau, A., Santelli-Rouvier, C., Santelli, M., Alibert-Franco, S., Mahamoud, A. and Barbe, J. (2000) Membrane permeation by multidrug-resistance-modulators and non-modulators: Effects of hydrophobicity and electric charge. *J. Pharm. Pharmacol.* **52**, 289–296.

Castro, A.F. and Altenberg, G.A. (1997) Inhibition of drug transport by genistein in multidrug-resistant cells expressing P-glycoprotein. *Biochem. Pharmacol.* **53**, 89–93.

Chan, M.M., Fong, D., Soprano, K.J., Holmes, W.F. and Heverling, H. (2003) Inhibition of growth and sensitisation to cisplatin-mediated killing of ovarian cancer cells by polyphenolic chemopreventive agents. *J. Cell Physiol.* **194**, 63–70.

Chang, L. and Karin, M. (2001) Mammalian, MAP kinase signaling casacades. *Nature* **410**, 37–40.

Chearwae, W., Anuchapreeda, S., Nandigama, K., Ambudkar, S.V. and Limtakul, P. (2004) Biochemical mechanism of modulation of human P-glycoprotein (ABCB1) by curcumin I, II and III purified from turmeric powder. *Biochem. Pharmacol.* **68**, 2043–2052.

Chieli, E., Romiti, N., Cervelli, F. and Tonigiani, R. (1995) Effects of flavonols on P-glycoprotein activity in cultures rat hepatocytes. *Life Sci.* **57**, 1741–1751.

Choi, J.A., Kim, J.Y., Lee, J.Y., Kang, C.M., Kwon, C.M., Yoo, Y.D., Kim, T.W., Lee, Y.S. and Lee, S.J. (2001) Induction of cell cycle arrest and apoptosis in human breast cancer cells by quercetin. *Int. J. Oncol.* **19**, 837–844.

Chu, Y.-F., Sun, J., Wu, X. and Liu, R.H. (2002) Antioxidants and antiproliferative activities of vegetables. *J. Agric. Food Chem.* **50**, 6910–6916.

Coley, H.M., Shotton, C.F., Ajose-Adeoqun, A., Modjtahedi, H. and Thomas, H. (2006) Receptor tyrosine kinase (RTK) inhibition is effective in chemosensitising EGFR-expressing drug resistant human ovarian cancer cell lines when used in combination with cytotoxic agents. *Biochem. Pharmacol.* **72**, 941–948.

Coley, T.H. (2003) Overcoming multidrug resistance in cancer: An update on the clinical strategy of inhibiting P-glycoprotein. *Cancer Cont.* **10**, 159–165.

Curphey, T.J., Kulhmann, E.T., Roebuck, B.B. and Longnecker, D.S. (1988) Inhibition of pancreatic and liver carcinogenesis in rats by retinoid- and selenium-supplemented diets. *Pancreas* **3**, 36–40.

Di Pietro, A., Conseil, G., Pérez-Victoria, J.M., Dayan, G., Baubichon-Cortay, H., Trompier, D., Steinfels, E., Jault, J.-M., de Wet, H., Maitrejean, M., Comte, G., Boumendjel, A., Mariotte, A.-M., Dumontet, C., McIntosh, D.B., Goffeau, A., Castanys, S., Gamarro, F. and Barron, D. (2002) Modulation by flavonoids of cell multidrug resistance mediated by P-glycoprotein and related ABC transporters. *Cell Mol. Life Sci.* **59**, 307–322.

Dorai, T. and Aggarwal, B.B. (2004) Role of chemopreventive agents in cancer therapy. *Cancer Lett.* **215**, 129–140.

Ejendal, K.F. and Hrycyna, C.A. (2002) Multidrug resistance and cancer: The role of the human ABC transporter ABCG2. *Curr. Protein Pept. Sci.* **3**, 503–511.

Elattar, T.M. and Virji, A.S. (1999) The effect of red wine and its components on growth and proliferation of human oral squamous carcinoma cells. *Anti-cancer Res.* **19**, 5407–5414.

Farivar-Mohenseni, H., Kandzari, S.J., Zaslau, S., Riggs, D.R., Jackson, B.J. and McFadden, D.W. (2004) Synergistic effects of COX-1 and -2 inhibition on bladder and prostate cancer *in vitro*. *Am. J. Surg.* **188**, 505–510.

Finley, J.W., Keck, A.S., Robbins, R.J. and Hintze, K.J. (2005) Selenium enrichment of broccoli: Interaction between selenium and secondary plant compounds. *J. Nutr.* **135**, 1236–1238.

Fisher, G.A., Bartlett, N.L., Lum, B.L., Brophy, N.A., Duran, G.E., Ehsan, M.N., Halsey, J. and Sikic, B.I. (1994) Phase I train of taxol (T) with high dose cyclosporine (CsA) as a modulator of multidrug resistance (MDR). *Proc. Am. Soc. Clin. Oncol.* **13**, 144.

Fong, W.-F., Wang, C., Zhu, G.-Y., Leung, C.-H., Yang, M.-S. and Cheung, H.-Y. (2007) Reversal of multidrug resistance in cancer cells by *Rhizome Alismatis* extract. *Phytomedicine* **14**, 160–165.

Fugiki, H., Suganuma, M., Kurusu, M., Okabe, S., Imayoshi, Y., Taniquchi, S. and Yoshida, T. (2003) New TNF-α releasing inhibitors as cancer preventive agents from traditional herbal medicine and combination cancer prevention study with EGCG and sulindac or tamoxifen. *Mutat. Res.* **523/524**, 119–125.

Guo, Z., Smith, T.J., Wang, E., Sadrieh, N., Ma, Q., Thomas, P.E. and Yang, C.S. (1992) Effects of phenylethylisothiocyanate, a carcinogenesis inhibitor, on xenobiotic-metabolizing enzymes and nitrosamine metabolism in rats. *Carcinogenesis* **13**, 2205–2210.

Horvath, P.M. and Ip, C. (1983) Synergistic effect of vitamin E and selenium in the chemoprevention of mammary carcinogenesis in rats. *Cancer Res.* **43**, 5335–5341.

Hu, Y.P., Pourquier, P., Doignon, F., Crouzet, M. and Robert, J. (1996) Effects of modulators of multidrug resistance on the expression of the MDR1 gene ion human KB cells in culture. *Anti-cancer Drug* **7**, 738–744.

Hwang, J.-T., Ha, J. and Park, J.O. (2005) Combination of 5-fluorouracil and genistein induces apoptosis synergistically in chemo-resistant cell through the modulation of AMPK and COX-2 signaling pathways. *Biochem. Biophys. Res. Commun.* **332**, 433–440.

Jayaram, H.N., Dion, R.L., Glazer, R.I., Johns, D.G., Robins, R.K., Srivastava, P.C. and Cooney, D.A. (1982) Initial studies in the mechanism of action of a new oncolytic thiazole nucleoside 2-β-D-ribofuranosyl thiazole-4-carboxamide NSC 266193. *Biochem. Pharmacol.* **31**, 2371–2380.

Kelley, M.K. and Bjeldanes, L.F. (1995) Modulation of glutathione S-transferase activity and isozyme pattern in liver and small intestine of rats fed goitrin- and T3-supplemented diets. *Food Chem. Toxicol.* **33**, 129–137.

Kensler, T.W., Groopman, J.D., Eaton, D.L., Curphey, T.J. and Roebuck, B.D. (1992) Potent inhibition of aflatoxin-induced hepatic tumorigenesis by the monofunctional enzyme inducer 1,2-dithiole-3-thione. *Carcinogenesis* **13**, 95–100.

Korutla, L., Cheung, J.Y., Mendelsohn, J. and Kumar, R. (1995) Inhibition of ligand induced activation of epidermal growth factor receptor tyrosine phosphorylation by curcumin. *Carcinogenesis* **16**, 1741–1745.

Krishna, R. and Mayer, L.D. (2000) Multidrug resistance (MDR) in cancer. Mechanisms, reversal using modulators of MDR and the role of MDR modulators in influencing the pharmacokinetics of anti-cancer drugs. *Eur. J. Pharm. Sci.* **11**, 265–283.

Liang, Y.C., Lin-shiau, S.Y., Chen, C.F. and Lin, J.K. (1997) Suppression of extracellular signals and cell proliferation through EGF receptor binding by (−)-epigallocatechin gallate in human A431 epidermoid carcinoma cells. *J. Cell Biochem.* **67**, 55–65.

Limtrakul, P., Anuchapreeda, S. and Buddhasukh, D. (2004) Modulation of human multidrug resistance MDR-1 gene by natural curcuminoids. *BMC Cancer* **4**, 13.

Liu, R.H. (2004) Potential synergy of phytochemicals in cancer prevention: Mechanism of action. *Am. Soc. Nutri. Sci.* 3479S–3485S.

Lum, B. and Gosland, M. (1995) MDR expression in normal tissues: Pharmacologic implications for the clinical use of P-glycoprotein inhibitors. *Hematol. Oncol. Clin. North Am.* **9**, 319–336.

Meijerman, I., Beijnen, J.H. and Schellens, J.H.M. (2006) Herb-drug interactions in Oncology: Focus on mechanisms of induction. *Oncologist* **11**, 742–752.

Mertens-Talcott, S.U. and Percival, S.S. (2005) Ellagic acid and quercetin interact synergistically with resveratrol in the induction of apoptosis and cause transient cell cycle arrest in human leukemia cells. *Cancer Lett.* **218**, 141–151.

Mouria, M., Gukovskaya, A.S., Jung, Y., Buechler, P., Hines, O.J., Reber, H.A. and Pandol, S.J. (2002) Food-derived polyphenols inhibit pancreatic cancer growth through mitochondrial cytochrome C release and apoptosis. *Int. J. Cancer* **98**, 761–769.

Nakagawa, H., Yamamoto, D., Kiyozuka, Y., Tsuta, K., Uemura, Y., Hioki, K., Tsutsui, Y. and Tsubura, A. (2000) Effects of genistein and synergistic action in combination with eicosapentaenoic acid on the growth of breast cancer cell lines. *J. Cancer Res. Clin. Oncol.* **126**, 448–454.

Nho, C.W. and Jeffery, E. (2001) Synergistic upregulation of phase II detoxification enzymes by glucosinolate breakdown products in cruciferous vegetables. *Toxicol. Appl. Pharmacol.* **174**, 146–152.

Notarbartolo, M., Poma, P., Perri, D., Dusonchet, L., Cervello, M. and Alessandro, N. (2005) Antitumor effects of curcumin, alone or in combination with cisplatin or doxorubicin on human hepatic cancer cells. Analysis of their possible relationship to changes in NF-κB activation and in IAP gene expression. *Cancer Lett.* **224**, 53–65.

Ohishi, T., Kushimoto, Y., Miura, N., Shiota, G., Kohri, T., Hara, Y., Haseqawa, J. and Isemura, M. (2002) Synergistic effects of (–)-epigallocatechin gallate with sulindac against colon carcinogenesis of rats treated with azomethane. *Cancer Lett.* **177**, 49–56.

Ozols, R.F., Cunnion, R.E., Klecker, R.W., Hamilton, T.C., Ostchega, Y., Parrillo, J.E. and Young, R.C. (1987) Verapamil and adriamycin in the treatment of drug-resistant ovarian cancer patients. *J. Clin. Oncol.* **5**, 641–647.

Sachinidis, A., Seul, C., Seewald, S., Ahn, H., Ko, Y. and Veter, H. (2000) Green tea compounds inhibit tyrosine phosphorylation of PDGF beta — receptor and transformation of A172 human glioblastoma. *FEBS Lett.* **471**, 51–55.

Sadava, D. and Winesburg, J. (2005) Contaminants of PC-SPES are not responsible for cytotoxicity in human small-cell lung carcinoma cells. *Cancer Lett.* **220**, 171–175.

Sakamoto, K. (2000) Synergistic effects of thearubigin and genistein on human prostate tumor cell (PC-3) growth via cell cycle arrest. *Cancer Lett.* **151**, 103–109.

Scambia, G., Ranelletti, F.O., Panici, P.B., De Vincenzo, R., Bonanno, G., Ferrandina, G., Piantelli, M., Bussa, S., Rumi, C., Cianfriqlia, M. *et al.* (1994) Quercetin potentiates the effect of adriamycin in multidrug-resistant MCF-7 human breast cancer cell line: P-glycoprotein as a possible target. *Cancer Chemother. Pharmacol.* **34**, 459–464.

Sen, S., Sharma, H. and Singh, N. (2005) Curcumin enhances vinorelbine mediated apoptosis in NSCLC cells by the mitochondrial pathway. *Biochem. Biophys. Res. Commun.* **331**, 1245–1252.

Senthilnathan, P., Padmavathi, R., Banu, S.M. and Sakthisekaran, D. (2006) Enhancement of antitumor effect of paclitaxel in combination with immunomodulatory *Withania somnifera* on benzo(a)pyrene induced experimental lung cancer. *Chem.-Biol. Interact.* **159**, 180–185.

Shapiro, A.B. and Ling, V. (1997a) Effect of quercetin on Hoechst 33342 transport by purified and reconstituted P-glycoprotein. *Biochem. Pharmacol.* **53**, 587–596.

Shapiro, A.B. and Ling, V. (1997b) Positively cooperative sites for drug transport by P-glycoprotein with distinct drug specificities. *Eur. J. Biochem.* **250**, 130–137.

Shen, F., Herenyiova, M. and Weber, G. (1999) Synergistic down-regulation of signal transduction and cytotoxicity by triazofurin and quercetin in human ovarian carcinoma cells. *Life Sci.* **64**, 1869–1876.

Sodhi, A., Montaner, S. and Gutkind, J.S. (2003) Molecular mechanisms of cancer. In: *Signal Transduction and Disease* (eds.) Finkel, T. and Gutkind, J.S. Wiley Interscience, New York, pp. 71–142.

Sparreboon, A. and Nooter, K. (2000) Does P-glycoprotein play a role in anti-cancer drug pharmacokinetics? *Drug Resist. Update* **3**, 357–363.

Sparreboon, A., Cox, M.C., Acharya, M.R. and Figg, W.D. (2004) Herbal remedies in the United States: Potential adverse interactions with anti-cancer agents. *J. Clin. Oncol.* **22**, 2489–2503.

Subbaramaiah, K. and Dannenberg, A.J. (2003) Cyclooxygenase-2: A molecular target for chemoprevention and treatment. *Trends Pharmacol. Sci.* **24**, 96–102.

Suganuma, M., Okabe, S., Kai, Y., Sueoka, N., Sueoka, E. and Fujiki, H. (1999) Synergistic effects of (–)-epigallocatechin gallate with (–)-epicatechin, sulindac or tamoxifen on cancer preventive activity in the human lung cancer cell line PC-9. *Cancer Res.* **59**, 44–47.

Suganuma, M., Ohkura, Y., Okabe, S. and Fujiki, H. (2001) Combination cancer prevention with with green tea extract and sulindac shown in intestinal tumor formation in Min mice. *J. Cancer Res. Clin. Oncol.* **127**, 69–72.

Surh, Y.-J. (1999) Molecular mechanisms of chemopreventive effects of selected dietary and medicinal phenolic substances. *Mutat. Res.* **428**, 305–327.

Suzuki, T., Nishio, K. and Tanabe, S. (2001) The MRP family and anti-cancer drug metabolism. *Curr. Drug Metab.* **2**, 367–377.

Tanos, V., Brzezinski, A., Drize, O., Strauss, N. and Peretz, T. (2002) Synergistic inhibitory effects of genistein and tamoxifen on human dysplastic and malignant epithelial breast cells *in vitro*. *Eur. J. Obstet. Gynecol. Reprod. Biol.* **102**, 188–194.

Teofili, L., Pierelli, L., Iovino, M.S., Leone, G., Scambia, G., De Vincenzo, R., Benedetti-Panici, P., Menichella, G., Macri, E., Piantelli, M., Ranelletti, F.O. and Larocca, L.M. (1992) The combination of quercetin and cytosine arabinoside synergistically inhibits leukemic cell growth. *Leuk. Res.* **16**, 497–503.

Yeh, Y.A., Herenyiova, M. and Weber, G. (1995) Quercetin: Synergistic action with carboxyamidotriazole in human breast carcinoma cells. *Life Sci.* **57**, 1285–1292.

Yoshida, M., Sakai, T., Hosokawa, N., Marui, N., Matsumoto, K., Fujioka, A., Nishino, H. and Aoike, A. (1990) The effect of quercetin on cell cycle progression and growth of human gastric cancer cells. *FEBS Lett.* **260**, 10–13.

Wallig, M.A., Kuchan, M.J. and Milner, J.A. (1993) Differential effects of cyanohydroxybutene and selenium on normal and neoplastic canine mammary cells *in vitro*. *Toxicol. Lett.* **69**, 97–105.

Wang, I.K., Lin-Shiau, S.Y. and Lin, J.K. (1999) Induction of apoptosis by apigenin and related flavonoids through cytochrome crelease and activation of caspase-9 and caspase-3 in leukaemia HL-60 cells. *Eur. J. Cancer* **35**, 1517–1525.

Weber, G., Shen, F., Prajda, N., Yang, H., Li, W., Yeh, A., Csokay, B., Olah, E. and Look, K.Y. (1997) Regulation of the signal transduction programs by drugs. *Adv. Enzyme Regul.* **37**, 35 55.

Williams, S.N., Pickwell, G.V. and Quottrochi, L.C. (2003) A combination of tea (*Camellia senensis*) catechins required for optimal inhibition of induced CYP1A expression by green tea extract. *J. Agric. Food Chem.* **51**, 6627–6634.

Wolff, M.S., Toniolo, P.G., Lee, E.W., Rivera, M. and Dubin, N. (1993) Blood levels of organochlorine residues and risk of breast cancer. *J. Nat. Cancer Inst.* **85**, 648–652.

Chapter 11

Ethnopharmacology Approaches for Botanical Immunomodulators and Chemoprotectants in Cancer Therapy

Patwardhan Bhushan & Gautam Manish

Abstract

Most of the cancer chemotherapeutic agents are associated with toxicity towards normal cells and tissues that share many characteristics with tumor cell, and in particular, high cell turnover. Optimal dosing of cancer chemotherapeutic agents is often limited because of severe non-myelosuppressive and myelosuppressive toxicities, therefore it is a continuing challenge to design therapy that is effective and also efficiently targeted towards tumor cells. Cytoprotective agents are expected to control or prevent these toxicities and include the use of synthetic and natural products. Specific chemoprotectants are emerging for cisplatin and anthracyclin antibiotics. None of the available agents satisfy criteria for an ideal chemoprotection. This has stimulated research for discovering natural resources with immunomodulatory and cytoprotective activities. Various botanicals and ethnopharmacological agents used in traditional medicine have been investigated by various workers for their chemoprotective, immunomodulating, adaptogenic and anti-tumor activities and have revealed promises towards developing into a potential drug for cancer treatment *per se* or as an adjuvant.

Keywords: Immunomodulation; Chemoprotection; Cancer; Chemotherapy; Adaptogens; Ayurveda.

11.1 Introduction

The importance of host immunity has been ignored for years in clinical oncology. Modulation of host immunity was previously attempted with glucocorticoids and cytotoxic drugs like cyclophosphamide however could not be established because of dose limiting toxicities. The routine therapy continued with the Big Three — surgery, chemotherapy and radiotherapy — all of which damaged host immunity. Most of the chemotherapeutic agents available today are cytotoxic and exert a variety of side-effects, mainly immunosuppression. However, recent advances in cellular and molecular immunology have allowed for an understanding of the complex interactions between immune system and tumor cells. Cancer vaccines are an outcome of these developments. In addition, the importance of host immunity and its relation to mean survival time has now been established in breast cancer. The same could be true for other solid epithelial tumors such as lungs, stomach, pancreas, colon and so forth. Similarly, the co-administration of immunomodulators such as IL-2 reverses the chemotherapy-associated lymphopenia and neutropenia. Neutropenia significantly impacts quality of life and is associated with immediate effects such as sepsis, while lymphocyte counts are detrimental to survival time. It is now recognized that immuno-modulatory therapy could provide a complement to conventional chemotherapy, especially where the host's defense mechanisms have to be activated under immunocompromised conditions. These trends emphasize the need to add the fourth modality to cancer treatment, *immunotherapy* (Elliot and Head, 2005). This has stimulated the interest in search for newer and safer immunomodulators for use in cancer therapy (Devi *et al.*, 1992; Patwardhan *et al.*, 1990). In addition, chemical agents preventing site-specific toxicity of cytotoxic drugs are among the current tools of cancer chemotherapy; however, their use is limited because of loco-regional protection offered. Traditional medicine offers many strategies to manage cancer treatments, including the use of anti-cancer therapeutic agents and adjuvants to chemotherapy (Patwardhan and Patwardhan, 2006). Traditional Chinese medicine and Indian Ayurveda represent two important great traditions. Both these systems have many commonalities, including basic principles and the use of botanical materials (Patwardhan *et al.*, 2005). Many such botanicals reported by various researchers as immuno-modulators, have exhibited promise as adjuvants for cancer therapy. We review here potential immunomodulators from botanicals, some of these mentioned in Ayurveda as *Rasayana*, i.e. exhibiting chemo- and radio-protection.

11.1.1 *Cancer therapy: a case for multitarget approach and the role of botanicals*

Considerable research effort that has gone into understanding the molecular and cell biological processes that give rise to cancer and has provided a wealth of information on various targets and mechanisms. Mechanism-based drugs that specifically target these cancer-specific mutations have undergone clinical exemplification. Gleevec (STI S71) inhibits the aberrant Abl tyrosine kinase activity in CML, and has demonstrated remarkable single-agent activity during CML blast crisis. However, the appearance of clinical resistance to Gleevec has begun to be a significant clinical problem (Druker and Karnofsky, 2003). Consequently, the traditional pharmacological paradigm of mono-target therapy is becoming increasingly compromised by the appearance of resistance to target- and mechanism-based drugs. This further reflects the redundancy in the pathways that govern signal transduction networks (Faivre *et al.*, 2006). Relevant combination therapies or multi-target approaches, where different mechanism-based agents are combined to control multiple aberrant pathways seen in the tumor, seem like a possible option. On the other hand, the development of multi-target molecules also appears to be an increasingly feasible and attractive option. In order to improvise on both these options, exploration of newer chemical diversity will be an utmost need (Kerr and La Thangue, 2004). Botanicals that are chemically complex will be important starting materials for the discovery of newer synergistic combinations and single agent multi-target drugs.

11.1.2 *Adjuvant therapy: newer avenues*

Adjuvant treatment is defined as additional therapy given in association with primary (initial) management. Previously, the adjuvant concept was limited to use after surgery or for locoregional chemoprotection. However with the success of tamoxifen in breast cancer, the discovery of safer and effective adjuvants is on the rise. Moreover, with increased understanding of cytotoxicity and host immune response, apoptosis and identification of targets for drug resistance, the scope of adjuvant concept and treatment has widened. The approach of "one size fits all" is no longer preferred now and more personalized regimens are being developed. In addition, various studies have shown positive correlations between immunocorrection during cancer therapy and increased chemoprotection, radioprotection and anti-tumor activity. Newer and safer adjuvants will be required for such regimens. The discovery of adjuvant currently relies on four important attributes:

(1) minimum interference with applied chemotherapy;
(2) adjuvant should minimize the risk of relapse with minimum side-effects;
(3) long-term safety; and
(4) cost-effectiveness.

Botanical immunomodulators especially based on ethnopharmacological approaches will offer a safer and cost-effective platform for the discovery of newer adjuvants.

11.1.3 *Natural products*: *discovery approaches*

There are two major ways of bioprospecting natural products for investigation. First, the classical method that relies on phytochemical factors, serendipity and random screening approaches. Second, uses traditional knowledge and practices as drug discovery engine. This is also known as ethnopharmacology approach, which is time- and cost-effective and may lead to better success than routine random screening. Various ethnopharma-cological agents are under investigation as immunomodulators. Traditional Chinese medicine, Japanese Kampo, Indian Ayurveda and such are becoming important bioprospecting tools. Ayurveda remains as one of the most ancient and yet living traditions practiced widely in India, Sri Lanka and other countries and has sound philosophical and experiential basis. India has about 45,000 plant species; medicinal properties have been assigned to many to several thousands. Ayurveda has detailed descriptions of over 700 herbs and 400,000-registered Ayurvedic practitioners routinely prescribe them particularly for treatment of chronic disease conditions. A considerable research on pharmacognosy, chemistry, pharmacology and clinical therapeutics has been carried out and Ayurvedic database has detailed descriptions of over 700 medicinal plants (Patwardhan, 2000; Patwardhan *et al.*, 2004).

11.1.4 *Ethnopharmacology*: *Ayurveda, Rasayana and immunomodulation*

Ayurveda gives a separate class of immunomodulating botanicals named *Rasayanas*. *Rasayanas* are non-toxic herbal preparations or individual herbs used to rejuvenate or attain the complete potential of healthy and or diseased individual in order to prevent diseases and degenerative changes that leads to disease. Pharmacodynamic studies on *Rasayana* botanicals have suggested many possible mechanisms such as non-specific and specific immunostimulation, free radicals quenching, cellular detoxification, cell proliferation and repair. Ayurveda (with particular reference to botanicals) may play an important role in modern health care, particularly where satisfactory treatment is not available. There is a need to evaluate the potential of Ayurvedic remedies as adjuvant to counteract side-effects of modern therapy and compare the cost-effectiveness of certain therapies *vis a vis* modern therapeutic schedules (Rege, 1999).

11.2 Material and Methods

11.2.1 *Scope of botanicals*

This is basically a review and we have used our own research as a basis for this article. In following paragraphs, we have reviewed the literature pertaining to botanicals (mainly from Ayurveda *Rasayana*) as agents for integrative oncology care. We have focused on three leading botanicals from the *Rasayana* class, namely *Withania somnifera*, *Tinospora cordifolia* and *Asparagus racemosus*, which have attracted interest of researchers globally for their potential as immunoadjuvants. At some places, we have also included some examples from non-Ayurveda botanicals that have shown similar kind of activities.

The reports obtained from MEDLINE databases have been organized and discussed under different facets of beneficial activities for anti-cancer therapy such as adaptogens, chemoprotectants, radioprotectants and anti-tumor activities. Finally, an overview of studies carried out by our institute has been discussed in purview of existing scenario of anti-cancer discovery.

11.3 Results

11.3.1 *Paraimmunity adjuvants*: *adaptogens or adjustive medicine*

Most of the synthetic chemotherapeutic agents available today are immunosuppressants, cytotoxic and exert a variety of side-effects. N. V. Lazarev; who phrased the concept of "a state of non-specifically increased resistance" of the organism (SNIR), laid down the theoretical basis for separation of a new group of medicinal substances. The medicinal substances causing SNIR were named "adaptogens" (Brekhman and Dardimov, 1969). Generally, adaptogens refer to those drugs that enable one to withstand stress and strain of life, impart immunity to give protection against diseases, postpone aging and improve vigor, vitality and longevity. They are also referred as adjustive medicine. The concept of "adjustive" remedies has been difficult to prove experimentally. A bi-functional information exchange network between the nervous and immune system is established by specific receptors for humoral substances on cells of nervous and immune systems. In particular, neuroregulators (neurotransmitters and neuromodulators) can modulate specific immune system function(s) and immunoregulators (immunomodulators) can modulate specific nervous system function(s). Acute and chronic inflammatory processes, malignancy, and immunological reactions stimulate the synthesis and release of immunomodulators in various cell systems. These immunomodulators have pivotal roles in the coordination of the host defense mechanisms and repair and induce a series of endocrine, metabolic, and neurologic response (Plata-Salaman, 1989). However with recent insight into the neuroendocrine immune system regulation, such adjustive effects on the homeostatic system of the body seem a very likely possibility.

11.3.1.1 Botanicals with adaptogenic activity

***Mistletoe lectin*:** Defined, non-toxic doses of the galactoside-specific mistletoe lectin (mistletoe lectin-I, a constituent of clinically approved plant extract) have immunomodulatory potencies. The obvious ability of certain lectins to activate non-specific mechanisms supports the assumption that lectin-carbohydrate interactions may induce clinically beneficial immunomodulation. Randomized multi-centre trials are being performed to evaluate the ability of complementary mistletoe lectin-I treatment to reduce the rate of tumor recurrences and metastases, to improve overall survival as well as the quality of life and to exert immunoprotection in cancer patients under tumor destructive therapy (Beuth, 1997). In a recent study on healthy human subjects, treatment with ML stimulates the production of GM-CSF, IL-5 and IFNgamma by PBMC, and this is accompanied by an increase of eosinophil- and granulocyte-counts (Huber *et al.*, 2005). In another clinical study on cancer patients, adjuvant potential of ML was established with BCG for superficial bladder cancer (Elsasser-Beile *et al.*, 2005). These observations may, therefore, open rational therapeutic indications for mistletoe extracts.

Panax ginseng: *Panax ginseng* (Araliaceae), a Korean/Chinese medicine employed for its putative medicinal properties in South Asia, stimulated basal natural killer (NK) cell-activity following sub-chronic exposure and helped stimulate recovery of NK function in cyclophosphamide-immunosuppressed mice but did not further stimulate NK activity in poly I:C treated mice, T and B cell responses were not affected. *Panax ginseng* provided a degree of protection against infection with *Listeria monocytogenes* but did not inhibit growth of transplanted syngenetic tumor cells. Increased resistance to *L. monocytogenes* was not detected in challenged mice previously given immunosuppressive doses of cyclophosphamide. These data suggest that *Panax ginseng* have some immunomodulatory properties, primarily associated with NK cell activity (Kim *et al.*, 1990). Ginseng alone, or in combination with vitamins and minerals, is mainly being promoted as general tonics, which increases non-specific resistance and sometimes even as an aphrodisiac. Ginseng on prolonged use shows a few adverse effects, notable of which is the "Ginseng abuse syndrome" (Siegel, 1979). In a recent study, Ginseng was found to enhance the anti-proliferation effect of 5-FU on HCT-116 human colorectal cancer cells (Wang *et al.*, 2007). In another study, Ginseng was found to reduce the genotoxic effect of cyclophosphamide (Wang *et al.*, 2006).

Achyranthes bidentata: *Achyranthes bidentata* polysaccharide (ABP), root extract (25–100 mg/kg, day –1 to 7), could inhibit tumor growth (S-180) by 31%–40%. Combination of cyclophosphamide and ABP increased the rate of tumor growth inhibition by 58%. ABP could potentiate LAK cell activity and increase the Con A induced production of tumor necrosis factor (TNF-β) from murine spleenocytes. The S-180 cell membrane content of sialic acid was increased and phospholipid decreased after ABP acting on cells for 24 hours. Data suggest that the anti-tumor mechanism of ABP may be related to potentiation of host immunosurveillance mechanism and the changes in cell membrane features (Yu and Zhang, 1995).

Viscum album **and** ***Echinacea purpurea*****:** Extracts of *Viscum album* (Plenosol) and *Echinacea purpurea* (Echinacin) are used clinically for their non-specific action on cell-mediated immunity. These two were shown to possess a stimulating effect on the production of lymphokines by lymphocytes and in the transformation test. A toxic effect on cells was produced only with very high, clinically irrelevant concentrations. Clinical application of these extracts can produce a stimulation of cell-mediated immunity (one therapeutic administration followed by a free interval of one week) or can have a depressive action (daily administration of higher doses). These observations were confirmed by lymphokine production and assay, 3H for at least three months, thymidine incorporation and a skin test with recall antigens (Coeugniet and Elek, 1987). In another experimental model, *Echinacea purpurea* extracts protected non-cancerous cells from apoptosis (Huntimer *et al.*, 2006). While, administration of Echinacea was found to have a significant effect on survival time of leukemia mice. These studies further support adjuvant potential of Echinacea (Miller, 2005).

11.3.1.2 Rasayana botanicals as adaptogens

Tinospora cordifolia**:** Treatment with aqueous, alcohol, acetone and petroleum ether extracts of stem of *Tinospora cordifolia* (TC) resulted in significant improvement in mice swimming time and body weights, petroleum ether extract showed significant protective effect against cyclophosphamide-induced immunosuppression. Prevention of cyclophosphamide-induced anemia was also reported (Patil *et al.*, 1997). TC was also found to promote thymic homeostasis via modulation of thymocyte proliferation and apoptosis resulting in higher survival in tumor-bearing animals (Singh *et al.*, 2005).

Withania somnifera**:** Pre-treatment with *Withania somnifera, Tinospora cordifolia, Asparagus racemosus*, induced a significant leucocytosis in cyclophosphamide-induced myelosuppressed animals. PMN functions, in terms of phagocytosis and intracellular killing were stimulated, as well as reticulo-endothelial system functions were greatly activated in treated animals. The phagocytic functions of peritoneal and alveolar macrophages were also stimulated with *Tinospora cordifolia*, *Asparagus racemosus* and *Emblica officinalis*. *Tinospora cordifolia*, *Asparagus racemosus*, *Emblica officinalis*, *Terminalia chebula*, *Bacopa monira* and *Withania somnifera* improved the carbon clearance, indicating stimulation of the reticulo endothelial system. A significant increase in the proliferative fraction in the bone marrow was observed in mice treated with *Tinospora cordifolia* as revealed in flow cytometry analysis (Dahanukar and Thatte, 1997). In a comparative pharmacological investigation of *Withania somnifera* (*Ashwagandha*) and Ginseng, showed a significant difference in anti-stress activity. Ginseng exhibited higher anti-stress activity, however gastric ulcers due to swimming stress were notably less in *Ashwagandha*. The anabolic study revealed that *Ashwagandha*-treated group had a greater gain in the body weight than the Ginseng group (Grandhi *et al.*, 1994).

11.3.2 *Chemoprotection*

Modern cancer therapy produces substantial acute and chronic toxicity, which impairs quality of life and limits the effectiveness of treatment. Recent clinical and laboratory data suggest that repair of treatment-related injury is a multiphase and continuous process providing multiple opportunities for pharmacologic intervention. A host of agents (toxicity antagonists) that modulate normal tissue response or interfere with mechanisms of toxicity are under development. Although significant challenges remain, the routine application of such agents promises to substantially reduce treatment-related morbidity and potentially allow treatment intensification in high-risk disease. The concept of site-specific inactivation of cytotoxic anti-cancer agents has been explored with numerous modalities. The goal of such chemoprotection is to improve the therapeutic ratio of an agent by selectively reducing its toxicity in non-tumor bearing tissue, which is target for dose-limiting toxicity. Furthermore, a chemoprotectant cannot add new toxicities that might otherwise limit the administration of maximally tolerated doses of chemotherapeutic agent (Dorr, 1991; Matthew and Craig, 1999).

11.3.2.1 Chemoprotection: drug targets and current trends

Chemoprotection and cytoprotection are studied under preventive oncology and are interchangeable terms in cancer chemotherapy. Preventive oncology applies pharmacological agents to reverse, retard, or halt progression of neoplastic cells to invasive malignancy (Krzystyniak, 2002). Cancer chemoprevention is one of newer approaches in the management of cancer. Epidemiological observations, pre-clinical animal pharmacology, knockout models, cancer cell lines and clinical trials have shown the efficacy of this approach. Many drug targets are under clinical development; prostaglandin pathway, estrogen receptor modulation, gluthathione peroxidase inhibition and immunomodulation appear promising. Celecoxib, tamoxifen, retinoids, rexinoids, selenium, tocopherols and mofarotene are some of the promising leads and are in clinical development (Krishnan *et al.*, 2003). New opportunities in clinical chemoprevention research include investigating the chemopreventive effects of phytochemicals (Kucuk, 2002). Safer immunomodulating agents suitable for long-term therapy remain an unmet therapeutic need.

11.3.2.2 Botanical immunomodulators as chemoprotectants

***Withania somnifera*:** It is an official drug mentioned in the Indian Herbal Pharmacopoeia and Ayurvedic Pharmacopoeia (Indian Herbal Pharmacopoeia, 1998). Studies indicate that *Withania somnifera* (Ashwagandha) (WS) modulated cyclophosphamide-induced toxicity. This reduction was in the terms of reversal of leuopenia, increase in bone marrow cellularity and reduction in CP-associated urotoxicity. Towards pharmacological mechanisms, WS was found to enhance interferon gamma (IFN-gamma), interleukin-2 (IL-2) and granulocyte macrophage colony stimulating factor (GM-CSF), which were lowered down by cyclo-phosphamide administration (Davis and Kuttan, 1999). These studies indicate *Withania somnifera* could reduce the cyclophosphamide toxicity is therefore useful in cancer chemotherapy (Davis and Kuttan, 1998). WS was also shown to prevent lipid peroxidation (LPO) in stress-induced animals indicating its adjuvant as well as chemoprotectant activity (Dhuley, 1998). In another mechanistic study, WS was found to be modulatory on O6-methylguanine-DNA methyltransferase (MGMT), which is important for chemoprevention from alkylating agent-induced O6 alkyl guananidines (Niture *et al.*, 2006). Glycowithanolides, consisting of equimolar con-centrations of sitoindosides VII-X and withaferin A, were isolated from the roots of WS and evaluated for protection in iron-induced hepatoxicity in rats. Ten days of oral administration of these active principles, in graded doses (10, 20 and 50 mg/kg), resulted in attenuation of hepatic lipid per-oxidation (LPO), the serum enzymes, alanine aminotransferase, aspartate aminotransferase and lactate dehydrogenase during iron-induced hepatoxicity (Bhattacharya *et al.*, 1987). In addition, anti-stress activity observed with *Withania somnifera* will be an additional benefit along with chemoprotectant activity.

***Tinospora cordifolia*:** It is widely used in Ayurvedic medicines and is known for its immunomodulatory, anti-hepatotoxic, anti-stress and antioxidant properties. It has been used in combination with other plant products to prepare a number of Ayurvedic preparations. The chemistry has been extensively studied and its chemical constituents can be broadly divided into alkaloids, diterpenoids, steroids, flavanoids and lignans. Reviews have appeared on quaternary alkaloids and biotherapeutic diterpene glucosides of *Tinospora* species. Much of the work has been carried out on berberine, jatrorrhizine, tinosporaside and columbin. Extracts of *Tinospora cordifolia* (TC) has been shown to inhibit the lipid peroxidation and superoxide and hydroxyl radicals *in vitro*. The extract was also found to reduce the toxic side-effects of cyclophosphamide (25 mg/kg, 10 days) in

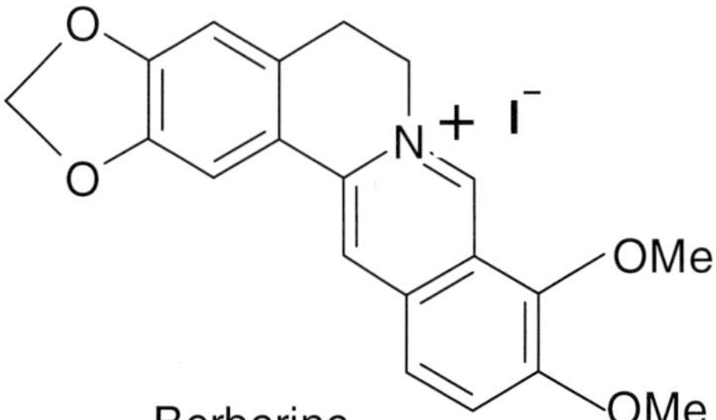

Berberine

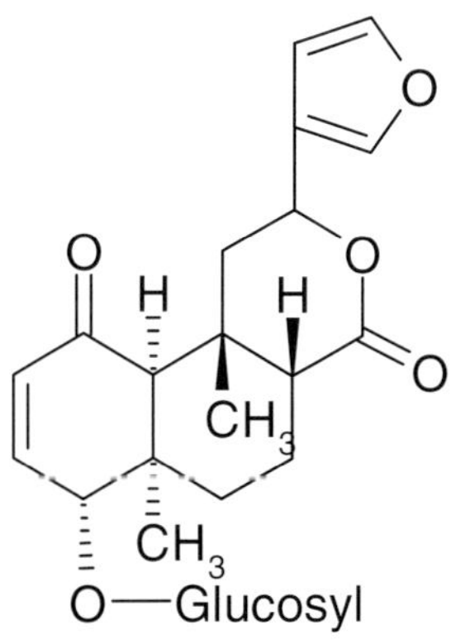

Tinosporaside

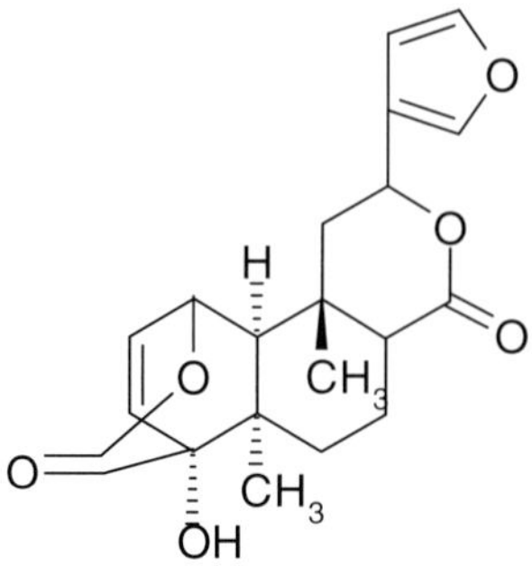

Columbin

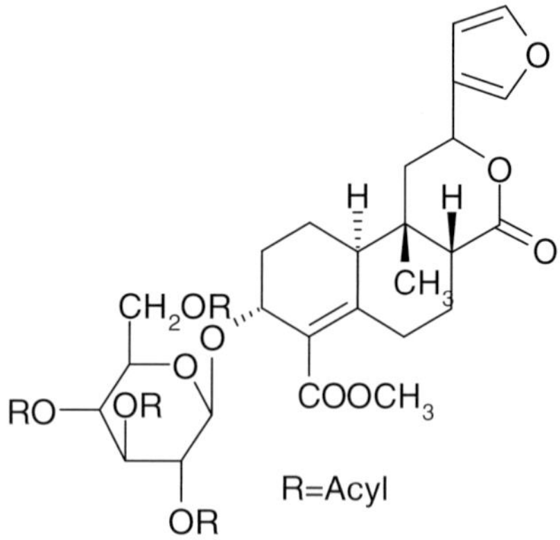

Cordifoliside A

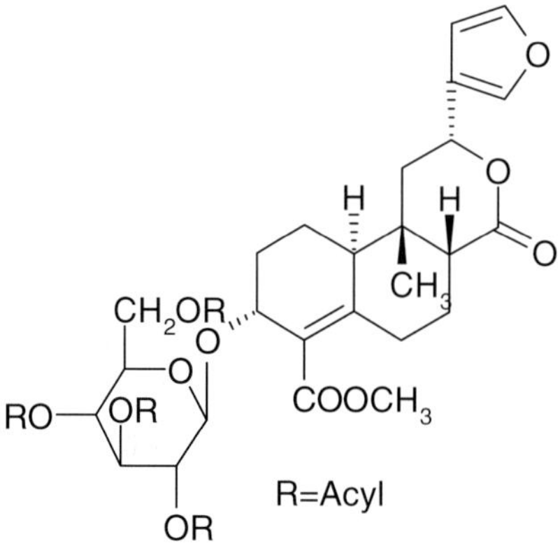

Cordifoliside B

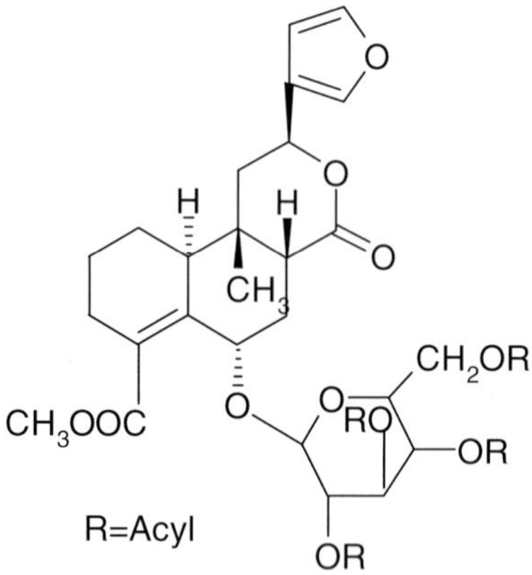

Cordifolioside C

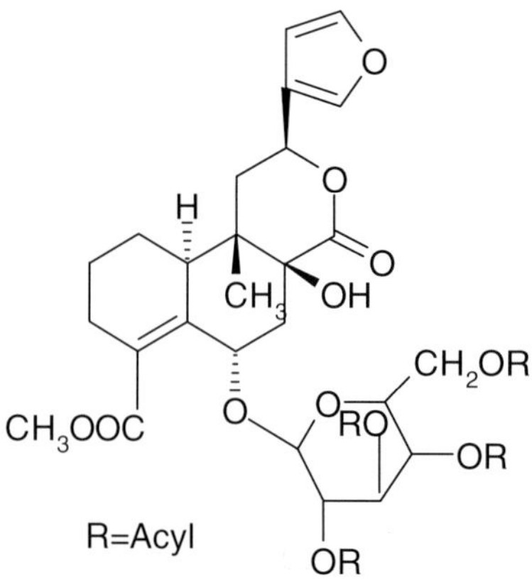

Cordioside

mice hematological system by the free radical formation as seen from total white cell count, bone marrow cellularity and α-esterase positive cells (Matthew and Kuttan, 1997). Extracts of *Tinospora cordifolia* have been shown to inhibit the lipid peroxidation and superoxide and hydroxyl radicals *in vitro*. The extract was also found to reduce the toxic side-effects of cyclophosphamide administration in mice. Moreover, administration of the extract partially reduced the elevated lipid peroxides in serum and liver as well as alkaline phosphatase and glutamine pyruvate transaminase, thus indicating the use of *Tinospora* extracts in reducing the chemotoxicity induced by free radical forming chemical (Matthew and Kuttan, 1997).

Active principles of TC were found to possess anti-complementary and immunomodulatory activities (Kapil and Sharma, 1997). TC is reported for its various immunopharmacological activities, e.g. inhibition of C3-convertase of the classical complement pathway. Humoral and cell-mediated immunity were reported for cardioside, cardifolioside A and cardiol and its activation were more pronounced with increasing incubation time (Patil, 1997). Extracts of *Tinospora cordifolia* has been shown to inhibit the lipid peroxidation and superoxide and hydroxyl radicals *in vitro*. The extract was also found to reduce the toxic side-effects of cyclophosphamide (25 mg/kg, 10 days) in mice hematological system by free radical formation as seen from total white cell count, bone marrow cellularity and α-esterase positive cells. In a recent clinical study, TC was found to protect against choloroqunine-induced spleenomegaly in slow responders, where 35%–50% regression of spleen size coupled with increase in Hb was observed, suggesting chemoprotection (Singh, 2005).

***Tinospora bakis*:** A dose-dependent cytoprotection by *Tinospora bakis*; a plant from Senegalese pharmacopoeia was observed the *in vitro* model. Lyophilized aqueous extract of plant roots decreased intracellular enzyme release (LDH and ASAT) from CCL_4-intoxicated hepatocytes isolated from rats. The cytoprotective effect was more effective for long course treatment (Diallo-Sall *et al.*, 1997).

***Asparagus racemosus*:** Chemically, *Asparagus racemosus* (AR) contains steroidal saponins, known as shatavarins, isoflavanones, isoflavones including 8-methoxy-5, 6,4′-trihydroxyisoflavone 7-O-beta-D-glucopyranoside, asparagamine, a polycyclic alkaloid, racemosol, a cyclic hydrocarbon

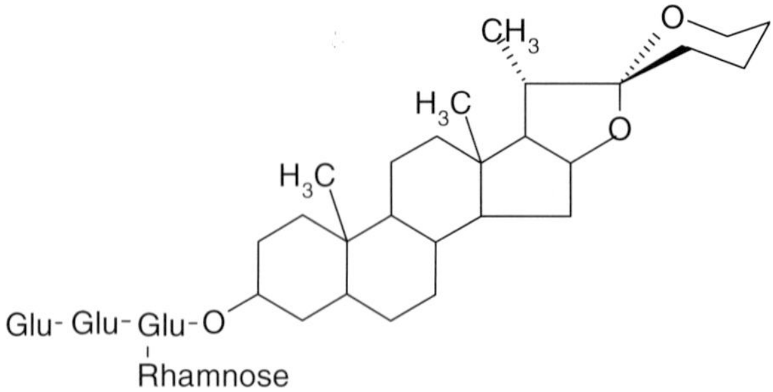

Shatavarin

(9,10-dihydrophenanthrene), polysaccharides and mucilage. It has been shown to stimulate macrophages and influence favorably long-term adaptation. It has been shown to stimulate macrophages and influence favorably long-term adaptation. Possible links between immunomodulatory and neuropharmacological activity have been suggested. Extracts of *Asparagus racemosus* were evaluated for its neuroendocrine immune modulating effect. It prevents stress-induced increase in plasma cortisol along with an activation of peritoneal macrophages and inhibition in gastric vascular damage (Dahanukar and Thatte, 1988). A comparative study between *Asparagus racemosus*, *Tinospora cordifolia*, glucan and lithium carbonate against the myelosuppressive effects of single (200 mg/kg, subcut.) and multiple doses (three doses, 30 mg/kg, *i.p.*) of cyclophosphamide in mice revealed all four drugs prevented, to varying degrees, leucopenia produced by cyclophosphamide (Thatte and Dahanukar, 1988). Treatment of *Asparagus racemosus* significantly inhibited Ochratoxin A-induced suppression of chemotactic activity and production of IL-1 and TNF-alpha by macrophages (Dhuley, 1997).

***Crocetin*:** A natural carotenoid, crocetin, at a dose of 50 mg/kg modulated the release of chloroaceteldehyde; a urotoxic metabolite of cyclophosphamide in the urine of mice given combined treatment. Crocetin at the same dose significantly elevated glutathione-S-transferase enzyme activity both in the bladder and the liver of mice treated with cyclophosphamide. In Sarcoma-180 tumor-bearing mice, crocetin has the ability to protect against cyclophosphamide-induced bladder toxicity without altering its anti-tumor activity (Chang *et al.*, 1996). Crocetin also inhibited benzo (a) pyrene induced

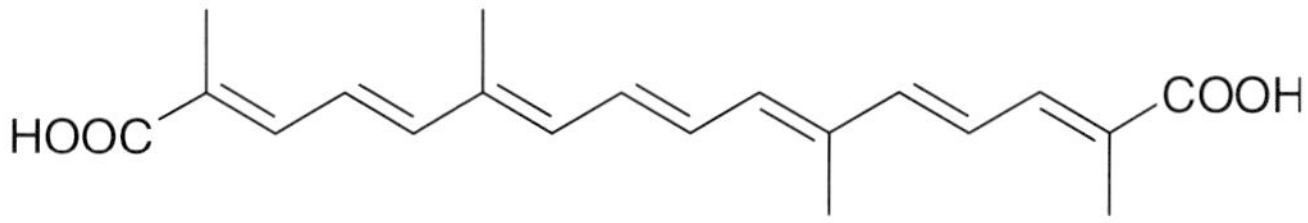

Crocetin

genotoxicity and neoplastic transformation in C3H10T1/2 cells. Crocetin was found to increase the activity of GST and decreases the formation of a benzo (a) pyrene-DNA adduct (Nair *et al.*, 1993).

***UL*-409:** Oral administration of UL-409, a herbal formulation at a dose of 600 mg/kg significantly prevented the occurrence of cold-resistant stress-induced ulcerations in Wistar rats, alcohol- and aspirin-induced gastric ulceration as well as cysteamine- and histamine-induced duodenal ulcers in rats and guinea pigs, respectively. The volume and acidity of gastric juice in pyloric-ligated rats was also reduced by UL-409. It also significantly, and dose-dependently, promoted gastric mucus secretion in normal as well as in stress-, drug- and alcohol-induced ulceration in animals (Mitra *et al.*, 1996).

***Mikania cordata*:** Induction of Phase 2 enzymes is an effective and sufficient strategy for achieving protection against the toxic and neoplastic effects of many carcinogens. Literature reports suggest that chemopreventive action of *Mikania chordata* is because of its effect on Phase 2 enzymes. *Mikani cordata* oral administration resulted in increased activities of microsomal uridine diphosphoglucose dehydrogenase, reduced nico-tinamide adenine dinucleotide (phosphate): quinine reductase and cytosolic glutathione s-transferases with a concomitant elevation in the contents of reduced glutathione. It was also found to increase total protein mass, fractional rate of protein synthesis, *Mikania chordata* ribosomal capacity and efficiency (rate/ribosome) and high turnover rate of protein (protein/DNA) on pre-treatment in CCL_4-treated hepatic tissue. This indicated the tissue repair leading to a functional improvement of the CCL_4 disorganized hepatocytes (Bishayee and Chatterjee, 1992). Oral administration of methanolic fraction of *Mikania cordata* (Burm., B. L. Robinson) significantly prevented occurrence of water immersion stress-induced gastric ulcers in a dose-responsive manner. The extract also dose-dependently inhibited gastric ulcers induced by ethanol, aspirin and phenylbutazone. The volume, acidity and peptic activity of the gastric juice in pylorus-ligated rates were not altered upon administration of the extract but significantly and dose-dependently promoted gastric mucus secretion in normal as well as stress- and ethanol-induced ulcerated animals. It was claimed that, the observed activity might be due to the modulation of defensive factors through an improvement of gastric cytoprotection (Mandal *et al.*, 1992).

Indigenous herbal drug formulations: *Brahma Rasayana* and *Ashwagandha Rasayana* were found to protect mice from cyclophosphamide-induced (50 mg/kg daily for 14 days) myelosuppression and subsequent leucopenia (Praveenkumar *et al.*, 1994). Treatment with *Asparagus racemosus*, *Tinospora cordifolia*, *Withania somnifera* and *Picrorhiza kurrooa* significantly inhibited carcinogen ochratoxin A (OTA)-induced suppression of chemotactic activity and production of interleukin-1 (IL-1) and tumor necrosis factor-alpha (TNF-α) by macrophages. Immu-21 poly herbal formulation that contains extracts of *Ocimum sanctum*, *Withania somnifera*, *Emblica officinalis* and *Tinospora cordifolia* at 100 mg/kg, daily, over seven days, and 30 mg/kg daily over 14 days, prevented cyclophosphamide-induced genotoxicity in mice (Jena *et al.*, 2003).

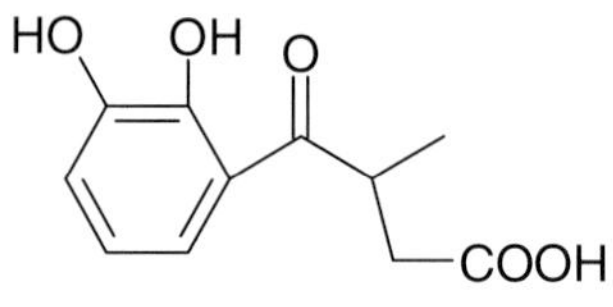

Plumbagin

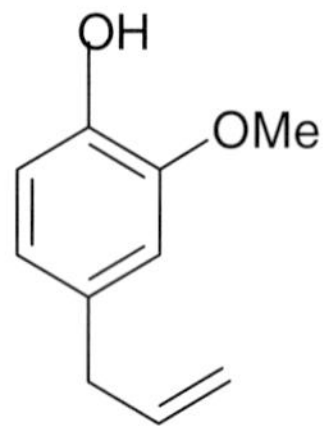

Eugenol

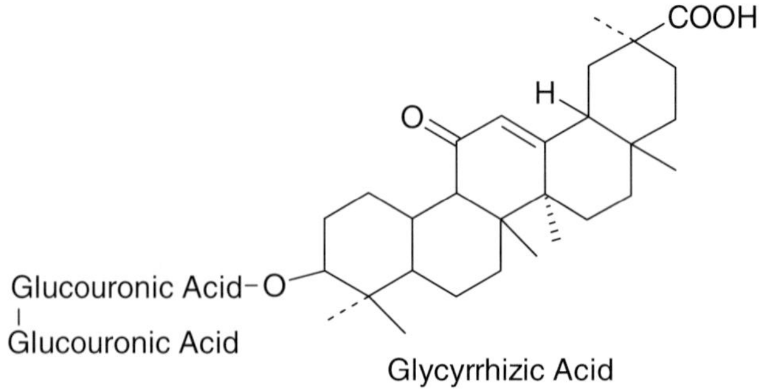

Glycyrrhizic Acid

11.3.2.3 Antioxidants in cytoprotection

A number of phytochemicals like caffeine, genistein, melatonin, silymarin, squalene, glycyrrhizic acid, plumbagin, eugenol, etc. have multiple physiological effects as well as antioxidant activity, which result in cyto-protection *in vivo*. Many antioxidants have additional immunomodulatory and anti-mutagenic properties and their modulation of cytotoxicity needs further examination and evaluation (Weiss and Landauer, 2003).

11.3.3 *Radioprotection*

Radiotherapeutics is still one of the major treatment modalities practiced for control of localized solid tumors. The major goal of therapy is the achievement of a total tumor control with limited toxicity and complications. Radiation doses that can be delivered without causing severe damage to surrounding normal tissues can be insufficient to eradicate a tumor. New strategies for the prevention of radiation injuries are currently being explored with the ultimate aim of developing globally radioprotective, non-toxic pharmacologics. This include development of agents as radiosensitizers, apoptosis inducers in tumor cells and radioprotectants, which can increase the radiosensitivity of such resistant tumors, reduce the radiation dose required and protect the normal tissue morbidity associated with tumoricidal radiation doses. Radioprotective agents, although widely studied in past four decades and include several thousand agents, have not reached the level of providing the agent that conforms to criteria of an optimal radio-protective, including effectiveness, specificity, availability, toxicity and tolerance. The prophylactic treatments under review encompass diverse pharmacological classes as novel immunomodulators, nutritional antioxidants, and cytokines (Weiss and Landauer, 2003).

With the advancement in understanding of tumor cell biology, many molecular mechanisms/targets have been identified for modulation of radiation response. Some important ones are COX-II, MMPs, TRAIL (TNFα–related apoptosis inducing ligand)/Apo2L, epidermal growth factor receptor (EGFR), etc. (Lammering, 2003; Marini and Belka, 2003; Petersen *et al.*, 2003). Substances reducing the radiation-induced toxicity by modulating the biological response to radiation injury may represent an alternative concept in radioprotection and hence there is interest and a need for new compounds that can protect tissues from radiation injury. Natural compounds may have an advantage, being more structurally diverse and safer, and hence more acceptable for human application.

11.3.3.1 Radioprotectants from botanicals

***Withaferin A*:** A steroidal lactone from *Withania somnifera* inhibited growth of Ehrlich ascites carcinoma in Swiss mice with increased survival and life-span. Anti-tumor and radiosensitizing effect was observed with combination treatment of abdominal gamma irradiation with withaferin A, resulting in increased tumor cure and tumor-free survival (Devi, 1996). Withaferin A showed growth inhibitory effect *in vitro* on both Chinese hamster V79 cells and HeLa cells. It reduced the survival of V79 cells in a dose-dependent manner (Sharada *et al.*, 1996). Combination treatment of alcoholic extract of *Withania somnifera* (500 mg/kg, i.p. 10 days) with one local exposure to gamma radiation (10 Gy) followed by hyperthermia (43°C for 30 minutes) significantly increased the tumor cure (Sarcoma 180 grown on the dorsum of adult BALB/c mouse), growth delay and animal survival. This combination was also significantly and synergistically depleted the tumor GSH level. Thus, *Ashwagandha*, in addition to having a tumor inhibitory effect, also acts as a radiosensitizer, and heat enhances these effects. The severe depletion in the tumor GSH content by the

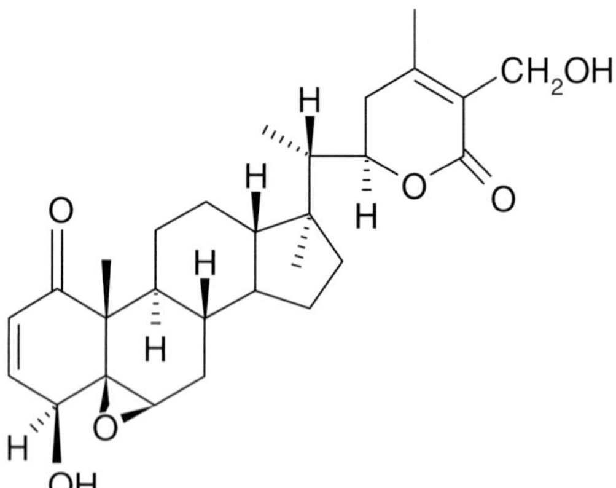

Withaferin A

combination treatment must have enhanced the tumor response, as the inherent protection by the thiol will be highly reduced (Devi *et al.*, 1993). The presence of a wide variety of effects such as hypotensive, anti-spasmodic, anti-tumor, anti-arthritic, anti-pyretic, analgesic, anti-inflammatory and hepatoprotective activities and anti-stress properties show that *Withania somnifera* may be acting by non-specifically increasing the resistance of the animals to various stressful conditions (Asthana and Raina, 1989).

11.3.4 *Botanical Immunomodulators as anti-tumor agents*

Plant products have contributed several novel compounds possessing promising anti-tumor activity. Crude extract of *Withania somnifera* root has a strong tumoricidal and tumor growth inhibitory activity. The combination of paclitaxel with *W. somnifera* could effectively treat the benzo(a)pyrene-induced lung cancer in mice by offering protection from reactive oxygen species damage and also by suppressing cell proliferation (Senthilnathan *et al.*, 2006a). Further, decreased activities of TCA cycle key enzymes such as isocitrate dehydrogenase (ICDH), succinate dehydrogenase (SDH), malate dehydrogenase (MDH) and alpha-ketoglutarate dehydrogenase (alpha-KGDH) in lung cancer bearing animals were observed (Senthilnathan *et al.*, 2006b) In a recent study, WS was inhibitory on vascular endothelium growth factor (VEGF), induced neo-vascularization was recorded (Mathur *et al.*, 2006). In another report, WS was found effective against forestomach and skin carcinogenesis and up to 60% and 92% inhibition in tumor incidence and multiplicity, respectively was observed. Towards immunological mechanisims, many reports including ours have confirmed up-regulation of Th1 response in various experimental models (Bani *et al.*, 2006; Khan *et al.*, 2006). A number of withanolides isolated from this plant have been reported in literature to possess both immunosuppressive and immunostimulatory properties. However, withaferin A has been claimed to attribute anti-cancer properties of WS. Withaferin A has been reported to show marked tumor inhibitory activity *in vitro* against cells derived from human carcinoma of nasopharynx and experi-mental mouse tumors. A single i.p. dose of withaferin A injection 24 or 48 hours after Ehrlich's ascites tumor transplantation produced an immediate growth reduction in 3%–80% of mice followed by complete disappearance of tumor cells in the peritoneal cavity of the surviving mice with no signs of tumor development. Further, withaferin A was found to inhibit proliferation in HUVECs (IC_{50} = 12 nM) at doses that are significantly lower than those required for tumor cell lines through a process associated with inhibition of cyclin D1 expression indicating angiogenesis inhibition. This phenomenon was also observed in WS extract, supporting withaferin A as the compound responsible for anti-cancer profile of WS (Mohan *et al.*, 2004). Towards pharmacological mechanisms, withaferin A was found to modulate NF Kappa B expression, which is an important target for inflammation and cancer (Kaileh *et al.*, 2007).

***Asparagus racemosus*:** Anti-tumor activity of the crude saponins obtained from shoots of *Asparagus racemosus* (asparagus crude saponins, ACS), was found to have anti-tumor activity. It inhibited the growth of human leukemia HL-60 cells in culture and macromolecular synthesis in a dose- and time-dependent manner. The ACS at 75–100 μgrams/ml range was cytostatic, at concentrations greater than 200 μgrams/ml was cytocidal to HL-60 cells. ACS at 6 and 50 μgrams/ml inhibited the synthesis of DNA, RNA and protein in HL-60 cells by 41%, 5% and 4% or by 84%, 68% and 59% respectively. The inhibitory effect of ACS on DNA synthesis was irreversible (Shao *et al.*, 1996).

11.4 Discussion

Critical analysis of these reports suggests that botanical immunomodulators have a strong and developing case for integration in cancer therapy. The analysis is based on the following observed facts/activities:

(1) significant modulation of chemotherapy-induced myelosuppression and reversal of cell counts (mainly, neutrophils and lymphocytes);
(2) modulation of host protective immunity resulting in higher survival percentages in tumor bearing animals (lag in tumor development and higher clearance-like effects resulting in tumor free survivals);
(3) evidences of efficacy as chemo and radioprotectants (modulation of genotoxicity also reported);
(4) evidences of synergism with chemotherapy in mediating higher anti-tumor activity;

(5) evidence of significant activity on relevant targets such as kinases, VEGF, COX, TNF-alpha and GM-CSF, etc.;
(6) modulation of host antioxidant enzyme systems such as isocitrate dehydrogenase (ICDH), succinate dehydrogenase (SDH), malate dehydrogenase (MDH) and alpha-ketoglutarate dehydrogenase (alpha-KGDH), suggesting their beneficial effect on chemotherapy-induced oxidative stress; and
(7) safety: these botanicals were found to be safe up to 2500 mg/kg levels on oral administration.

Clearly, these reports are also supportive towards the potential of ethnopharmacology approaches in drug discovery and the use of botanicals as novel sources for discovery of curative synergistic combinations and/or multi-target molecules for cancer therapy. However, significant bottlenecks remain for following up these observations to clinic, limited information on efficacy of these botanicals in tumor models; little information on cellular targets; and tissues relating to quality control and standardization (Diwanay *et al.*, 2004b).

We have been studying *Rasayana* botanicals namely *Withania somnifera*, *Tinospora cordifolia*, and *Asparagus racemosus*. Our studies on these plants revealed that these plants have significant immunomodulatory activity that varies according to biological stimuli. Given that, we tried to explore the efficacy of these botanicals in three different conditions such as cancer, inflammation and infection. In cancer study, we followed a system pharmacology approach, where the effect of test materials was studied on three different aspects of anti-cancer therapy in a similar model. We studied the effect of these test materials on chemotherapy-induced myelo-suppression, anti-tumor and effect on host immunity in tumor-bearing animals. We observed that treatment of ascitic sarcoma bearing mice with formulation of total extracts of WS and TC and alkaloid free polar extract of WS resulted in protection towards cyclophosphamide-induced myelo- and immuno-suppression, while some polar fractions from WS showed anti-tumor activity. Further, WS, TC and AR extracts were found to potentiate antigen-specific immunity in chemotherapy-treated tumor-bearing animals. WS and TC had significant effects on cellular immunity whereas AR modulated humoral immunity preferentially (Diwanay *et al.*, 2004a). Taking lead from these observations, AR, WS and TC were evaluated for their immunoadjuvant potential in the *pertussis* model, where these plants reduced the dose of vaccine required to confer protection against *pertussis* intracerebral challenge, increasing survival percentage and significant increase in *pertussis* antibody titers. The same trend was repeated where higher humoral immunity was observed with AR whereas TC and WS showed preference towards cellular immunity (Gautam *et al.*, 2004a and b). In the inflammation model, WS has shown moderate analgesic, anti-inflammatory and disease-modifying activity in experimental animals and arthritis patients (Saraf *et al.*, 1989; Ziauddin *et al.*, 1996; Agarwal *et al.*, 1999). Towards clinical efficacy, formulation containing same WS extract, showed disease-modifying activity in arthritis patients (Chopra *et al.*, 2004). These trends indicated that these plants have relevant targets for addressing cancer, inflammation and infection. This can be further supported by recent evidence of common immunological targets in these three indications (Dalgleish, 2005; Lucia and Torkko, 2004). Towards pharmacological mechanisms, we hypothesized that these test materials have significant effect on immune-homeostasis. Our hypothesis is supported by studies on CpG oligonucleitides that modulated targets relevant to cancer, inflammation and infection and which was shown to have modulatory influence on immune homeostasis or Th1-Th2 balance (Yang, 2003; Weiner, 2000). Taking lead, we explored the effect of TC, WS and AR on Th1-Th2 balance in normal and immune suppressed states using flow cytometry. Levamisole was used as positive control. The studies indicated that while WS and TC have a significant effect on Th1 (cellular target for CMI immunity), AR showed mixed Th1/Th2 activity. The correlations of Th1 and mixed Th1/Th2 activity with cellular and humoral immunity respectively are well established. Moreover, these plants exhibited modulatory effects on cytotoxic lymphocyte ($CD8^+$ T cells) production leading to reduced tumor growth (Senthilnathan *et al.*, 2006a). In a comparative pharmacological investigation of WS and Ginseng, the WS-treated group showed better anabolic and anti-stress activity than Ginseng with additional anti-inflammatory activity (Singh *et al.*, 2005). Towards standardization, the active groups in TC (terpenoids), AR (saponins) and WS (withanolides) were identified and effective ratios were established. The studies towards further identification of synergistic moieties following the same approach are in progress.

In summary, there are clear trends to show that ethnopharmacology knowledge and experiential base have potential to offer a safer and cost-effective approach towards discovery of newer chemical diversity for such newer multi-target approaches (Wermuth, 2004; Patwardhan, 2005). A golden triangle consisting of Traditional Knowledge, Modern Medicine and Modern Science with systems orientation will converge to form an innovative discovery engine for newer, safer, affordable and effective therapies (Mashelkar, 2005; Patwardhan and Gautam, 2005). In India, efforts in these directions are underway to establish pharmacoepidemiological and experimental evidence base for new chemical/molecular entities and development of standardized herbal formulations under the Council for Scientific and Industrial Research and Government of India's New Millennium Indian Technology Leadership Initiative (CSIR, 2006) and Department of Science and Technology and Government of India's Drugs and Pharmaceutical Research Program (DST, 2004).

11.4 Conclusion

Many chemical agents are used as chemoprotectants for conventional cancer chemotherapy and/or radiation therapy. However, their effect is locoregional and is dependent on dose and time of administration in contest to anti-cancer drugs. The limitations and inconvenience of their use has stimulated research for discovering natural resources with immunological activity. Various botanicals and ethnopharmacological agents of traditional medicine are under investigation for chemoprotective and immunomodulatory activities. The results are encouraging. Chemoprofiling of these botanicals have been reported but most of the activity reports are on crude, semi-processed extracts and or fractions. Several reports suggest cytostatic, cytotoxic properties along with enhanced immune function in extract and/or polyherbal formulations. Nevertheless, any single component isolated from extract or formulation may not retain all the three desired properties. There have been attempts to isolate and characterize active moieties with limited success. Many authors have hypothesized the presence of synergism and buffering in extracts, however, systematic scientific investigations on pharmacodynamics, kinetics, dosing and interactions need to be undertaken to study these principles. Furthermore, studies are required to better understand the molecular and biochemical mechanisms involved in immunoregulation and its role in cytoprotection and radioprotection. Such efforts might lead to effective integration of botanical medicine in cancer therapy. This review will be useful in the bioprospecting exercises for developing newer, safer and effective agents for therapeutic management of cancer.

References

Agarwal, R., Diwanay, S., Patki, P.S. and Patwardhan, B. (1999) Studies on immunomodulatory activity of *Withania somnifera* in experimental immune inflammation. *J. Ethnopharmacol.* **67**, 27–35.

Asthana, R. and Raina, M.K. (1989) Pharmacology of *Withania somnifera* (Linn) Dunal — A review. *Indian Drug* **26**(5), 199–205.

Bani, S., Gautam, M., Sheikh, F.A., Khan, B., Satti, N.K., Suri, K.A., Qazi, G.N. and Patwardhan, B. (2006) Selective Th1 up-regulating activity of *Withania somnifera* aqueous extract in an experimental system using flow cytometry. *J. Ethnopharmacol.* **107**(1), 107–115.

Beuth, J. (1997) Clinical relevance of immunoactive mistletoe lectin-I. *Anti-cancer Drug* **8**(1), S53–S55.

Bhattacharya, A., Ramanathan, M., Ghosal, S. and Bhattacharya, S.K. (1987) Anti-stress activity of sitoindosides VII and VIII: New acylsterylglucosides from *Withania somnifera*. *Phytother. Res.* **1**, 32–37.

Bishayee, A. and Chatterjee, M. (1994) Anticarcinogenic biological response of *Mikania cordata*. Reflections in hepatic biotransformation systems. *Cancer Lett.* **81**(2), 193–200.

Brekhman, I.L. and Dardimov, I.V. (1969) New substances of plant origin which increase non-specific resistance. *Ann. Rev. Pharmacol.* **21,** 419–426.

Chang, W.C., Lin, Y.L., Lee, M.J., Shiow, S.J. and Wang, C.J. (1996) Inhibitory effect of crocetin on benzo (a) pyrene genotoxicity and neoplastic transformation in C3H10T1/2 cells, *Anti-cancer Res.* **16**(6B), 3603–3608.

Chopra, A., Levin, P., Patwardhan, B. and Chitre, D. (2004) A 32-week randomized, placebo controlled clinical evaluation of RA 11, an ayurvedic drug for treatment of osteoarthritis of knees. *J. Clin. Rheumatol.* **10**, 236–245.

Coeugniet, E.G. and Elek, E. (1987) Immunomodulation with *Viscum album* and *Echinacea purea* extracts. *Onkologie* **10**(3), 27–33.

CSIR (2006) www.csir.res.in/csir/external/heads/collaborations/NM.pdf

Dahanukar, S.A. and Thatte, U.M. (1988) *Rasayana* concept of Ayurveda myth or reality: An experimental study. *Indian Pract.*, pp. 245–252.

Dahanukar, S.A. and Thatte, U.M. (1997) Current status of Ayurveda in phytomedicine. *Phytomedicine* **4**(4), 359–368.

Dalgleish, A.G. (2005) Cancer and Inflammation. *Br. J. Cancer* **92**, 792–793.

Davis, L. and Kuttan, G. (1998) Suppressive effect of cyclophosphamide-induced toxicity by *Withania somnifera* extract in mice. *J. Ethnopharmcol.* **62**(3), 209–214.

Davis, L. and Kuttan, G. (1999) Effect of *Withania somnifera* on cytokine production in normal and cyclophosphamide treated mice. *Immunopharmcol. Immunotoxicol.* **21**(4), 695–703.

Devi, P.U. (1996) *Withania somnifera* Dunal (Ashwagandha): Potential plant source of a promising drug for cancer chemotherapy and radiosensitization. *Indian J. Exp. Biol.* **34**(10), 927–932.

Devi, P.U., Sharada, A.C., Solomon, F.E. and Kamath, M.S. (1992) *In vivo* growth inhibitory effect of *Withania somnifera* (*Ashwagandha*) on a transplantable mouse tumor, Sarcoma 180. *Indian J. Exp. Biol.* **30**, 169–172.

Devi, P.U., Sharada, A.C. and Soloman F.E. (1993) Anti-tumor and radiosensitizing effects of *Withania somnifera* (*Ashwagandha*) on a transplantable mouse tumor, Sarcoma-180. *Indian J. Exp. Biol.* **31**(7), 607–611.

Dhuley, J.N. (1997) Effect of some Indian herbs on macrophage functions in ochratoxin A treated mice. *J. Ethnopharmacol.* **58**(1), 15–20.

Dhuley, J.N. (1998) Effect of Ashwagandha on lipid peroxidation in stress-induced animals. *J. Ethnopharmacol.* **60**(2), 173–178.

Diallo-Sall, A., Niang-Ndiaye, M., Ndiaye, A.K. and Dieng, C.F. (1997) Hepatoprotective effect of a plant from the *Senegalese pharmacopoeia*: *Tinospora bakis* (*Menispermaceae*) using an *in vitro* model. *Dakar. Med.* **42**(1), 15–18.

Diwanay, S., Chitre, D. and Patwardhan, B. (2004a) Immunoprotection by botanical drugs in cancer chemotherapy. *J. Ethnopharmacol.* **90**, 49–55.

Diwanay, S., Gautam, M. and Patwardhan, B. (2004b) Cytoprotection and immunomodulation in cancer therapy. *Curr. Med. Chem.* **4**, 479–490.

Dorr, R.T. (1991) Chemoprotectants for cancer chemotherapy. *Semin. Oncol.* **18**(1), 48–58.

Druker, B.J. and Karnofsky, D.A. (2003) Award Lecture. Imatini as a paradigm of targeted therapies. *J. Clin. Oncol.* **21**(23 Suppl), 239s–245s.

DST (2004) http://www.dst.gov.in/scientific-programme/td-drugs.htm

Elliott, R.L. and Head, J.F. (2005) Host immunity ignored in clinical oncology: A medical opinion. *Cancer Biother. Radiopharm.* **20**(2), 123–125.

Elsasser-Beile, U., Leiber, C., Wolf, P., Lucht, M., Mengs, U. and Wetterauer, U. (2005) Adjuvant intravesical treatment of superficial bladder cancer with a standardized mistletoe extract. *J. Urol.* **174**(1), 76–79.

Faivre, S., Djelloul, S. and Raymond, E. (2006) New paradigms in anti-cancer therapy: Targeting multiple signaling pathways with kinase inhibitors. *Semin Oncol.* **33**(4), 407–420.

Gautam, M., Diwanay, S., Gairola, S., Shinde, Y.S., Jadhav, S.S. and Patwardhan, B.K. (2004a) Immune response modulation to DPT vaccine by aqueous extract of *Withania somnifera* in experimental system. *Int. Immunopharmacol.* **4**, 841–849.

Gautam, M., Diwanay, S., Gairola, S., Shinde, Y.S., Patki, P. and Patwardhan, B.K. (2004b) Immunoadjuvant potential of *Asparagus racemosus* aqueous extract in experimental system. *J. Ethnopharmacol.* **91**, 251–255.

Grandhi, A., Mujumdar, A.M. and Patwardhan, B. (1994) A comparative pharmacological investigation of Ashwagandha and Ginseng. *J. Ethnopharmacol.* **44**, 131–135.

Huber, R., Rostock, M., Goedl, R., Ludtke, R., Urech, K., Buck, S. and Klein, R. (2005) Mistletoe treatment induces GM-CSF- and IL-5 production by PBMC and increases blood granulocyte and eosinophil counts: A placebo controlled randomized study in healthy subjects. *Eur. J. Med. Res.* **18**(10), 411–418.

Huntimer, E.D., Halaweish, F.T. and Chase, C.C. (2006) Proliferative activity of *Echinacea angustifolia* root extracts on cancer cells: Interference with doxorubicin cytotoxicity. *Chem. Biodivers.* **3**(6), 695–703.

Indian Herbal Pharmacopoeia. (1998) Joint publication of Indian Drugs Manufacturer's Association and Regional Research Laboratory Jammu-Tawi, pp. 165–173.

Jena, G.B., Nemmani, K.V., Kaul, C.L. and Ramarao, P. (2003) Protective effect of a polyherbal formulation (Immu-21) against cyclophosphamide-induced mutagenicity in mice. *Phytother. Res.* **17**(4), 306–310.

Kaileh, M., Vanden Berghe, W., Heyerick, A., Horion, J., Piette, J., Libert, C., De Keukeleire, D., Essawi, T. and Haegeman, G. (2007) Withaferin A strongly elicits IKappaβ kinase beta hyperphosphorylation concomitant with potent inhibition of its kinase activity. *J. Biol. Chem.* **282**, 4253–4264.

Kapil, A. and Sharma, S. (1997) Immunopotentiating compounds from *Tinospora cordifolia*. *J. Ethnopharmacol.* **58**(2), 89–95.

Kerr, D.J. and La Thangue, N.B. (2004) Signal transduction blockade and cancer: Combination therapy or multi-targeted inhibitors? *Ann. Oncol.* **15**(12), 1727–1729.

Khan, B., Ahmad, S.F., Bani, S., Kaul, A., Suri, K.A., Satti, N.K., Athar, M. and Qazi, G.N. (2006) Augmentation and proliferation of T lymphocytes and Th-1 cytokines by *Withania somnifera* in stressed mice. *Int. Immunopharmacol.* **6**(9), 1394–1403.

Kim, J.Y., Germolee, D.R. and Luster, M.I. (1990) *Panax ginseng* as a potential immunomodulator: Studies in mice. *Immunopharmacol. Immunotoxicol.* **12**(2), 257–276.

Krishnan, K., Campbell, S., Abdel-Rahman, F., Whaley, S. and Stone, WL. (2003) Cancer chemoprevention drug targets. *Curr. Drug Target* **4**(1), 45–54.

Krzystyniak, K.L. (2002) Current strategies for anti-cancer chemoprevention and chemoprotection. *Acta Pol. Pharm.* **59**(6), 473–478.

Kucuk, O. (2002) New opportunities in chemoprevention research. *Cancer Invest.* **20**(2), 237–245.

Lammering, G. (2003) Anti-epidermal growth factor receptor strategies to enhance radiation action. *Curr. Med. Chem.* **3**(5), 327–333.

Lucia, M.S. and Torkko, K.C. (2004) Inflammation as a target for prostate cancer chemoprevention: Pathological and laboratory rationale. *J. Urol.* **172**(6 Pt 1), 2483–2484.

Mandal, P.K., Bishayee, A. and Chatterjee, M. (1992) Stimulation of hepatic protein synthesis in response to *Mikania cordata* root extract in carbon tetrachloride-induced hepatotoxicity in mice. *Ital. J. Biochem.* **41**(6), 345–351.

Marini, P. and Belka, C. (2003) New strategies for combined treatment with ionizing radiation. *Curr. Med. Chem.* **3**(5), 334–342.

Mashelkar, R.A. (2005). Global voices of science: India's R&D. Reaching for the top. *Science* **307**, 1415–1417.

Mathur, R., Gupta, S.K., Singh, N., Mathur, S., Kochupillai, V. and Velpandian, T. (2006) Evaluation of the effect of *Withania somnifera* root extracts on cell cycle and angiogenesis. *J. Ethnopharmacol.* **105**(3), 336–341.

Mathew, S. and Kuttan, G. (1997) Antioxidant activity of *Tinospora cordifolia* and its usefulness in the amelioration of cyclophosphamide activity. *J. Exp. Clin. Cancer. Res.* **16**(4), 407–411.

Matthew, L. and Craig, L. (1999) Chemoprotectants: A review of their clinical pharmacology and therapeutic efficacy. *Drug* **57**, 293–308.

Miller, S.C. (2005) Echinacea: A miracle herb against aging and cancer? Evidence *in vivo* in mice. *Evid. Complement. Altern. Med.* **2**(3), 309–314.

Mitra, S.K., Gopumadhavan, S., Hemavathi, T.S., Muralidhar, T.S. and Venkataranganna, M.V. (1996) Protective effect of UL-409, a herbal formulation against physical and chemical factor induced gastric and duodenal ulcers in experimental animals. *J. Ethnopharmacol.* **52**(3), 165–169.

Mohan, R., Hammers, H.J., Bargagna-Mohan, P., Zhan, X.H., Herbstritt, C.J., Ruiz, A., Zhang, L., Hanson, A.D., Conner, B.P., Rougas, J. and Pribluda, V.S. (2004) Withaferin A is a potent inhibitor of angiogenesis. *Angiogenesis* **7**(2), 115–122.

Nair, S.C., Panikar, K.R. and Parthod, R.K. (1993) Protective effect of crocetin on bladder toxicity induced by cyclophosphamide. *Cancer Biother.* **8**(4), 339–343.

Niture, S.K., Rao, U.S. and Srivenugopal, K.S. (2006) Chemopreventative strategies targeting the MGMT repair protein: Augmented expression in human lymphocytes and tumor cells by ethanolic and aqueous extracts of several Indian medicinal plants. *Int. J. Oncol.* **29**(5), 1269–1278.

Patil, M., Patki, P., Kamath, H.V. and Patwardhan, B. (1997) Antistress activity of *Tinospora cordifolia* (Wild) Miers. *Indian Drug* **34**(4), 211–215.

Patwardhan, B. (2000) Ayurveda: The designer medicine. Review of ethnopharmacology and bioprospecting research. *Indian Drug* **37**, 213–227.

Patwardhan, B. (2005) Ethnopharmacology and drug discovery. *J. Ethnopharmacol.* **100**, 50–52.

Patwardhan, B. and Gautam, M. (2005) Botanical immunodrugs: Scope and opportunities. *Drug Discov. Today* **10**, 495–502.

Patwardhan, B. and Patwardhan, A. (2006) Traditional medicine: Modern approach for affordable global health, *Report for World Health Organization's Commission on Intellectual Property Innovation & Public Health*, Ancient Science of Life, Supplement to Silver Jubilee issue, Jan–July.

Patwardhan, B., Kalbag, D., Patki, P.S. and Nagasampagi, B.A. (1990) Search of immunoregulatory agent — a review. *Indian Drug* **28**(2), 56–63.

Patwardhan, B., Vaidya, A. and Chorgade, M. (2004) Ayurveda and natural products drug discovery. *Curr. Sci.* **86**, 789–799.

Patwardhan, B., Warude, D., Pushpangadan, P. and Bhatt, N. (2005) Ayurveda and traditional Chinese medicine: A comparative overview. *Evid. Complement. Altern. Med.* **2**(4), 465–473.

Petersen, C., Baumann, M. and Petersen, S. (2003) New targets for the modulation of radiation response — selective inhibition of the enzyme cyclooxygenase 2. *Curr. Med. Chem.* **3**(5), 354–359.

Plata-Salaman, C.R. (1989) Immunomodulators and feeding regulation: A humoral link between the immune and nervous systems. *Brain Behav. Immun.* **3**(3), 193–213.

Praveenkumar, V., Kuttan, R. and Kuttan, G. (1994) Chemoprotective action of Rasayanas against cyclophosphamide toxicity. *Tumori* **80**, 306–308.

Rege, N.N. (1999) Adaptogenic properties of six Rasayana herbs in ayurvedic medicine. *Phytother. Res.* **13**, 275–291.

Saraf, M.N., Ghooi, R.B. and Patwardhan, B. (1989) Studies on mechanism of action of *S. anacardium* in rheumatoid arthritis. *J. Ethnopharmacol.* **25**, 159–164.

Senthilnathan, P., Padmavathi, R., Magesh, V. and Sakthisekaran, D. (2006a) Chemotherapeutic efficacy of paclitaxel in combination with *Withania somnifera* on benzo(a)pyrene-induced experimental lung cancer. *Cancer Sci.* **97**(7), 658–664.

Senthilnathan, P., Padmavathi, R., Magesh, V. and Sakthisekaran, D. (2006b) Modulation of TCA cycle enzymes and electron transport chain systems in experimental lung cancer. *Life Sci.* **78**(9), 1010–1014.

Shao, Y., Chin, C.K., Ho, C.T., Ma, W., Garrison, S.A. and Huang, M.T. (1996) Anti-tumor activity of the crude saponins obtained from asparagus. *Cancer Lett.* **104**(1), 31–36.

Sharada, A.C., Soloman, F.E., Devi, P.U., Udupa, N. and Srinivasan, K.K. (1996) Anti-tumor and radiosensitizing effects of withaferin A on mouse Ehrlich ascites carcinoma *in vivo*. *Acta Oncol.* **35**(1), 95–100.

Siegel, R.K. (1979) Ginseng abuse syndrome — problems with the Panacea. *J. Am. Med. Assoc.* **241**(15), 1614–1615.

Singh, R.K. (2005) *Tinospora cordifolia* as an adjuvant drug in the treatment of hyper-reactive malarious splenomegaly — case reports. *J. Vector Borne Dis. Mar.* **42**(1), 36–38.

Singh, N., Singh, S.M., Prakash and Singh, G. (2005) Restoration of thymic homeostasis in a tumor-bearing host by *in vivo* administration of medicinal herb *Tinospora cordifolia*. *Immunopharmacol. Immunotoxicol.* **27**(4), 585–599.

Tam, Y.K. (2003) Immunostimulatory oligonucleotides: Ready for immunotherapy prime time! *J. Hematother. Stem Cell Res.* **12**, 467–471.

Thatte, U.M. and Dahanukar, S.A. (1988) Comparative study of immuno-modulating activity of Indian medicinal plants, lithium carbonate and glucan. *Methods Find. Exp. Clin. Pharmacol.* **10**, 639–644.

Wang, C.Z., Luo, X., Zhang, B., Song, W.X., Ni, M., Mehendale, S., Xie, J.T., Aung, H.H., He, T.C. and Yuan, C.S. (2007) Notoginseng enhances anti-cancer effect of 5-fluorouracil on human colorectal cancer cells. *Cancer Chemother. Pharmacol.* **60**(1), 69–70.

Wang, Z., Zheng, Q., Liu, K., Li, G. and Zheng, R. (2006) Ginsenoside Rh(2) enhances antitumour activity and decreases genotoxic effect of cyclophosphamide. *Basic Clin. Pharmacol. Toxicol.* **98**(4), 411–415.

Weiner, G.J. (2000) Immunostimulatory DNA sequences and cancer therapy. *Semin. Immunopathol.* **22**, 107–116.

Weiss, J.F. and Landauer, M.R. (2003) Protection against ionizing radiation by antioxidant nutrients and phytochemicals. *Toxicology* **189**(1–2), 1–20.

Wermuth, C.G. (2004) Multitargeted drugs: The end of the 'one target-one disease' philosophy? *Drug Discov. Today* **9**, 826–827.

Yu, S. and Zhang, Y. (1995) Effect of Achyranthes bidenta polysaccharide (ABP) on anti-tumor activity and immune function of S-180 bearing mice. *Chung Hua Chung Liu Tsa Chih* (*China*) **17**(4), 275–278.

Ziauddin, M., Phansalkar, N., Patki, P.S., Diwanay, S. and Patwardhan, B. (1996) Studies on immunomodulatory effects of *Ashwagandha*. *J. Ethnopharmacol.* **50**, 69–76.

Chapter 12

Bioactive Polysaccharides from TCM Herbs as Anti-Cancer Adjuvants

Raymond Chang

Abstract

Purpose: To review the nature, extent, bioactivities and clinical application of bioactive polysaccharides in Traditional Chinese Medicine (TCM), especially as adjuvants in cancer treatment.

Methodology: Literature Review.

Findings: Many fungal and plant derived bioactive polysaccharides with a broad range of immunomodulatory activities are found in TCM. Some such polysaccharides have been developed into drugs and showed clinical efficacy in controlled trials while the majority of such compounds remain as nutraceuticals with only preliminary research. Such polysaccharides are generally non-toxic and also possess other bioactivities such as inducing differentiation, stimulating hematopoiesis, anti-metastasis, and anti-angiogenesis, which make them ideal adjuvants in modern cancer therapy.

Conclusion: Bioactive polysaccharides occur extensively in TCM herbs and is the basis of potential useful application of TCM as adjuvant in cancer therapies.

Keywords: Polysaccharides; Medicinal Plants; Traditional Chinese Medicine; Cancer.

12.1 Introduction

As a major class of biomolecules, carbohydrates are the most complex and least appreciated for their bioactivity (Stryer, 1995). In the past three decades, an increasing number of reports describing the isolation and bioactivity of polysaccharide glucans and proteoglucans from plant and other sources highlight the potential role of this class of molecules in cancer therapy as a result of its immunostimulatory properties (Wong *et al.*, 1994). More recently, other biological mechanisms such as apoptotic and anti-angiogenic effects including its effects on the c-Myc, c-Fos, and vascular endothelial growth factor (VEGF) expression (Yang, 2005) highlight the potential broad spectrum bioactivity of this class of compounds as anti-cancer adjuvants.

12.2 Bioactive Polysaccharides in Chinese Herbs

Known bioactive polysaccharides are found in fungi, lichens, higher plants, marine as well as animal sources throughout the world, but some of the most well characterized and clinically relevant polysaccharides are found in Traditional Chinese Medicine (TCM) (Ooi and Liu, 2000), especially those herbs from the TCM materia medica classically characterized as tonic in nature or having "Fu-Zhen" (Sun *et al.*, 1981) properties. Many such tonic Chinese herbs have been found to possess immunomodulatory and other anti-tumor bioactivities and are potentially useful in cancer therapy (Sun, 1986). As such, the search and characterization of novel, safe and effective natural compounds from Chinese herbs is a significant goal for anti-cancer research.

12.3 Immunomodulatory Property of Polysaccharides and the β-Glucan Receptor

Naturally derived polysaccharides including heteroglycans and proteoglycans of certain molecular weight and structure have specific broad-ranged immunomodulatory properties which have been recognized for several decades. Such immunomodulating activity includes activation of macrophages (Adachi *et al.*, 1990), monocytes (Czop and Austen, 1985a), natural killer cells (Peter *et al.*, 1988), lymphocyte activated killer cells (Yamasaki *et al.*, 1989), dendritic cells (Kim, 2007), tumor-infiltrating lymphocytes (Kariya *et al.*, 1991) and other lymphocytes (Kumazawa *et al.*, 1985). The stimulated release of various cytokines including interferons (Kandefer-Szerszen and Kawecki, 1973), interleukins (Sakagami *et al.*,

1988), tumor necrosis factor (Abel and Czop, 1992) and colony stimulating factors (Hashimoto *et al.*, 1990) have also been well documented. Such polysaccharides are thus considered multi-cytokine inducers and this is probably due to induction of gene expression of various immunomodulatory cytokines and cytokine receptors (Liu *et al.*, 1999).

An important feature of the bioactivity of immunomodulatory polysaccharides is the importance of its structure-function relationship. Differences in molecular weight, tertiary structure or conformation, and composition all affect polysaccharide bioactivity. In general, polysaccharides in a configuration with β1–3, 1–4, or 1–6 branch chains are necessary for activity and complex branch-chained polysaccharides with anionic structures and higher molecular weights have greater immunostimulating activities (Cleary *et al.*, 1999). Differences in bioactivity may be due to differences in receptor affinity or receptor-ligand interaction on the cell surface (Mueller *et al.*, 2000).

The description of a beta-glucan receptor on monocytes by Czop and Austen (1985b) served as a basis to understand the immunopotentiating bioactivity of polysaccharides and explained why herbs and materials from different sources with similarly structured polysaccharide content share similar immunomodulatory activity.

12.4 Immunomodulatory Property of Polysaccharides and the Toll-Like Receptor (TLR) System

The toll-like receptor (TLR) system constitutes a pylogenetically ancient, evolutionary conserved, archetypal pattern recognition system, which is the basis of antigen recognition by and activation of the immune system. Toll-like receptor agonists have long been used as immunoadjuvants in anti-cancer immunotherapy and increasing evidence suggests that cancer may progress via subversion of the TLR signalling pathways (Killeen *et al.*, 2006). Natural as well as synthetic ligands of TLR receptors such as lipid A analogs, poly(I:C), loxoribine, oligodeoxynucleotides have all been shown to be effective in regulating immune response (Fasciano and Li, 2006). The TLRs are expressed on macrophages and dendritic cells which are key in newly developed immunotherapeutic protocols against cancer (Buchsel and Demeyer, 2006). Immunomodulatory polysaccharides from single TCM herbs (Lin *et al.*, 2005) as well as TCM/Kampo herbal formulae (Chino *et al.*, 2005) have recently been found to modulate TLR receptors thus opening a new avenue to understand the biological basis of potential usefulness of polysaccharides from TCM in cancer therapies.

12.5 Polysaccharides as Anti-tumor Adjuvants

The usefulness of bioactive polysaccharides found in TCM with a β1–3 β1–4 or β1–6 configuration in enhancing the immune system and therefore indirectly reducing tumorigenesis as well as tumor growth has been extensively demonstrated in animals while prolonged survival as a result of treatment with polysaccharide derived nutraceuticals and drugs have been noted in a number of controlled clinical trials carried out in Japan and China.

12.6 Immunomodulatory and Anti-tumor Polysaccharides in TCM

Immunopotentiating traditional Chinese herbs with proven anti-tumor activity may be broadly considered as fungals or botanicals. Almost 200 species of such fungi have demonstrable anti-tumor activity, although not all such fungi are in the TCM pharmacopeia (Borchers *et al.*, 1999). Fungals especially from the Basidiomycetes family have been found to possess bioactive polysaccharides (Wasser and Weis, 1999). According to a survey by Jong and Donovick (1989), 109 anti-tumor subsances from fungi were from Basidiomycetes, and 51 of these were glucans or polysaccharide compounds from no less than 26 different species. Some of these fungal polysaccharides have been systematically studied as well as developed into nutraceuticals [e.g. *Agaricus blazei* (Itoh *et al.*, 1994), *Cordyceps sinensis* (Kuo *et al.*, 1996), *Ganoderma sp.* (Chang, 1996), *Grifola frondosa* (Hishida *et al.*, 1988)] or drugs [e.g. Krestin from *Coriolus versicolor* (Kondo and Torisu, 1985), Lentinan from *Lentinus edodes* (Chihara *et al.*, 1987), Schizophyllan from *schizophyllum communes* (Komatsu *et al.*, 1963)], but others have also been preliminarily studied (see Table 12.1).

As a representative agent, Lentinan from *Lentinus edodes* was identified in the late 1960s by Chihara *et al.* (1970). It is a branched

Table 12.1. Select medicinal fungi reported to contain bioactive polysaccharides.

Agaricus blazei (Ohno *et al.*, 2001)
Auricularia auricula (Misaki, 1981)
Flammulina velutipes (Leung *et al.*, 1997)
Hericium erinaceum (Mizuno *et al.*, 1992)
Inonotus sp. (Ohtsuka *et al.*, 1977)
Phellinus sp. (Han *et al.*, 1999)
Pleurotus sp. (Chenghua *et al.*, 2000)
Polyporus sp. (Zhang *et al.*, 1991)
Poria sp. (Kanayama *et al.*, 1986)
Tricholoma aggregatum (Komatsu *et al.*, 1973)
Tremella sp. (Xia and Lin, 1989)

chain molecule with a backbone of 1–3 β-D-glucan and side chains of β1–3 and β1–6 D-glucose residues. It has been demonstrated to elicit anti-tumor activity by the stimulation of host-mediated immune responses and thus inhibit the growth of implanted tumors in laboratory animals (Chihara, 1983). Lentinan has also been demonstrated to be active as a parenteral agent in prolonging survival in recurrent and metastatic gastric and colorectal cancer when given in combination with chemotherapy in controlled clinical trial (Nimura *et al.*, 2006; Wakui *et al.*, 1986). Recent advances in the biological understanding of polysaccharide function identifies the effect of Lentinan on dendritic cells to perhaps be a key factor for its anti-tumor effect in chemoimmunotherapy (Mushiake *et al.*, 2005).

Another representative agent is Krestin [PSK], which is a protein-bound polysaccharide extracted from the CM-101 strain of *Coriolus versicolor* (Kondo and Torisu, 1985). Unlike Lentinan, PSK is a β1–4 glucan containing 10% protein and is active orally. PSK has also been statistically demonstrated to prolong survival in clinical trials involving gastric (Nakazato *et al.*, 1994), colorectal (Mitomi *et al.*, 1992) esophageal (Ogoshi *et al.*, 1995), nasopharyneal (Go and Chung, 1989), non-small cell lung (Hayakawa *et al.*, 1993), and breast cancer (Toi *et al.*, 1992). The polysaccharide peptide (PSP) isolated from the COV-1 strain mycelia of *Coriolus versicolor* has proven benefits in clinical trials in China for esoplageal, gastric and lung cancers (Ng, 1998).

Table 12.2. Representative traditional Chinese/Kampo herbs reported to contain bioactive polysaccharides.

Acanthopanax Giraldii Harms (Wang *et al.*, 1992)
Achyranthes bidentata (Li and Li, 1997)
Aloe sp. (Zhang and Tizard, 1996)
Atractylodes (Inagaki *et al.*, 2001)
Beniscasa cerifera (Kumazawa *et al.*, 1985)
Cinnamomum cortex (Haranaka *et al.*, 1985)
Curcuma zedoaria (Kim *et al.*, 2000)
Codonopsis pilosula (Wang *et al.*, 1996)
Dipsacus asperoides (Zhang *et al.*, 1997)
Epimedium sagittatum (Liu *et al.*, 1991)
Imperata cylindrica (Pinilla and Luu, 1999)
Isatis indigotica (Xu and Lu, 1991)
Malva verticillata (Gonda *et al.*, 1990)
Panax notoginseng (Gao *et al.*, 1996)
Pseudostellaria heterophylla (Wang *et al.*, 1992)
Radix bupleuri (Geng and Chen, 1989)
Radix glycyrrhizia (Nose *et al.*, 1998)
Radix hadysari (Lan *et al.*, 1987)
Radix Rehmannia (Xu, 1992)
Salvia miltiorrhiza (Hromakova *et al.*, 1999)
Zizyphi fructus (Yamaoka *et al.*, 1996)

Besides fungals, many so called "Fu-Zhen" (tonifying) traditional Chinese herbs contain bioactive polysaccharides and have been studied for their immunomodulatory and anti-tumor activity. All of these are catalogued in a comprehensive and public online database on anti-cancer Asian materials developed and maintained by the Insitute of East-West Medicine in New York (www.asiancancerherb.info). These botanicals include common herbs such as *Actinidia chinensis* (Lin, 1988), *Angelica sinensis* (Choy *et al.*, 1994), *Astralgalus membranaceus* (Huang *et al.*, 1982), *Ligustrum lucidum* (Lau *et al.*, 1994), *Panax ginseng* (Lee *et al.*, 1997) as well as others (see Table 12.2).

TCM usually employs herbal formulae and most useful TCM formulae for cancer patients contain herbs with immunopotentiating activity from its polysaccharide content (Ito and Shimura, 1985a and b). Examples of standard TCM (and Kampo) formulae with published experimental results demonstrating such immunostimulatory properties include *Xiao-Chai-Hu-Tang* [*Sho-saiko-to*] (Nagatsu *et al.*, 1989), *Shi-quan-da-bu-tang* [*Juzen-taiho-to*] (Zee-Cheng, 1992) and *Bu-zhong-yi-qi-tang* [*Hochu-ekki-to*] (Li *et al.*, 1999).

12.7 Clinical Observations on Polysaccharides as Anti-cancer Adjuvants

It is important to realize that although TCM herbs that contain bioactive polysaccharides may derive some of their anti-cancer efficacy via immunopotentiation, many such herbs contain other complementary anti-neoplastic substances.

Conversely, such bioactive polysaccharides may have other anti-tumor actions beyond immunopotentiation. Such anti-tumor mechanisms include induction of cellular differentiation (Chen *et al.*, 1997), anti-angiogenesis (Kanoh *et al.*, 1994), and anti-metastasis (Kobayashi *et al.*, 1995). Furthermore, the polysaccharides have other applications beyond anti-tumor in cancer patients. Such agents may also be useful in enhancing hematopoiesis (Liu *et al.*, 1991), ameliorating side-effects of chemotherapy and radiation as well as generally improving the well-being of the cancer patient.

Most clinical trials of bioactive polysaccharides in cancer have used the agents with conventional treatments such as chemotherapy and radiation. It is important to note that such polysaccharides have been found to be clinically useful across a spectrum of solid-tumors, including colorectal, gastric, lung, and breast cancers, with the overall result of enhancing survival.

Regarding the issues of side-effects, besides the report of a low incidence of allergic reactions to individual herbs or polysaccharide drugs, major complications and/or organ toxicity has not so far been reported with this family of agents.

As there is always a concern of potential adverse interaction with conventional therapy with herbal or nutraceutical products, it is important to note that there have been no studies to suggest negative interactions with polysaccharide derived agents and chemotherapy or radiation.

Not all polysaccharides are comparable and it is not prudent to entirely rely on *in vitro* data on one aspect of a polysaccharide's effectiveness (e.g. NK cell stimulation) as a basis of comparing various different polysaccharide derived agents. While clinical trial data may not be available for many such agents, clinical decision should be guided by trial data if available, or by the extent and quality of available medical literature on each agent. Furthermore, it is important to carefully consider the choice of polysaccharide agent as there can be significant differences in bioactivity secondary to differences in species, cultivation, method of extraction, formulation, as well as route and amount of dosage. Practically, availability of agent, cost, and potential efficacy are the main clinical considerations when choosing a suitable polysaccharide to prescribe to a patient.

12.8 Future Directions in the Development of Polysaccharides as Cancer Adjuvants

From existing laboratory and clinical evidence, it is certain that bioactive polysaccharides in TCM herbs are multifaceted and useful adjuncts in cancer care. However, lack of standardization and pharmacokinetic data among a spectrum of popular polysaccharide based nutraceuticals, limited controlled trial data in the West on such agents, and relative lack of knowledge about these herbal agents among conventional cancer care professionals hamper the wide application of this unique class of agents. It is hoped that standardization as well as further clinical studies will be a basis for advancement in our knowledge and use of such agents.

References

Abel, G. and Czop, J.K. (1992) Stimulation of human monocyte beta-glucan receptors by glucan particles induces production of TNF-alpha and IL-1 beta. *Int. J. Immunopharmacol.* **14**, 1363–1373.

Adachi, Y., Ohno, N., Ohsawa, M., *et al.* (1990) Macrophage activation *in vitro* by chemically cross-linked (1->3)-beta-D-glucans. *Chem. Pharm. Bull.* **38**, 988–992.

Borchers, A.T., Stern, J.S., Hackman, R.M., *et al.* (1999) Mushrooms, tumors, and immunity. *Proc. Soc. Exp. Biol. Med.* **221**, 281–293.

Buchsel, P.C. and Demeyer, E.S. (2006) Dendritic cells: Emerging roles in tumor immunotherapy. *Clin. J. Oncol. Nurs.* **10**, 629–640.

Chang, R.Y. (1996) Potential application of Ganoderma polysaccharides in the immune surveillance and chemoprevention of cancer. In: *Mushroom Biology and Mushroom Products* (ed.) Royse, D.J. Pennsylvania State, University Park, pp. 153–159.

Chen, Y.J., Shiao, M.S., Lee, S.S. and Wang, S.Y. (1997) Effect of *Cordyceps sinensis* on the proliferation and differentiation of human leukemic U937 cells. *Life Sci.* **60**, 2349–2359.

Chenghua, D., Xingliang, Y., Xiaoman, G., *et al.* (2000) A beta-D-glucan from the sclerotia of pleurotus tuber-regium (Fr.) Sing. *Carbohydr. Res.* **328**, 629–633.

Chihara, G. (1983) Preclinical evaluation of lentinan in animal models. *Adv. Exp. Med. Biol.* **166**, 189–197.

Chihara, G., Hamuro, J., Maeda, Y., Arai, Y. and Fukuoka, F. (1970) Fractionation and purification of the polysaccharides with marked anti-tumor activity, especially lentinan, from *Lentinus edodes* (Berk.) Sing. (an edible mushroom). *Cancer Res.* **30**, 2776–2781.

Chihara, G., Hamuro, J., Maeda, Y.Y., *et al.* (1987) Anti-tumor and metastasis-inhibitory activities of lentinan as an immunomodulator: An overview. *Cancer Detect. Prev. Suppl.* **1**, 423–443.

Chino, A., Sakurai, H., Choo, M.K., *et al.* (2005) *Juzentaihoto*, a Kampo medicine, enhances IL-12 production by modulating Toll-like receptor 4 signaling pathways in murine peritoneal exudate macrophages. *Int. Immunopharmacol.* **5**, 871–882.

Choy, Y.M., Leung, K.N., Cho, C.S., *et al.* (1994) Immunopharmacological studies of low molecular weight polysaccharide from *Angelica sinensis*. *Am. J. Chin. Med.* **22**, 137–145.

Cleary, A., Kelly, G.E. and Husband, A.J. (1999) The effect of molecular weight and beta 1,6 linkages on priming of macrophage function in mice by (1–3)-beta-D-glucan. *Immunol. Cell. Biol.* **77**, 395–403.

Czop, J.K. and Austen, K.F. (1985a) Generation of leukotrienes by human monocytes upon stimulation of their beta-glucan receptor during phagocytosis. *Proc. Natl. Acad. Sci.* **82**, 2751–2755.

Czop, J.K. and Austen, K.F. (1985b) A β-glucan inhibitable receptor on human monocytes. *J. Immunol.* **134**, 2588–2593.

Fasciano, S. and Li, L. (2006) Intervention of Toll-like receptor-mediated human innate immunity and inflammation by synthetic compounds and naturally occurring products. *Curr. Med. Chem.* **13**, 1389–1395.

Gao, H., Wang, F., Lien, E.J. and Trousdale, M.D. (1996) Immunostimulating polysaccharides from Panax notoginseng. *Pharm. Res.* **13**(8), 1196–1200.

Geng, J.X. and Chen, S.R. (1989) Isolation and identification of polysaccharides from Radix Bupleuri. *Zhongguo Zhong Yao Za Zhi* **14**(1), 37–40, 63.

Go, P. and Chung, C.H. (1989) Adjuvant PSK immunotherapy in patients with carcinoma of the nasopharynx. *J. Int. Med. Res.* **17**, 141–149.

Gonda, R., Tomoda, M., Kanari, M., Shimizu, N. and Yamada, H. (1990) Constituents of the seed of *Malva verticillata* VI. Characterization and immunological activities of a novel acidic polysaccharide. *Chem. Pharm. Bull.* **38**, 2771–2774.

Han, S.B., Lee, C.W., Jeon, Y.J., *et al.* (1999) The inhibitory effect of polysaccharides isolated from *Phellinus linteus* on tumor growth and metastasis. *Immunopharmacology* **41**, 157–164.

Haranaka, K., Satomi, N., Sakurai, A., *et al.* (1985) Anti-tumor activities and tumor necrosis factor producibility of traditional Chinese medicines and crude drugs. *Cancer Immunol. Immunother.* **20**(1), 1–5.

Hashimoto, K., Suzuki, I., Ohsawa, M., Oikawa, S. and Yadomae, T. (1990) Enhancement of hematopoietic response of mice by intraperitoneal administration of a beta-glucan, SSG, obtained from *Sclerotinia sclerotiorum. J. Pharmacobiodyn.* **13**, 512–517.

Hayakawa, K., Mitsuhashi, N., Saito, Y., *et al.* (1993) Effect of Krestin (PSK) as adjuvant treatment on the prognosis after radical radiotherapy in patients with non-small cell lung cancer. *Anti-cancer Res.* **13**, 1815–1820.

Hishida, I., Nanba, H. and Kuroda, H. (1988) Anti-tumor activity exhibited by orally administered extract from fruit body of *Grifola frondosa* (*Maitake*). *Chem. Pharm. Bull.* **36**, 1819–1827.

Hromadkova, Z., Ebringerova, A. and Valachovic, P. (1999) Comparison of classical and ultrasound-assisted extraction of polysaccharides from *Salvia officinalis L. Ultrason. Sonochem.* **5**, 163–168.

Huang, Z.S., Lu, G.B. and Guo, J.H. (1982) Studies on the polysaccharides of *Huang Qi* (Astralgalus). *Acta. Pharm. Sin.* **17**, 200–204.

Inagaki, N., Komatsu, Y., Sasaki, H., *et al.* (2001) Acidic polysaccharides from rhizomes of *Atractylodes lancea* as protective principle in Candida-infeced mice. *Planta Med.* **67**, 428–431.

Itoh, H. and Shimura, K. (1985a) Studies on the anti-tumor activity of traditional Chinese medicines (I). *Gan To Kagaku Ryoho* **12**, 2145–2148 (in Japanese).

Itoh, H. and Shimura, K. (1985b) Studies on the anti-tumor activity of traditional Chinese medicines (II). The anti-tumor mechanism of traditional Chinese medicines. *Gan To Kagaku Ryoho* **12**, 2149–2154 (in Japanese).

Itoh, H., Amano, H. and Noda, H. (1994) Inhibitory action of a (1–>6)-beta-D-glucan-protein complex (FIII-2-b) isolated from *Agaricus blazei Murill* (*'himematsutake'*) on Meth A fibrosarcoma-bearing mice and its anti-tumor mechanism. *Jpn. J. Pharmacol.* **66**, 265–271.

Jong, S.C. and Donovick, R. (1989) Anti-tumor and antiviral substances from fungi. *Adv. Appl. Microbiol.* **34**, 183–262.

Kanayama, H., Togami, M., Adachi N., Fukai Y. and Okumoto, T. (1986) Studies of the anti-tumor active polysaccharides from the mycelia of *Poria cocos Wolf.* III. Anti-tumor activity against mouse tumors. *Yakugaku Zasshi* **106**, 307–312 (in Japanese).

Kandefer-Szerszen, M and Kawecki, Z. (1973) Water extracts of fungi as interferon inducers. *Acta Microbiol. Pol. Acad.* **5**, 163–168.

Kanoh, T., Matsunaga K., Saito K. and Fujii, T. (1994) Suppression of *in vivo* tumor-induced angiogenesis by the protein-bound polysaccharide PSK. *In Vivo* **8**, 247–250.

Kariya, K., Okamoto, N., Fujimoto, T., *et al.* (1991) Lysis of fresh human tumor cells by autologous peripheral blood lymphocytes and tumor-infiltrating lymphocytes activated by PSK. *Jpn. J. Cancer Res.* **82**, 1044–1050.

Killeen, S.D., Wang, J.H., Andrews, E.J. and Redmond, H.P. (2006) Exploitation of the Toll-like receptor system in cancer: A double-edged sword? *Br. J. Cancer* **95**, 247–252.

Kim, J.Y., Yoom, Y.D., Ahn, J.M., *et al.* (2007) Angelan isolated from *Angelica gigas Nakai* induces dendritic cell maturation through toll-like receptor 4. *Int. Immunopharmacol.* **7**(1), 78–87.

Kim, K.I., Kim, J.W., Hong, B.S., *et al.* (2000) Anti-tumor, genotoxicity and anticlastogenic activities of polysaccharide from *Curcuma zedoaria*. *Mol. Cell* **10**, 392–398.

Kobayashi, H., Matsunaga K. and Oguchi, Y. (1995) Antimetastatic effects of PSK (Krestin), a protein-bound polysaccharide obtained from basidiomycetes: An overview. *Cancer Epidemiol. Biomarkers Prev.* **4**, 275–281.

Komatsu, N., Okubo, S., Kikumoto, S., *et al.* (1963) Host mediated anti-tumor action of *Schizophyllum commune*. *Gann* **60**, 137–144.

Komatsu, N., Komatsu, N., Kikumoto, S., *et al.* (1973) *Process for Manufacture of Polysaccharides with Anti-tumor Action*. US Patent 4, 221, 705.

Kondo, M. and Torisu, M. (1985) Evaluation of anti-cancer activity of a protein-bound polysaccharide PS-K (Krestin). In: *Basic Mechanisms and Clinical Treatment of Tumor Metastasis* (eds.) Torisu, M. and Yoshida, T. Academic Press, New York, pp. 623–636.

Kumazawa, Y., Nakatsuru, Y., Fujisawa, H., *et al.* (1985) Lymphocyte activation by a polysaccharide fraction separated from hot water extracts of *Angelica acutiloba Kitagawa. J. Pharmacobiodyn.* **8**, 417–424.

Kuo, Y.C., Tsai, W.J., Shiao, M.S., *et al.* (1996) *Cordyceps sinensis* as an immunomodulatory agent. *Am. J. Chin. Med.* **24**, 111–125.

Lan, Z.F., Zhang, Z.L., Cheng, G.Q., *et al.* (1987) Effects of Radix Hadysari polysaccharide on immunological function and transplanted tumors in mice. *Zhongguo Yao Li Xue Bao* **8**(3), 275–277 (in Chinese).

Lau, B.H., Ruckle, H.C., Botolazzo, T. and Lui, P.D. (1994) Chinese medicinal herbs inhibit growth of murine renal cell carcinoma. *Cancer Biother.* **9**, 153–161.

Lee, Y.S., Chung, I.S., Lee, I.R., *et al.* (1997) Activation of multiple effector pathways of immune system by the antineoplastic immunostimulator acidic polysaccharide ginsan isolated from *Panax ginseng. Anti-cancer Res.* **17**, 323–331.

Leung, M.Y., Fung, K.P. and Choy, Y.M. (1997) The isolation and characterization of an immunomodulatory and anti-tumor polysaccharide preparation from *Flammulina velutipes. Immunopharmacology* **35**, 255–263.

Li, T., Tamada, K., Abe, K., *et al.* (1994) The restoration of the anti-tumor T cell response from stress-induced suppression using a traditional Chinese herbal medicine *Hochu-ekki-to* (TJ-41:*Bu-Zhong-Yi-Qi-Tang*). *Immunopharmacology* **43**, 11–21.

Li, Z.K. and Li D.D. (1997) The immunomodulatory effect of *Achyranthes bidentata* polysaccharides. *Yao Xue Xue Bao* **32**, 881–887 (in Chinese).

Lin, P.F. (1988) Anti-tumor effect of *Actinidia chinensis* polysaccharide on murine tumor. *Zhonghua Zhong Liu Za Zhi* **10**(6), 441–444 (in Chinese).

Lin, Y.L., Liang, Y.C., Lee, S.S. and Chiang, B.L. (2005) Polysaccharide purified from *Ganoderma lucidum* induced activation and maturation of human monocyte-derived dendritic cells by the NF-kappaB and p38 mitogen-activated protein kinase pathways. *J. Leukoc. Biol.* **78**, 533–543.

Liu, F., Ding, G. and Li, J. (1991) Effects of *Epimedium sagittatum Maxim.* Polysaccharides on DNA synthesis of bone marrow cells of "yang deficiency"animal model caused by hydroxyurea. *Zhongguo Zhong Yao Za Zhi* **16**, 620–622 (in Chinese).

Liu, F., Ooi, V.E. and Fung, M.C. (1999) Analysis of immunomodulating cytokine mRNAs in the mouse induced by mushroom polysaccharides. *Life Sci.* **64**, 1005–1011.

Misaki, A., Kakuta, M., Sasaki, T.M., Tanaka, M. and Miyahi, H. (1981) Studies on interrelation of structure and anti-tumor effects of polysaccharides:

Anti-tumor action of periodate-modified, branched (1–3)-β-D-glucan of *Auricularia auricula-judae* and other polysaccharides containing (1,3)-glycoside. *Carbohydr. Res.* **92**, 115–129.

Mitomi, T., Tsuchiya, S., Iijima, N., *et al.* (1992) Randomized controlled study on adjurant immunochemotherapy with PSK in curatively resected colorectal cancer. The Cooperative Study Group of Surgical Adjuvant Immunochemotherapy for Cancer of Colon and Rectum (Kanagawa). *Dis. Colon. Rectum* **35**(2), 123–130.

Mizuno, T., Wasa, T., Ito, H., Suzuki, C. and Ukai, N. (1992) Anti-tumor-active polysaccharides isolated from the fruiting body of *Hericium erinaceum*, an edible and medicinal mushroom called *yamabushitake* or *houtou. Biosci. Biotechnol. Biochem.* **56**, 347–348.

Mueller, A., Raptis, J., Rice, P.J., *et al.* (2000) The influence of glucan polymer structure and solution conformation on binding to (1–>3)-beta-D-glucan receptors in a human monocyte-like cell line. *Glycobiology* **10**, 339–346.

Mushiake, H., Tsunoda, T., Nukatsukia, M., *et al.* (2005) Dendritic cells might be one of key factors for eliciting anti-tumor effect by chemoimmunotherapy *in vivo. Cancer Immunol. Immunother.* **54**, 120–128.

Nagatsu, Y., Inoue, M. and Ogihara, Y. (1989) Modification of macrophage functions by *Shosaikoto* (kampo medicine) leads to enhancement of immune response. *Chem. Pharm. Bull.* **27**, 1540–1542.

Nakazato, H., Koike, A., Saji, S., *et al.* (1994) Efficacy of immunochemotherapy as adjuvant treatment after curative resection of gastic cancer. *Lancet* **343**, 1122–1126.

Ng, T.B. (1998) A review of research on the protein-bound polysaccharide (polysaccharopeptide, PSP) from the mushroom *Coriolus versicolor* (*Basidiomycetes*: *Polyporaceae*). *Gen. Pharmacol.* **30**, 1–4.

Nimura, H., Mitsumori, N., Takahashi, N., *et al.* (2006) S-1 combined with lentinan in patients with unresectable or recurrent gastric cancer. *Gan To Kagaku Ryoho* **33**(Suppl. 1), 106–109 (in Japanese).

Nose, M., Terawaki, K., Oguri, K., *et al.* (1998) Activation of macrophages by crude polysaccharide fractions obtained from shoots of *Glycyrrhiza glabra* and hairy roots of *Glycyrrhiza uralensis in vitro. Biol. Pharm. Bull.* **21**, 1110–1112.

Ogoshi, K., Satou, H., Isono, K., *et al.* (1992) Postoperative long-term immunochemotherapy for esophageal carcinoma. *Jpn. J. Surg.* **12**, 249–256.

Ohno, N., Furukawa, M., Miura, N.N., *et al.* (2001) Anti-tumor neta glucan from the cultured fruit body of *Agaricus blazei. Biol. Pharm. Bull.* **24**, 820–828.

Ohtsuka, S., Uneo, S., Yoshikumi, C., *et al.* (1997) *Polysaccharides and Method of Producing Same*. US Patent 4, 051, 314.

Ooi, V.E. and Liu, F. (2000) Immunomodulation and anti-cancer activity of polysaccharide-protein complexes. *Curr. Med. Chem.* **7**, 715–729.

Peter, G., Karoly, V., Imre, B., *et al.* (1988) Effects of Lentinan on cytotoxicity of human lymphocytes. *Immunopharmacol. Immunotoxicol.* **10**, 157–163.

Pinilla, V. and Luu, B. (1999) Isolation and partial characterization of immunostimulating polysaccharides from *Imperata cylindrica. Planta Med.* **65**, 549–552.

Sakagami, Y., Mizoguchi, Y., Shin, T., *et al.* (1988) Effects of an anti-tumor polysaccharide, schizophyllan, on interferon-gamma and interleukin 2 production by peripheral blood mononuclear cells. *Biochem. Biophys. Res. Comm.* **155**, 650–655.

Stryer, L. (1995) Carbohydrates. In: *Biochemistry* (ed.) Stryer, L. W.H. Freeman and Co., New York, pp. 447–477.

Sun, Y. (1986) Chinese medicinal herbs as biological response modifiers. In: *Natural Immunity, Cancer, and Biological Response Modification* (eds.) Lotzova, E. and Herberman, R. Karger, Basel, pp. 206–211.

Sun, Y., Zhang, Y.H., Yu, G.Q., *et al.* (1981) Effect of Fu-zheng therapy in the management of malignant diseases. *Chin. Med. J.* **61**, 97–101.

Toi, M., Hattori, T., Akagi, M., *et al.* (1992) Randomized adjuvant trial to evaluate the addition of tamoxifen and PSK to chemotherapy in patients with primary breast cancer. *Cancer* **70**, 2475–2483.

Wakui, A., Kasai, M., Konno, K., Abe, R., Kanamaru, R., *et al.* (1986) Randomized study of Lentinan on patients with advanced gastric and colorectal cancer. *Gan To Kagaku Ryoho* **13**, 1050–1059 (in Japanese).

Wang, J.Z., Tsumura, H., Shimura, K. and Ito, H. (1992) Antitumor activity of polysaccharide from a Chinese medicinal herb, *Acanthopanax giraldii* Harms. *Cancer Lett.* **65**(1), 79–84.

Wang, Z.T., Ng, T.B., Yeung, H.W. and Xu, G. (1996) Immunomodulatory effect of a polysaccharide-enriched preparation of *Codonopsis pilosula* roots, *Pharmacology* **27**, 1347–1350.

Wasser, S.P. and Weis, A.L. (1999) Therapeutic effects of substances occurring in higher Basidiomycetes mushrooms: A modern perspective. *Crit. Rev. Immunol.* **19**, 65–96.

Wong, C.K., Leung, K.N., Fung, K.P. and Choy, Y.M. (1994) Immunomodulatory and anti-tumor polysaccharides from medicinal plants. *J. Int. Med. Res.* **22**, 229–312.

Xia, D. and Lin, Z.B. (1989) Effects of Tremella polysaccharides on immune function in mice. *Zhongguo Yao Li Xue Bao* **10**, 453–457.

Xu, J.P. (1992) Research on liu wei Rehmannia oral liquid against side-effect of drugs of anti-tumor chemotherapy. *Zhongguo Zhong Si Yi Jie He Za Zhi* **12**, 734–737, 709–710 (in Chinese).

Xu, Y.M. and Lu, P.C. (1991) Experimental studies on immunostimulatory effects of *Isatis indigotica* polysaccharides. *Zhong Xi Yi Jie He Za Zhi* **6**, 357–359 (in Chinese).

Yamaoka, Y., Kawakita, T., Kaneko, M. and Nomoto, K. (1996) A polysaccharide fraction of *Ziziphi fructus* in augmenting natural killer activity by oral administration. *Biol. Pharm. Bull.* **19**, 936–939.

Yamasaki, K., Sono, S., Yamashita, T., *et al.* (1989) Synergistic induction of lymphokine-activated killer activity by IL-2 and the polysaccharide Lentinan and therapy of spontaneous pulmonary metastases. *Cancer Immunol. Immunother.* **29**, 871–892.

Yang, J., Zhang, W., Shi, P., *et al.* (2005) Effects of exopolysaccharide fraction (EPSF) from a cultivated *Cordyceps sinensis* fungus on c-Myc, c-Fos, and VEGF expression in B16 melanoma-bearing mice. *Pathol. Res. Pract.* **201**(11), 745–750.

Zee-cheng, R.K. (1992) *Shi-quan-da-bu-tang*, SQT. A potent Chinese biological response modifier in cancer immunotherapy, potentiation and detoxification of anti-cancer drugs. *Methods Find. Exp. Clin. Pharmacol.* **14**, 725–736.

Zhang, L. and Tizard, I.T. (1996) Activation of a mouse macrophage cell line by acemannan: The major carbohydrate fraction from Aloe vera gel. *Immunopharmacology* **35**, 119–128.

Zhang, Y., Kiyohara, H., Matsumoto, T. and Yamada, H. (1997) Fractionation and chemical properties of immunomodulating polysaccharides from roots of *Dipsacus asperoides*. *Planta Med.* **63**, 393–399.

Zhang, Y.H., Liu, Y.L. and Yan, S.C. (1991) Effect of *Polyporus umbellatus* polysaccharide on function of macrophages in the peritoneal cavities of mice with liver lesions. *Zhong Xi Yi Jie He Za Zhi* **11**, 225–226 (in Chinese).

Chapter 13

Clinical Evaluation of Herbal Formula Decoction in Treating Non-Small Cell Lung Cancer by Various Rating Scales

Jie You & Zhi-Ming Shi

Abstract

Objective: To comprehensively evaluate the clinical effect of Herbal Formula decoction in treating patients with non-small cell lung cancer by various rating scales.

Methods: One hundred and two cases of non-small lung cancer were randomly divided into two groups, namely the combination group (which consisted of 61 cases and treated by both Herbal Formula decoction and chemotherapy) and the control group (41 cases receiving chemotherapy only). A total of two therapeutic courses were observed. The efficacy was evaluated by using various scales, including two international quality of life scales — the European Organization for Research and Treatment of Cancer Lung Cancer Quality of Life Questionnaire (EORTC QLQ-LC43) and the Functional Assessment of Cancer Therapy General and Lung (FACT-L); and Karnofsky's index of Performance Status (KPS) and the Eastern Cooperative Oncology Group (ECOG) performance status scales; and the Primary Lung Cancer Symptoms Scale of Traditional Chinese Medicine (LCSL-TCM).

Result: The quality of life scores in the combination group were significantly improved after treatment in various fields, including the functional symptomatic sub-fields, whereas those of the chemotherapy group significantly decreased. The difference between them was statistically significant ($P < 0.05$). For the combination group patients, most symptoms were alleviated after treatment, whereas most symptoms were aggravated in the control group, and their quality of life scores decreased in many fields. ECOG and KPS scoring showed similar results. The gastrointestinal reactions and bone marrow suppression of the combination group were less than those of the control group ($P < 0.05$). The clinical remission rates were not significantly different between the two groups ($P > 0.05$).

Conclusion: Herbal Formula decoction can improve the quality of life in non-small cell lung cancer patients, alleviate the disease or therapy-related symptoms, reduce the side-effects of chemotherapy, and improve the performance status.

Keywords: Herbal Formula Decoction; Non-Small Cell Lung Cancer; Quality of Life; Rating Scales; Efficacy Assessment.

13.1 Introduction

Quantitative rating measures have been widely used in lung cancer treatment to assess the clinical efficacy. In this present study, we evaluated the effectiveness of Herbal Formula decoction on improving the quality of life and alleviating the symptoms in patients with non-small cell lung cancer by a variety of scales, including two well-rated international quality of life scales: the European Organization for Research and Treatment of Cancer Quality of Life Questionnaire — Lung Cancer (EORTC QLQ-LC43) and the Functional Assessment of Cancer Therapy — General and Lung (FACT-L); and two performance status scales: Karnofsky's index of Performance Status (KPS) and the Eastern Cooperative Oncology Group (ECOG); and the TCM primary lung cancer symptoms scale (LCSL-TCM).

13.2 Material and Methods

13.2.1 *Case selection criteria*

13.2.1.1 Inclusion criteria

(1) Accordance with the diagnostic (Chinese Anti-Cancer Association, 1997) and staging criteria of primary bronchogenic carcinoma (AJCC/UICC, 1997);
(2) confirmed by pathological diagnostic;
(3) aged between 18–75 years old;
(4) first time chemotherapy;

(5) KPS > 70;
(6) no abnormal liver and kidney functions;
(7) expected survival > 5 months; and
(8) willing to participate in the clinical trial.

13.2.1.2 Exclusion criteria

(1) Serious complications;
(2) severe systematic disease requiring special treatment;
(3) mental disease;
(4) tuberculosis and other specific infectious diseases; and
(5) poor compliance.

13.2.1.3 Omission criteria

Cases would be asked to leave the program if one of the following occurred:

(1) Serious complications or acute deterioration requiring intensive care during the treatment course;
(2) moratorium on chemotherapy and/or change to other therapies and chemotherapy was not completed for two cycles due to the disease situation; or
(3) questionnaires were not completed due to various reasons.

13.2.2 *Clinical data*

From January to December 2003, we observed 125 non-small cell lung cancer patients with first-time chemotherapy, of which 23 cases lost contact due to various reasons and 102 cases (74.5%) completed the observation. All the cases were recruited in Longhua Hospital, affiliated to Shanghai University of Traditional Chinese Medicine and Shanghai Chest Hospital. The patients were randomly divided into combination and chemotherapy groups — 61 cases in the combination group and 41 cases in the chemotherapy group completed the trial, as shown in Table 13.1. In the combination group, 45 cases were male and 16 cases were female. The average

Table 13.1. Clinical data of the combination and chemotherapy groups.

Group	n	Gender		Ave. Age	Marriage		Tumor type	
		M	F		Married	Unmarried	Central	Peripheral
Combination	61	45	16	57.4	56	5	19	42
Chemotherapy	41	29	12	57.4	40	1	18	23

Group	Stage				Pathology		Surgery	
	Iib	IIIa	IIIb	IV	Squamous	Adeno-carcinoma	With surgery	W/O surgery
Combination	5	14	17	25	24	37	26	35
Chemotherapy	5	12	12	14	21	20	16	25

age was 57.4 years. Five cases were unmarried while 56 cases were married; 19 cases were central type and 42 cases were peripheral type of primary carcinoma; five cases were in stage IIb, 14 cases were in stage IIIa, 17 cases were in stage IIIb, and 25 cases were in stage IV; 24 cases were squamous cell carcinoma and 37 cases were adenocarcinoma; 26 cases underwent surgical operation while 35 cases did not receive surgical operation. In the chemotherapy group, 29 cases were male and 12 cases were female. The average age was 57.4 years. One case were unmarried while 40 cases were married; 18 cases were central type and 23 cases were peripheral type of primary carcinoma; five cases were in stage IIb stage, 12 cases were in stage IIIa, 12 cases were in stage IIIb, and 14 cases were in stage IV; 21 cases were squamous cell carcinoma and 20 cases were adeno-carcinoma; 16 cases underwent surgical operation while 25 cases did not receive surgical operation. The clinical data were not significantly different between the two groups ($P > 0.05$).

13.2.3 *Treatment methods*

Both groups of patients received general and symptomatic treatments. For example, a painkiller (acesodyne) was given to patients based on the principle of the World Health Organization's (WHO) three-step method of relieving pain; federal cough syrup was given to treat dry cough; licorice mixture was given to treat expectoration; codeine was given to treat serious cough; G-CSF was used when the bone marrow was suppressed to level II; and anti-emetic was given prior to chemotherapy. The combination group was treated by both Herbal Formula decoction and chemotherapy while the chemotherapy group received chemotherapy only. Both groups received NP chemo-therapy regimen, on which vinorebine was given by intraveneous injection at 25 mg/m^2 on days 1 and 8, cisplatin was given by intraveneous infusion at 80 mg/m^2 on day 1. One cycle was 28 days and patients received two cycles of treatment in total. Herbal Formula decoction was composed of the following Chinese medicinal herbs: *Sheng Huang Qi* (*Astragalus membranacens*) 30 g, *Sheng Bai Zhu* (*Atractylodes Rhizome*) 15 g, *Bei Sha Sen* (*Radix glehniae*) 15g, *Shi Shang Bai* (*Selaginella doederleinii*) 30 g, *Qi Ye Yi Zhi Hua* (*Paris polyphylla* var. *chinensis*) 24 g, *Bing Qiu Zi* (*Oreorchis patens*) 30 g, *Shan Yu Rou* (*Determining*) 12 g, *Xian Ling Pi* (*Epimedium*) 15 g, etc. It was continuously given from the third day of the first cycle of chemotherapy to the 28th day of the second cycle of chemotherapy.

13.2.4 *Observation parameters and assessment criteria*

13.2.4.1 Short-term therapeutic assessment

Short-term therapeutic efficacy was assessed before treatment and after completion of two cycles of chemotherapy using the product of the lesion's longest diameter and its longest vertical diameter as criteria. It was divided as complete remission (CR), partial remission, non-change (NC), and progressive development (PD), according to the WHO efficacy criteria on solid tumors (Sun, 2001).

13.2.4.2 Quality of life

International quality of life scales: Quality of life was evaluated one day prior to the first therapeutic cycle and 28 days after completion of the second cycle of chemotherapy. The questionnaires were self-rated by the patients. Total quality of life score and the scores on all fields were calculated using an international standard scoring method (Wan, 1999).

Performance status: Performance status was evaluated before and after treatment simul-taneously with quality of life.

13.2.4.3 Symptoms

TCM symptoms scale: TCM primary lung cancer symptoms scale (LCSL-TCM) in the Guiding Principles of Clinical Research on New Drugs of TCM was used for assessment (Zheng, 2002). The scale uses scoring method, in which non-symptoms are scored 0, slight symptoms are scored 1, moderate symptoms are scored 2, and serious symptoms are scored 3.

EORTC QLQ-LC43 symptoms scale and lung cancer specific sub-modules: EORTC QLQ-LC43 and EORTC QLQ-LC3 were evaluated using an international standard scoring system (Wan, 1999).

13.2.4.4 Toxicity and side-effects of chemotherapy

Toxicity and side-effects were graded once every therapeutic cycle using the WHO criteria on general toxicity and side-effects of anti-cancer drugs.

13.2.5 *Statistics*

Data were analyzed by SPSS 11.5 statistical software. The *t*-test and analysis of variance were used to analyze quantitative and qualitative data, respectively. Grading data were analyzed by Wilcoxon Rank test. Comparison of difference was applied as it was significantly different between the body field of EORTC QLQ-LC43 and the baseline of lung cancer LC13 before treatment.

13.3 Results

13.3.1 *Short-term therapeutic effect*

As shown in Table 13.2, the remission rates of non-surgical patients were not significantly different between the combination and the chemotherapy

Table 13.2. Comparison of the remission rate between combination and chemotherapy group.

Group	Without surgery				With surgery		
	n	Partial remission	Non-change	Progressive development	*n*	Non-change	Progressive development
Combination	35	6 (17.1)	26 (74.3)	3 (8.6)	26	25 (96.2)	1 (3.8)
Chemotherapy	25	2 (8.0)	20 (80.0)	3 (12.0)	16	12 (75.0)	4 (25.0)

groups, whereas the remission rate of surgical patients in the combination group was higher than that in the chemotherapy group.

13.3.2 *Quality of life*

13.3.2.1 EORTC QLQ-LC43 scores in the combination and chemotherapy groups before and after treatment

As shown in Table 13.3, after treatment the EORTC QLQ-LC43 scores of the combination group increased in the following fields, including role, emotional, and cognitive function, general health, and social function, whereas it decreased in physical field. This indicated the quality of life had improved in the above fields after treatment. In the symptom sub-scales, scores on fatigue, pain, dyspnoea, insomnia, and appetite loss were significantly lower than those of pre-treatment ($P < 0.05$), while nausea and vomiting, constipation, and diarrhea did not change after treatment. By summarizing all the symptoms as general symptom sub-scales and calculating the total score, it was found that the total score was significantly lower than that of pre-treatment ($P < 0.05$), which suggested that the symptoms were alleviated after treatment in general.

After treatment, EORTC QLQ-LC43 scores of the chemotherapy group increased in body field, while they decreased in the fields of role, emotional, and cognitive function, general health, and social function ($P < 0.05$). In the symptom sub-scales, scores on nausea and vomiting, fatigue, pain, appetite loss, and constipation were significantly higher than those of pre-treatment ($P < 0.05$), while dyspnoea, diarrhea, insomnia did not change after treatment. Total symptom sub-scales score was

Table 13.3. EORTC QLQ-LC43 scores in the combination and chemotherapy groups before and after treatment.

Field	Combination group			Chemotherapy group		
	Pre-treatment	Post-treatment	Margin	Pre-treatment	Post-treatment	Margin
Physical function	84.81 ± 7.32	$80.44 \pm 6.54^*$	$4.37 \pm 7.97^\dagger$	81.62 ± 7.27	$88.29 \pm 7.57^*$	6.67 ± 8.03
Role function	51.64 ± 24.67	$66.39 \pm 22.87^*$	$14.75 \pm 29.04^\dagger$	56.91 ± 22.04	$43.90 \pm 20.33^*$	−13.01 ± 22.21
Emotional function	62.70 ± 22.80	$82.38 \pm 19.73^*$	$19.67 \pm 27.64^\dagger$	67.28 ± 16.29	$60.16 \pm 16.82^*$	−7.11 ± 19.24
Cognitive function	65.85 ± 20.43	$80.87 \pm 17.96^*$	$15.03 \pm 23.90^\dagger$	67.07 ± 22.51	$59.76 \pm 20.74^*$	−7.32 ± 23.58
Social function	52.19 ± 24.43	63.66 ± 20.30	$11.48 \pm 26.45^\dagger$	58.94 ± 21.44	$44.31 \pm 18.11^*$	−14.63 ± 21.79
General health	55.33 ± 19.43	$68.17 \pm 16.77^*$	$12.84 \pm 22.03^\dagger$	51.83 ± 15.08	$41.46 \pm 17.53^*$	−10.73 ± 19.26
Symptom subscales	294.35 ± 123.74	$179.33 \pm 113.51^*$	$115.03 \pm 133.34^\dagger$	194.35 ± 136.32	$439.43 \pm 111.93^*$	109.21 ± 133.94
Fatigue	57.74 ± 22.21	$36.98 \pm 17.06^*$	$20.77 \pm 23.61^\dagger$	52.85 ± 18.39	$65.31 \pm 16.52^*$	12.47 ± 23.73
Nausea and vomiting	12.02 ± 17.51	8.20 ± 14.15	$-3.83 \pm 20.04^\dagger$	11.79 ± 17.58	$32.11 \pm 17.63^*$	20.33 ± 25.42
Pain	30.05 ± 21.04	$15.58 \pm 18.97^*$	$14.49 \pm 24.05^\dagger$	31.30 ± 16.75	$40.24 \pm 17.47^*$	8.94 ± 19.04
Dyspnoea	32.79 ± 23.95	$22.40 \pm 22.54^*$	$10.38 \pm 23.21^\dagger$	26.02 ± 22.99	34.96 ± 23.51	8.94 ± 29.84
Insomnia	47.54 ± 26.15	25.68 ± 28.15	$21.86 \pm 31.56^\dagger$	39.84 ± 28.11	47.97 ± 25.87	8.13 ± 33.98
Loss of appetite	41.53 ± 24.84	$19.13 \pm 22.33^*$	$22.40 \pm 28.36^\dagger$	34.96 ± 31.58	$52.28 \pm 17.65^*$	20.33 ± 37.92
Constipation	18.03 ± 24.02	13.11 ± 18.54	$-4.92 \pm 24.22^\dagger$	19.51 ± 26.85	$39.02 \pm 27.79^*$	19.51 ± 26.85
Diarrhea	7.10 ± 15.05	3.83 ± 10.71	−3.28 ± 17.96	6.50 ± 22.63	5.69 ± 12.70	−0.81 ± 26.34
Financial difficulties	46.9 ± 24.63	$34.43 \pm 27.19^*$	$13.11 \pm 30.60^\dagger$	75.61 ± 40.16	$65.04 \pm 31.58^*$	11.38 ± 31.28
Lung Cancer specific subscales	22.24 ± 8.13	$14.70 \pm 8.01^*$	−7.54 ± 10.05	$18.05 \pm 7.77^*$	$26.02 \pm 10.03^*$	7.97 ± 11.17

Note: Compared to the same group before treatment, $^*P < 0.05$; compared to chemotherapy group, $^\dagger P < 0.05$.

Table 13.4. FACT-L scores in the combination and chemotherapy groups before and after treatment.

Group	Case	Time	Physical	Community & Family	Emotional	Functional	Relationship with doctor	Lung cancer additional care	Total score
Combination	61	Pre-treatment	23.61 ± 4.00	18.33 ± 3.19	20.10 ± 4.06	11.72 ± 4.51	6.92 ± 1.00	29.77 ± 3.71	110.44 ± 14.82
		Post-treatment	$27.57 \pm 4.47^*$	$19.85 \pm 3.16^*$	$23.63 \pm 3.51^*$	$15.60 \pm 4.88^*$	7.13 ± 1.11	$34.02 \pm 3.92^*$	$127.80 \pm 16.48^*$
		Difference	$3.97 \pm 5.17^\dagger$	1.58 ± 3.81	$3.58 \pm 4.95^\dagger$	$3.90 \pm 5.02^\dagger$	2.69 ± 4.31	$8.80 \pm 15.55^\dagger$	$17.57 \pm 18.61^\dagger$
Chemotherapy	41	Pre-treatment	23.95 ± 4.86	17.32 ± 3.04	19.02 ± 4.79	11.61 ± 4.13	6.88 ± 1.03	30.10 ± 4.12	109.05 ± 15.73
		Post-treatment	$18.76 \pm 3.88^*$	17.30 ± 2.56	18.31 ± 4.19	$9.66 \pm 4.41^*$	6.66 ± 1.11	$27.27 \pm 3.45^*$	$98.46 \pm 14.84^*$
		Difference		0.49 ± 3.59	-0.88 ± 5.15	-1.95 ± 5.50	-0.22 ± 3.60	-2.83 ± 3.43	10.59 ± 17.90

Note: Compared to the same group before treatment, $^*P < 0.05$; compared to the difference with chemotherapy group, $^\dagger P < 0.05$.

significantly higher ($P < 0.05$), which suggested the symptoms tended to get worse.

13.3.2.2 FACT-L scores in the combination and chemotherapy groups before and after treatment

As listed in Table 13.4, for the combination group, except the score on the relationship with doctor did not change obviously after treatment, scores on all other fields increased significantly compared to pre-treatment ($P < 0.05$). The scores on all fields in the chemotherapy group were significantly lower after treatment compared to those of pre-treatment. The scores on the fields of relationship with doctor, society, and emotion did not show any significant change after treatment.

13.3.3 *Changes in symptoms between the combination and chemotherapy groups before and after treatment*

13.3.3.1 Comparison of symptoms between the combination and chemotherapy groups before and after treatment

As there was no difference in the total symptom sub-scales score between the two groups before and after treatment, whereas there was difference in the total score of lung cancer modules between the two groups, the margin of pre- and post-treatment scores was compared (Table 13.5). After treatment, the scores on various fields in the com-bination group tended to decrease, which indicated the symptoms were alleviated. In contrast, the scores on various fields in the chemotherapy group increased, indicating the symptoms were aggravated. After treat-ment, in the combination group except the scores on constipation, diarrhea, dysphagia, peripheral neuropathy, alopecia, other site's pain, scores on all other symptoms were significantly lower than those of pre-treatment. In the chemotherapy group after treatment, scores on fatigue, nausea and vomiting, pain, appetite loss, arm or shoulder pain were significantly higher, which indicated the symptoms were getting worse, with the exception was that the scores on the fields of diarrhea, hemoptysis, oral ulcer, and other site's pain between the combination and chemotherapy group showed no difference, scores on all other fields in the combination

Table 13.5. Comparison of symptoms between the combination and chemotherapy group before and after treatment.

Symptom	Combination group		Chemotherapy group	
	Pre-treatment	Post-treatment	Pre-treatment	Post-treatment
Symptom sub-scales	294.35 ± 123.74	$179.33 \pm 113.51^{\dagger,\S}$	294.35 ± 136.32	$439.43 \pm 111.93^{\dagger}$
Fatigue	57.74 ± 22.21	$36.98 \pm 17.06^{\dagger,\S}$	52.85 ± 18.39	$65.31 \pm 16.52^{\dagger}$
Nausea and vomiting	12.02 ± 17.51	$8.20 \pm 14.15^{\dagger,\S}$	11.79 ± 17.58	$32.11 \pm 17.63^{\dagger}$
Pain	30.05 ± 21.04	$15.58 \pm 18.97^{\dagger,\S}$	31.30 ± 16.75	$40.24 \pm 17.47^{\dagger}$
Dyspnoea	32.79 ± 23.95	$22.40 \pm 22.54^{\dagger,\S}$	26.02 ± 22.99	34.96 ± 23.51
Insomnia	47.54 ± 26.15	$25.68 \pm 28.15^{\dagger,\S}$	39.84 ± 28.11	47.97 ± 25.87
Diarrhea	7.10 ± 15.05	3.83 ± 10.71	6.50 ± 22.63	5.69 ± 12.70
Constipation	18.03 ± 24.02	$13.11 \pm 18.54^{\S}$	19.51 ± 26.85	39.02 ± 27.79
Lung cancer module	$22.24 \pm 8.13^{\ddagger}$	$14.70 \pm 8.01^{\dagger,\S}$	18.05 ± 7.77	$26.02 \pm 10.03^{\dagger}$
Dyspnoea resting	18.51 ± 21.54	$8.89 \pm 19.28^{\dagger,\S}$	17.07 ± 22.52	24.39 ± 23.60
Walking	40.98 ± 25.38	$23.33 \pm 18.72^{\S}$	34.96 ± 23.51	48.78 ± 25.92

Note: Compared to pre-treatment, $^{*}P < 0.05$, $^{\dagger}P < 0.01$; compared to the chemotherapy group after treatment, $^{\ddagger}P < 0.05$, $^{\S}P < 0.01$.

Table 13.5. *(Continued)*

Symptom	Combination group		Chemotherapy group	
	Pre-treatment	Post-treatment	Pre-treatment	Post-treatment
Ascending stairs	56.28 ± 22.39	42.22 ± 28.04†,§	17.07 ± 25.59	18.75 ± 27.94
Cough	46.45 ± 24.58	20.00 ± 23.12†,§	39.02 ± 22.24	39.22 ± 20.24
Hemoptysis	7.10 ± 17.34	4.44 ± 16.77†	28.39 ± 20.59	47.49 ± 34.20
Oral ulcer	6.01 ± 14.28	6.67 ± 23.61*	4.88 ± 14.07	9.76 ± 17.07
Dysphagia	14.75 ± 28.88	3.33 ± 10.08	13.01 ± 19.55	19.51 ± 21.05
Peripheral neuropathy	7.65 ± 14.13	2.78 ± 11.13‡	27.77 ± 20.26	15.45 ± 21.21
Alopecia	29.51 ± 29.25	35.56 ± 30.60	21.61 ± 29.38	32.48 ± 29.11
Chest pain	33.33 ± 20.18	13.89 ± 17.67†,‡	11.38 ± 17.65	10.57 ± 18.91
Arm/shoulder pain	20.22 ± 20.44	9.83 ± 20.50†,§	19.55 ± 9.80	49.59 ± 34.33†
Other site's pain	2.40 ± 15.78	23.33 ± 16.58	29.17 ± 24.09	26.67 ± 22.90

Note: Compared to pre-treatment, $^{*}P < 0.05$, $^{\dagger}P < 0.01$; compared to the chemotherapy group after treatment, $^{\ddagger}P < 0.05$, $^{\S}P < 0.01$.

Table 13.6. Comparison of KPS and ECOG scores between the combination and chemotherapy group before and after treatment.

			KPS (score)				ECOG (score)					
Group	Case	Time	60–69	70–79	80–89	90–100	0	1	2	3	4	5
Combination	61	Pre-treatment	0	20	35	6	0	3	46	12	12	0
		Post-treatment	0	2	28	31	0	26	34	1	1	0
Chemotherapy	41	Pre-treatment	0	2	25	14	0	4	37	0	0	0
		Post-treatment	1	23	15	2	0	0	18	23	23	0

group were significantly lower than those of the chemotherapy group after treatment.

13.3.3.2 TCM symptoms scale

The score of TCM symptom scale in the combination group after treatment was 6.05 ± 5.50, which was lower than pre-treatment score (11.31 ± 6.13) ($P < 0.05$). In contrast, the score of TCM symptom scale in the chemotherapy group after treatment was higher than pre-treatment score (16.21 ± 6.64 vs. 10.73 ± 5.71) ($P < 0.01$). It was significantly different between the two groups after treatment ($P < 0.05$).

13.3.4 *Comparison of KPS and ECOG scores between the combination and chemotherapy group before and after treatment*

As shown in Table 13.6, the number of cases which KPS scores increased and meanwhile ECOG decreased after treatment in the combination group were more than those in the chemotherapy group ($P < 0.01$).

13.3.5 *Comparison of side-effects between the combination and chemotherapy groups*

As shown in Table 13.7, side-effects in the combination group were lower than those in the chemotherapy group and what is more its reaction period was shorter ($P < 0.05$, Wilcoxon rank test).

Table 13.7. Comparison of side-effect between the combination and chemotherapy groups.

			Gastrointestinal reactions				Bone marrow suppression				Days of bone marrow suppression			
Group	Case	Therapeutic cycle	Non	I	II	III or higher	Non	I	II	III or higher	0	< 1W	1–2W	> 2W
Combination	61	1	8	35	17	1	10	23	22	6	9	42	10	0
		2	21	27	13	0	20	23	15	3	20	39	2	0
Chemotherapy	41	1	7	24	9	1	9	7	10	15	9	15	17	0
		2	2	24	10	5	4	9	17	11	4	14	21	0

13.4 Discussion

Lung cancer is a chronic disease with poor prognosis (Frost *et al.*, 2002). Especially in the advanced stage, due to the serious disease-related symptoms such as cough, pain, fatigue, and dyspnoea, etc. patients with lung cancer always suffer from psychological distress and physical pain and their quality of life is affected. Although chemotherapy is one of the main therapeutic approaches for advanced lung cancer, many patients cannot endure chemotherapy due to various reasons. Even for those who can tolerate chemotherapy, the median survival time only increased two to four months (Breathnach *et al.*, 2001; Cella, 2003); furthermore, the pain caused by the toxicity and side-effect of chemotherapy may offset the clinical advantages of tumor shrinkage or stability. Codey *et al.* (2003) found that in 177 lung cancer patients who received chemotherapy, the symptoms of fatigue, pain, constipation, loss of appetite, and vomiting were aggravated and might last for six months.

Quality of life is one of the independent factors for prognosis and survival expectation. Due to the limited survival period of lung cancer patients, alleviating of disease-related or therapeutic-related symptoms is the main aim of treatment for lung cancer, especially in advanced stages. Therefore, currently alleviation of symptoms and improvement of life quality have been one of the end points of lung cancer therapy (Paris, 1996). Especially for those with metastatic or advanced disease, and mainly treated by palliation, the combination of the traditional clinical efficacy and quality of life which is mainly based on patients' subjective feelings will provide more comprehensive criteria for justification when evaluating the risk and advantages of the treatment.

With Herbal Formula decoction as the basic recipe, we evaluated the quality of life and symptom changes in lung cancer patients treated by the combination of chemotherapy and Herbal Formula decoction before and after treatment using two international quality of life questionnaires, and compared with treatment by chemotherapy only. The results showed that after two cycles of treatment, in the chemotherapy group scores of quality of life on all fields (including sub-scales) and total score decreased significantly, indicating the quality of life was lower than that of pre-treatment. This was in accordance with the clinical observations. Clinically, aggravation or occurrence of the chemotherapy-related toxic and side-effect reactions such as vomiting, nausea, constipation, and fatigue, etc. could be observed. Furthermore, our results indicated scores on the fields of physical, emotional, social, and role functions and self-review health status decreased in chemotherapy patients. This was also supported by Morita *et al.*'*s* results (2003). Osoba *et al.* (1994) studied 160 lung cancer patients using QLQ-C30 and found that after chemotherapy scores on the fields of social and role function and total score on quality of life decreased, fatigue, nausea and vomiting became more serious than those before chemotherapy, which was similar to what we observed on the chemotherapy group in our study. Although Bonomi (2003) and Anderson *et al.* (2000) pointed out that chemotherapy could alleviate patients' clinical symptoms and improve their quality of life, we found only in a few cases the symptoms were alleviated after two months' observation in our study, and there were new symptoms occurrence or the existing symptoms were aggravated for most patients. The variance could be due to different cycles of observation.

The combination group received chemotherapy and meanwhile was treated with Herbal Formula decoction site according to symptoms. After treatment, scores on most symptoms tended to decrease. The margin between pre- and post-treatment was significantly different, indicating the symptoms were alleviated. Our results indicated that combination of chemotherapy and Herbal Formula decoction can alleviate the disease and chemotherapy-related symptoms.

During the chemotherapy course, inhibition and remission of its toxicity and side-effects will benefit patients in improving their quality of life in the early stage of chemotherapy, strengthen their confidence, and help them tolerate and accomplish the whole course of chemotherapy. Our results showed that scores on the physical region, symptom sub-scales, and lung cancer specific modules decreased in the patients treated by both chemotherapy and Herbal Formula decoction, indicating the symptoms were alleviated and their physical status became better; meanwhile scores on the fields of social, role, and emotional function increased, suggesting that the general quality of life was improved. The disease-related symptoms such as cough, dyspnoea, pain, and fatigue tended to be alleviated while the chemotherapy-related symptoms such as nausea and vomiting were not aggravated. The total scores on the whole symptom and the scores on various symptoms were significantly lower than those in the chemotherapy group. Assessment through TCM symptoms scale, KPS and ECOG scales also showed similar results.

In chemotherapy, toxicity and side-effects athough it was not different with regard to gastrointestinal reaction and bone marrow suppression between the combination and chemotherapy groups in the first therapeutic cycle, the number of days of bone marrow suppression in the combination group was less than in the chemotherapy group. In the second cycle of chemotherapy, the level and duration of gastrointestinal reaction and bone marrow suppression of the combination group were less than those of the chemotherapy group, which objectively further demonstrated Herbal Formula decoction could alleviate the disease and chemotherapy-related symptoms in patients with non-small cell lung cancer and improved their quality of life. Although the short-term therapeutic effect was not significantly different between the two groups, the remission rate of the combination group was higher than that of the chemotherapy group. As the non-surgical cases were few and the observation was only for two treatment courses, the above results need to be further confirmed in the future.

Quantitative measures have been widely used by the international lung oncology field to assess clinical therapeutic efficacy, of which the quality of life scale, its symptoms sub-scale and all the items of the mainly symptom-composed specific modules were screened and selected based on wide epidemiological survey and through fixed scale-making procedures. It has been tested for ten years in the clinic and amended three times. Due to their normalized and quantitative chara-cteristics, these scales have been gradually accepted by the international lung oncology field as assessment tools; furthermore, they are completed by patients, which then reflect patients' sensation more objectively and hence make assessments more accurate.

Clinical studies have demonstrated that TCM can alleviate patients' symptoms and improve their quality of life. However, well-recognized normalized and quantitative measures have been lacking for a long time. The application of the symptom sub-scale of the international quality of life scale provided a new approach for research in this field. In this study, we evaluated the effect of Herbal Formula decoction on alleviating the symptoms in patients with non-small cell lung cancer using the symptoms sub-scale, lung cancer specific scale, and TCM primary lung cancer symptoms scale. We evaluated this decoction by normalized and quantitative measures. The results indicated the data measured via the above scales were consistent.

References

American Joint Committee on Cancer (AJCC)/International Union against Cancer (UICC) (1999) Staging system for lung cancer. In: *Practical Oncology* (ed.) Zhou, J.C. People's Medical Publishing House, Beijing, pp. 23.

Anderson, H., Hopwood, P., Stephens, R.J., *et al.* (2000) Gemcitabine plus best supportive care (BSC) vs. BSC in inoperable non-small cell lung cancer: A randomized trial with quality of life as the primary outcome. *Br. J. Cancer* **83**(4), 447–453.

Bonomi, P. (2003) New approaches to symptom improvements in lung cancer patients. *J. Lung Cancer* **41**(Suppl. 4), 32–36.

Breathnach, O.S., Freidlin, B., Conley, B., *et al.* (2001) Twenty-two years of phase 111 trials for patients with advanced non-small cell lung cancer: Sobering results. *J. Clin. Oncol.* **19**(6), 734–742.

Cella, D. (2003) Impact of ZD1839 on non-small cell lung cancer related symptoms as measured by the functional assessment of cancer therapy-lung scale. *Semin. Oncol.* **30**(1 Suppl. 1), 39–48.

Chinese Anti-Cancer Association. (1997) *New Criterion of Diagnosis and Treatment of Malignant Tumor*, 9th Vol. Chinese Academy of Medical Science and Peking Union Medical College Press, Beijing, pp. 737–781.

Cooley, M.E., Short, T.H. and Moriarty, H.J. (2003) Symptom prevalence, distress, and change over time in patients receiving treatment for lung cancer. *Psycho-Oncology* **12**(7), 694–708.

Frost, M.H., Bonomi, A.E., Ferrans, C.E., *et al.* (2002) Patient, clinician, and population perspectives on determining the clinical significance of quality-of-life scores. *Mayo Clin. Proc.* **77**(5), 488–494.

Morita, S., Kobayashi, K., Eguchi, K., *et al.* (2003) Influence of clinical parameters on quality of life during chemotherapy in patients with advanced non-small cell lung cancer: Application of a general linear model. *Jpn. J. Clin. Oncol.* **33**(9), 470–476.

Osoba, D., Zee, B., Pater, J., *et al.* (1994) Psychometric properties and responsiveness of the EORTC quality of life questionnaire (QLQ-C30) in patients with breast, ovarian and lung cancer. *Qual. Life Res.* **3**(5), 353–364.

Paris, K. (1996) Quality of life as a new end point. *Chest* **109**(5), 110–112.
Sun, Y. (ed.) (2001) *Oncology*. People's Medical Publishing House, Beijing, pp. 994.
Wan, C.H. (1999) *The Methods of Measurement and Evaluation of Quality of Life*. Yunnan University Press, Kunming, pp. 225.
Zheng, X.Y. (ed.) (2002) *Guiding Principles of Clinical Research on New Drugs of TCM*. China Medical Pharmaceutical Science and Technology Publishing House, Beijing, pp. 219.

Chapter 14

New Approach for Evaluating the Anti-Breast Cancer Activity of Traditional Chinese Medicine

John M. Pezzuto, Richard C. Moon, Charles K.-H. Chang & Ching-Jer Chang

Abstract

Traditional Chinese medicine includes thousands of formulations, largely based on mixtures of terrestrial plants, and these formulations are administered for essentially all types of human diseases including cancer. Nonetheless, there are no generally accepted pre-clinical models for assessing the potential clinical efficacy of traditional Chinese medicines for treating cancer. Based on extensive analyses of traditional use for the potential treatment of human breast cancer, and systematic evaluations of the literature reports indicating mediation of well-defined bioactivities or biochemical markers consistent with control of proliferation or differentiation of cancer cells, 18 different traditional Chinese medicines have been selected as prime examples of promising leads. For the first step of the experimental approach, the herbs need to be properly identified. Next, complex formulations are produced by traditional methods under cGMP conditions and characterized by means of HPLC-fingerprints. Finally, anti-tumor or cancer preventive response can be assessed with (1) transgenic mice engineered to develop mammary adenocarcinoma, and (2) Sprague-Dawley rats bearing *N*-methyl-*N*-nitrosourea-induced mammary tumors. Animals with intact immune systems are used since this may be intimately related to the mechanism of action of traditional Chinese medicine. As a result of these procedures, a good indication of the true biologic potential of these traditional medicines should be established, and sufficient chemical and botanical information should be available to permit a smooth transition for more advanced translational studies.

Keywords: Traditional Chinese Medicine; Breast Cancer; Mammary Tumor; Transgenic Mice; *N*-Methyl-*N*-Nitrosourea.

14.1 Introduction

Breast cancer is the most predominant cancer in women worldwide. An estimated 11 million new breast cancer cases were reported worldwide in 2002 (Kamangar *et al.*, 2006), and approximately 178,480 new cases are expected in the US in 2007 (Jemal *et al.*, 2007). Although significant progress in breast cancer treatment has been made in recent years (Winchester *et al.*, 2006; Popat and Smith, 2006; Ruso and Ruso, 2004), in the US, approximately 40,460 breast cancer deaths are anticipated in 2007. It is thus extremely critical to explore new treatment modalities for breast cancer. In addition, however, an effective approach for the control of breast cancer is prevention (Popat and Smith, 2006; Ruso and Ruso, 2004; Chan and Morris, 2006; Veronesi and Bonanni, 2005; Hanf and Gonder, 2005; Forman *et al.*, 2003; Chemoprevention Working Group, 1999). Our current understanding of multi-step carcinogenesis provides many opportunities to block or inhibit the initiation, promotion and progression of breast cancer. As a result, several clinical trials for breast cancer prevention are ongoing (Cuzick *et al.*, 2003; Arun and Hortobagyi, 2002; International Breast Cancer Intervention Study Investigators, 2002).

Conventional cancer chemotherapy often induces serious adverse effects. In addition, the prognosis for advanced breast cancer is dismal. In part, due to this situation, it is common for cancer patients to explore alternative therapies. For example, according to a survey reported by Adler (1999), the usage of an alternative modality by women with breast cancer in San Francisco indicates that 72% used one form of alternative modality for two to four months. Traditional Chinese medicine (Cohen *et al.*, 2002) or botanical remedies (Chemoprevention Working Group, 1999; Cuzick *et al.*, 2003; Arun and Hortobagyi, 2002; International Breast Cancer Intervention Study Investigators, 2002; Adler, 1999; Cohen *et al.*, 2002; Manson, 2003; Park and Pezzuto, 2002; Reddy *et al.*, 2003) are the most frequently used modality. Both low (Tang *et al.*, 2003a) and high molecular weight (Tang *et al.*, 2003b) compounds from Chinese herbal medicines have been developed as anti-tumor agents. Most pre-clinical studies have focused on the discovery and development of active components from one single herb/diet as potential therapeutic or preventive agents. However, traditional Chinese medical practice rarely utilizes one single herb for the treatment of disease. The essence of traditional Chinese medicine rests on the harmony and balance of two key energy sources, "Yin" and "Yang". The physiological balance is accomplished by combination of multiple medicinal herbs. The synergistic and additive effects of multiple ingredients and multiple pharmacological targets result in the ultimate efficacy of traditional Chinese medicine. The traditional decoction method for the preparation of the complex formulae is designed to yield optimal formulation for absorption, distribution, metabolism, excretion and toxicity. The complex formula may thus provide a distinct complemental and alternative modality to the conventional treatment and prevention of breast cancer. Consequently, it is important to focus on the complex formula instead of one single herb.

Numerous anecdotal case studies on the intervention of breast cancer with traditional Chinese medicine in Chinese women have been reported (Cohen *et al.*, 2002; Xie, 1997; Cheung, 1999; Hsu, 1982; Lang and Mung, 1992). Most of these studies were not well controlled. The selection of the herbal ingredients for each individualized formula was not clearly defined. In this report, we have critically evaluated numerous complex formulas of traditional Chinese medicine for the treatment of cancer based on 12 highly relevant bioactivities for the prevention and treatment of cancer. These complex formulas will then be evaluated by two animal models:

(1) rat mammary adenocarcinoma induced by *N*-methyl-*N*-nitrosourea; and
(2) transgenic mouse mammary adenocarcinoma transformed by a recombinant gene expressing the SV 40 large tumor antigen with a hormone responsive promoter.

These *in vivo* efficacy results will provide essential justifications for further clinical trials to establish the evidence-based anti-breast cancer activity of traditional Chinese medicine.

14.2 Selection of Traditional Chinese Medicine

For the purpose of this presentation, the selection of complex formulas in traditional Chinese medicine were initially based on clinical case reports compiled by Hsu (1982) and Lang and Mung (1992), mainly for the treatment of breast cancer. In addition, any formula containing a protected species was excluded. The final selection of the sample formulas rests on an extensive literature review of the plant genera and species. As a result, 18 Chinese medicinal formulas were chosen. Each formula must be composed of medicinal herbs of which more than 75% have been reported to demonstrate at least one of the following bioactivities:

(1) anti-carcinogenicity/anti-mutagenicity;
(2) *in vivo* anti-tumor efficacy;
(3) *in vitro* anti-tumor cytotoxicity;
(4) immunomodulation activity;
(5) modulation of oncogenic signal transduction;
(6) induction of apoptosis or differentiation;
(7) inhibition of metastasis or angiogenesis;
(8) phytoestrogen activity;
(9) attenuation of the side effects of cancer chemotherapy or radiotherapy;
(10) inhibition of cyclooxygenase-2;
(11) modulation of nitric oxide synthase activity/expression; or
(12) antioxidation activity.

The Chinese medicinal formulas meeting these criteria are listed below. Only one to two representative references for the above bioactivities for each herb are cited.

(1) **Hai-zao-zhen-yin-tang:** *Cassia tora* (seed, 30 g) (Hong *et al.*, 2002; Koyama *et al.*, 2002), *Citrus tangerina* (peel, 15 g) (Kris-Etherton *et al.*, 2002; Nangia-Makker *et al.*, 2002), *Dendrobium nobile* (stem, 2 g) (Ye *et al.*, 2002), *Laminaria japonica* (whole plant, 30 g) (Teas, 1983), *Ligustrum lucidum* (fruit, 15 g) (Lau *et al.*, 2002; Niikawa *et al.*, 1993), *Lonicera japonica* (flower, 15 g) (Shi *et al.*, 1999), *Lucium chinese* (seed, 12 g) (Gan *et al.*, 2001; Chin *et al.*, 2003), *Pseudostellaria heterophylla* (rhizome, 9 g) (Wong *et al.*, 1994), *Poria cocos* (dry body, 12 g) (Ukiya *et al.*, 2002), *Rehmannia*

glutinosa (steamed root, 15 g) (Kim *et al.*, 1999; Liang *et al.*, 1999), *Salvia miltiorrhiza* (root, 15 g) (Chen *et al.*, 2001; Gali Muhtasib and Affara, 2000), and *Sargassum fusiforme* (whole plant, 30 g) (Stevan *et al.*, 2001; Itoh *et al.*, 1995).

(2) **Tian-lou-tang:** *Ampelopsis japonica* (root, 9 g) (Park *et al.*, 2000; Lee and Lin, 1988), *Brassica campestris* (seed, 30 g) (van Poppel *et al.*, 1999; Brignall, 2001), *Caragana sinica* (flower, 9 g) (Zhu and Xu, 2003), *Echinop latifolius* (root, 15 g) (Lam *et al.*, 1991; Kim *et al.*, 1998), *Podophyllum* (*Dysosma*) *pleianthum* (root, 9 g) (Gordaliza *et al.*, 2004; Yin and Chen, 1989), *Eupolyphaga sinensis* (whole body, 9 g), *Ficus pumila* (flower ovary, 30 g) (Peraza-Sanchez *et al.*, 2002; Simon *et al.*, 2001), and *Semiaquilegia adoxoides* (root, 30 g).

(3) **Zhou-shi-ru-xian-ai-fang:** *Bupleurum chinense* (root, 10 g) (Tsai *et al.*, 2002b; Matsuda *et al.*, 1997), *Citrus trangerina* (green peel, 15 g) (Kris-Etheron *et al.*, 2002; Nangia-Makker, 2002), *Cyperus rotundus* (root, 15 g), *Curcuma aromatica* (rhizome, 15 g) (Aggarwal *et al.*, 2003), *Oldenlandia diffusa* (whole plant, 50 g) (Yoshida *et al.*, 1997; Chung *et al.*, 2002), *Prunus persica* (semen, 7.5 g) (Heo *et al.*, 2001), *Scutellaria barbata* (whole plant, 30 g) (Lee *et al.*, 2002a; Chan *et al.*, 2002), and *Vaccaria segetalis* (seed, 25 g) (Morita *et al.*, 1997).

(4) **Er-dan-tang:** *Angelica dahurica* (root, 9 g) (Kapadia *et al.*, 2002; Pae *et al.*, 2002), *Angelica sinensis* (root, 45 g) (Kapadia *et al.*, 2002; Pae *et al.*, 2002), *Bombyx mori* (dry body, 6 g), *Citrus tangerina* (seed, 12g) (Kris-Etheron *et al.*, 2002; Nangia-Makker *et al.*, 2002), *Justicia procumbens* (whole plant, 30 g) (Day *et al.*, 2002; Navarro *et al.*, 2001), *Paeonia suffruitocosa* (root bark, 6 g) (Lee *et al.*, 2002b; Oh *et al.*, 2001), *Prunella vulgaris* (flower, 45 g) (Heo *et al.*, 2001), and *Salvia miltiorrhiza* (root, 15 g) (Chen *et al.*, 2001; Gali Muhtasib and Affara, 2000).

(5) **Chai-hu-ching-kan-tang:** *Angelica sinensis* (root, 1.5 g) (Kapadia *et al.*, 2002; Pae *et al.*, 2002), *Artium lappa* (fruit, 1.5 g) (Hirose *et al.*, 2000; Morita *et al.*, 1984), *Bupleurum chinense* (root, 2 g) (Tsai *et al.*, 2002b; Matsuda *et al.*, 1997), *Cnidium officinale* (root, 1.5 g) (Kwak *et al.*, 2002), *Coptis chinensis* (root, 1.5 g) (Schinella

et al., 2002; Fukuda *et al.*, 1999), *Forsythia suspensa* (fruit, 1.5 g) (Schinella *et al.*, 2002), *Gardenia jasminoides* (fruit, 1.5 g) (Chang *et al.*, 2002; Tuchinda *et al.*, 2002), *Glycyrrhiuza uralensis* (root, 1.5 g) (Watanabe *et al.*, 2002; Wang and Nixon, 2001), *Mentha haplocalyx* (whole plant, 1.5 g) (Villasenor *et al.*, 2002; Zheng *et al.*, 1993), *Paeonia lactiflora* (root, 1.5 g) (Lee *et al.*, 2002b; Oh *et al.*, 2001), *Phellodendron chinense* (bark, 1.5 g) (Gray *et al.*, 1988; Kishi *et al.*, 1992), *Platycodon grandiflorum* (root, 1.5 g), *Rehmannia glutinosa* (root, 1.5 g) (Kim *et al.*, 1999; Liang *et al.*, 1999), *Scutellaria baicalensis* (root, 1.5 g) (Lee *et al.*, 2002a; Chan *et al.*, 2002), and *Trichosanthe kirilowii* (root, 1.5 g) (Kong *et al.*, 1998; le Mai *et al.*, 2002).

(6) **Chai-hu-kuei-chih-tang:** *Bupleurum chinense* (root, 5 g) (Tsai *et al.*, 2002b; Matsuda *et al.*, 1997), *Cinnamomum cassia* (bark, 2.5 g) (Hong *et al.*, 2002), *Glycyrrhiza uralensis* (root, 1.5 g) (Watanabe *et al.*, 2002; Wang and Nixon, 2001), *Paeonia lactiflora* (root, 2.5 g) (Lee *et al.*, 2002b; Oh *et al.*, 2001), *Panax ginseng* (root, 2 g) (Yun, 2003; Bespalov *et al.*, 2001), *Pinella ternata* (rhizome, 4 g), *Scutellaria baicalensis* (root, 2 g) (Lee *et al.*, 2002a; Chan *et al.*, 2002), and *Zingiber officinale* (root, 1 g) (Murakami *et al.*, 2002; Vimala *et al.*, 1999).

(7) **Chai-hu-shu-kan-san:** *Bupleurum chinense* (root, 4 g) (Tsai *et al.*, 2002b; Matsuda *et al.*, 1997), *Citrus aurantium* (fruit, 2 g) (Kris-Etherton *et al.*, 2002; Nangia-Makker *et al.*, 2002), *Citrus tangerina* (green peel, 2 g) (Kris-Etherton *et al.*, 2002; Nangia-Makker *et al.*, 2002), *Cnidium officinale* (root, 3 g) (Kwak *et al.*, 2002), *Cyperus rotundus* (root, 3 g), *Gardenia jasminoides* (fruit, 3 g) (Chang *et al.*, 2002; Tuchinda *et al.*, 2002), *Glycyrrhiza uralensis* (root, 2 g) (Watanabe *et al.*, 2002; Wang and Nixon, 2001), *Paeonia lactiflora* (root, 4 g) (Lee *et al.*, 2002b; Oh *et al.*, 2001), and *Zingiber officinale* (root, 1 g) (Murakami *et al.*, 2002; Vimala *et al.*, 1999).

(8) **Chia-wei-hsiao-yao-san:** *Angelica sinensis* (root, 3 g) (Kapadia *et al.*, 2002; Pae *et al.*, 2002), *Atractylodes macrocephala* (root, 3 g) (Yu *et al.*, 2001), *Bupleurum chinense* (root, 3 g), (Tsai *et al.*, 2002b; Matsuda *et al.*, 1997), *Gardenia jasminoides* (fruit, 2 g) (Chang *et al.*, 2002; Tuchinda *et al.*, 2002), *Glycyrrhiza uralensis*

(root, 2 g) (Watanabe *et al.*, 2002; Wang and Nixon, 2001), *Mentha haplocalyx* (whole plant, 1 g) (Villasenor *et al.*, 2002; Zheng *et al.*, 1993), *Paeonia lactiflora* (root, 3 g) (Lee *et al.*, 2002b; Oh *et al.*, 2001), *Paeonia suffruitocosa* (root bark, 2 g) (Lee *et al.*, 2002b; Oh *et al.*, 2001), and *Poria cocos* (dry body, 3 g) (Ukiya *et al.*, 2002).

(9) **Hsiang-pei-yang-jung-tang:** *Angelica sinensis* (root, 9 g) (Kapadia *et al.*, 2002; Pae *et al.*, 2002), *Atractylodes macrocephala* (root, 12 g) (Yu *et al.*, 2001), *Citrus aurantium* (fruit, 6 g) (Kris-Etherton *et al.*, 2002; Nangia-Makker *et al.*, 2002), *Cnidium officinale* (root, 6 g) (Kwak *et al.*, 2002), *Cyperus rotundus* (root, 9 g), *Fritillaria cirrhosa* (rhizome, 6 g), *Glycyrrhiza uralensis* (root, 4.5 g) (Watanabe *et al.*, 2002; Wang and Nixon, 2001), *Platycodon grandiflorum* (root, 9 g), *Poria cocos* (dry body, 12 g) (Ukiya *et al.*, 2002), *Rehmannia glutinosa* (root, 12 g) (Kim *et al.*, 1999; Liang *et al.*, 1999), *Salvia miltiorrhiza* (root, 9 g) (Chen *et al.*, 2001; Gali Muhtasib and Affara, 2000), *Zingiber officinale* (fresh root, 3 g) (Murakami *et al.*, 2002; Vimala *et al.*, 1999), and *Zizyphus jujuba* (fruit, 4 g) (Su *et al.*, 2002; Aliev *et al.*, 2002).

(10) **Hsiao-chai-hu-tang:** *Bupleurum chinense* (root, 7 g) (Tsai *et al.*, 2002b; Matsuda *et al.*, 1997), *Glycyrrhiza uralensis* (root, 2 g) (Watanabe *et al.*, 2002; Wang and Nixon, 2001), *Panax ginseng* (root, 3 g) (Yun, 2003; Bespalov *et al.*, 2001), *Pinella ternata* (root, 5 g), *Scutellaria baicalensis* (root, 3 g) (Lee *et al.*, 2002a; Chan *et al.*, 2002), *Zingiber officinale* (root, 4 g) (le Mai *et al.*, 2002; Morita *et al.*, 1997), and *Zizyphus jujuba* (fruit, 3 g) (Su *et al.*, 2002; Aliev *et al.*, 2002).

(11) **Hsiao-yan-san:** *Angelica sinensis* (root, 3 g) (Kapadia *et al.*, 2002; Pae *et al.*, 2002), *Atractylodes macrocephala* (root, 3 g) (Yu *et al.*, 2001), *Bupleurum chinense* (root, 3 g) (Tsai *et al.*, 2002b; Matsuda *et al.*, 1997), *Glycyrrhiza uralensis* (root, 1.5 g) (Watanabe *et al.*, 2002; Wang and Nixon, 2001), *Mentha haplocalyx* (whole plant, 1 g) (Villasenor *et al.*, 2002; Zheng *et al.*, 1993), *Paeonia lactiflora* (root, 3 g) (Lee *et al.*, 2002b; Oh *et al.*, 2001), *Poria cocos* (dry body, 3 g) (Ukiya *et al.*, 2002), and *Zingiber officinale* (fresh root, 2 g) (le Mai *et al.*, 2002; Morita *et al.*, 1997).

(12) **Hua-yen-tang:** *Astragalus membranaceus* (root, 30 g) (Hsieh *et al.*, 2002; Wong *et al.*, 1992), *Atractylodes macrocephala* (root, 60 g) (Yu *et al.*, 2001), *Brassica juncea* (seed, 6 g) (van Poppel *et al.*, 1999; Brignall, 2001), *Lonicera japonica* (stem, 30 g) (Shi *et al.*, 1999), *Panax ginseng* (root, 30 g) (Yun, 2003; Bespalov *et al.*, 2001), *Poria cocos* (dry body, 9 g) (Ukiya *et al.*, 2002), and *Rubia cordifolia* (root, 6 g) (Wakita *et al.*, 2001; Adwankar and Chitnis, 1982).

(13) **Huang-lien-chieh-tu-tang:** *Coptis chinensis* (root, 2 g) (Schinella *et al.*, 2002; Fukuda *et al.*, 1999), *Gardenia jasminoides* (fruit, 2 g) (Chang *et al.*, 2002; Tuchinda *et al.*, 2002), *Phellodendron chinense* (bark, 2 g) (Gray *et al.*, 1988; Kishi *et al.*, 1992), and *Scutellaria baicalensis* (root, 3 g) (Lee *et al.*, 2002a; Chan *et al.*, 2002).

(14) **I-chi-yang-jung-tang:** *Angelica sinensis* (root, 6 g) (Kapadia *et al.*, 2002; Pae *et al.*, 2002), *Astragalus membranaceus* (root, 6 g) (Hsieh *et al.*, 2002; Wong *et al.*, 1992), *Atractylodes macrocephala* (root, 6 g), *Fritillaria cirrhosa* (rhizome, 6 g), *Glycyrrhiza uralensis* (root, 1.5 g) (Watanabe *et al.*, 2002; Wang and Nixon, 2001), *Paeonia lactiflora* (root, 6 g) (Lee *et al.*, 2002b; Oh *et al.*, 2001), *Panax ginseng* (root, 6 g) (Yun, 2003; Bespalov *et al.*, 2001), *Platycodon grandiflorum* (root, 1.5 g), *Poria cocos* (dry body, 6 g) (Ukiya *et al.*, 2002), *Rehmannia glutinosa* (steamed root, 6 g) (Kim *et al.*, 1999; Liang *et al.*, 1999), *Zingiber officinale* (root, 3 g) (Murakami *et al.*, 2002; Vimala *et al.*, 1999), and *Zizyphus jujuba* (fruit, 2 g) (Su *et al.*, 2002; Aliev *et al.*, 2002).

(15) **Kuei-chih-fu-ling-wan:** *Cinnamomum cassia* (bark, 4 g) (Hong *et al.*, 2002), *Paeonia lactiflora* (root, 4 g) (Lee *et al.*, 2002b; Oh *et al.*, 2001), *Paeonia suffruticosa* (root bark, 4 g) (Lee *et al.*, 2002b; Oh *et al.*, 2001), *Poria cocos* (dry body, 4 g) (Ukiya *et al.*, 2002), and *Prunus persica* (semen, 4 g).

(16) **Kuei-pi-tang:** *Angelica sinensis* (root, 2 g) (Kapadia *et al.*, 2002; Pae *et al.*, 2002), *Astragalus membranaceus* (root, 2 g) (Hsieh *et al.*, 2002; Wong *et al.*, 1992), *Atractylodes macrocephala* (root, 3 g) (Yu *et al.*, 2001), *Euphoria longana* (fruit, 3 g) (Minakata

et al., 1985), *Glycyrrhiza uralensis* (root, 1 g) (Watanabe *et al.*, 2002; Wang and Nixon, 2001), *Panax ginseng* (root, 3 g) (Yun, 2003; Bespalov *et al.*, 2001), *Platycodon grandiflorum* (root, 1 g), *Poria cocos* (dry body, 3 g) (Ukiya *et al.*, 2002), *Saussurea lappa* (root, 1.5 g) (Jeong *et al.*, 2002; Duan *et al.*, 2002), *Zingiber officinale* (root, 1 g) (Murakami *et al.*, 2002; Vimala *et al.*, 1999), *Zizyphus jujuba* (fruit, 1 g) (Su *et al.*, 2002; Aliev *et al.*, 2002), and *Zizyphus jujuba var. spinosa* (seed, 3 g) (Su *et al.*, 2002; Aliev *et al.*, 2002).

(17) **Shih-liu-wei-liu-chi-yin:** *Angelica dehurica* (root, 2 g) (Kapadia *et al.*, 2002; Pae *et al.*, 2002), *Angelica sinensis* (root, 3 g) (Kapadia *et al.*, 2002; Pae *et al.*, 2002), *Areca catechu* (seed, 2 g), *Astragalus membranaceus* (root, 2 g) (Hsieh *et al.*, 2002; Wong *et al.*, 1992), *Cinnamomum cassia* (bark, 3 g) (Hong *et al.*, 2002), *Citrus aurantium* (seed, 2 g) (Kris-Etherton *et al.*, 2002; Nangia-Makker *et al.*, 2002), *Cnidium officinale* (root, 6 g) (Kwak *et al.*, 2002), *Glycyrrhiza uralensis* (root, 2 g) (Watanabe *et al.*, 2002; Wang and Nixon, 2001), *Lindera strychnifolia* (root, 2 g) (Tsai *et al.*, 2002a), *Magnolia officinale* (bark, 2 g) (Yang *et al.*, 2002), *Paeonia lactiflora* (root, 3 g) (Lee *et al.*, 2002b; Oh *et al.*, 2001), *Panax ginseng* (root, 3 g) (Yun, 2003; Bespalov *et al.*, 2001), *Perilla frutescens var. crispa* (leaf, 2 g) (Crowell *et al.*, 1994), *Platycodon grandiflorm* (root, 3 g), *Saposhnikovia divaricata* (root, 2 g) (Wang *et al.*, 2000), and *Saussurea lappa* (root, 2 g) (Jeong *et al.*, 2002; Duan *et al.*, 2002).

(18) **Tzu-ken-mu-li-tang:** *Angelica sinensis* (root, 6 g) (Kapadia *et al.*, 2002; Pae *et al.*, 2002), *Astragalus membranaceus* (root, 2 g) (Hsieh *et al.*, 2002; Wong *et al.*, 1992), *Cimicifuga foetida* (root, 2 g) (Muños and Pluchino, 2003), *Cnidium officinale* (root, 6 g) (Kwak *et al.*, 2002), *Glycyrrhiza uralensis* (root, 1 g) (Watanabe *et al.*, 2002; Wang and Nixon, 2001), *Lithospermum erythrorhizon* (root, 3 g) (Kim *et al.*, 2002), *Lonicera japonica* (flower, 1.5 g) (Shi *et al.*, 1999), *Otrea rivularis* (shell, 4 g), *Paeonia lactiflora* (root, 3 g) (Lee *et al.*, 2002b; Oh *et al.*, 2001), and *Rheum palmatum* (rhizome, 1.5 g) (Shi *et al.*, 2001; Wang *et al.*, 2002).

14.3 Preparation and Quality Control of Complex Medicinal Formula

Mingtong Pharmaceutical (MTP) Company, an integrated member of this research team, has procured more than 300 herbs from different suppliers. MTP routinely utilizes approximately 200 herbs each year for the production of a variety of Chinese medicinal formulas under cGMP regulations. All procured herbs are visually/microscopically examined and matched with authentic herbarium samples. Thin-layer chromatographic profiles are determined to verify the herb identity. MTP has also initiated a program to establish the HPLC profiles for the most frequently used herbs. In the future, DNA fingerprinting of all active herbs will be utilized to validate the authenticity of the procured materials. All selected Chinese medicinal formulas are prepared by a decoction method by MTP using a standard cGMP processes.

As listed above, the traditional Chinese medicinal formulas under discussion consist of four to 16 herbs. However, none of the herbal constituents for the prevention or treatment of breast cancer has been determined. Thus, standard quality control methods used for single active ingredients are not going to be directly applicable to the quality control of these complex formulas (Tsai, 2001), but results should be useful for helping to assure reproducibility. Toward this end, water extracts of the formula can be fractionated by a solid phase extraction method using a C_{18} silica gel cartridge, and then sequentially washed with water and ethanol. Both water and ethanol fractions can be analyzed by reversed phase HPLC using a photodiode arrayed UV or evaporative light scattering detector. These chromatograms will serve as fingerprints for the initial quality control of these materials. In the next phase of work with active formulas, further refined HPLC systems can be developed for the quantitative determination of potentially active compounds.

14.4 Animal Models for Breast Cancer

Animal models for human breast cancer have been used to test the anti-carcinogenic or anti-tumor efficacy of newly developed compounds, to study interactions among anti-carcinogenic or anti-tumor agents, and to investigate possible mechanisms by which these chemopreventive or anti-tumor drugs may act to inhibit carcinogenesis or growth of breast cancer cells (Matulka and Wagner, 2005). Among the various *in vivo* and *in vitro* models of breast cancer, the most widely used in chemoprevention studies have been the mammary adenocarcinoma induced by chemical carcinogens in the female Sprague-Dawley rat. Data obtained from studies using the rat mammary adenocarcinoma model system have been supplemented by the results of experiments conducted in several mouse models for breast cancer. Most notable among the latter are mouse mammary tumors, induced by exposure to mouse mammary tumor virus (MMTV) or 7,12-dimethylbenz(*a*)anthracene (DMBA) and, more recently, several mouse transgenic models.

14.4.1 *Maximum tolerated dose*

The importance of selecting agent dose levels which do not suppress body weight gain or induce gross signs of toxicity cannot be over-emphasized in all animal models. Many investigators have noted an inhibition of carcinogenesis that can be associated with a reduced rate of body weight gain. Should an agent be found to have significant anti-cancer activity, it is imperative that this activity be disassociated from both the induction of toxicity and the reduction of caloric intake that may be associated with ingestion of that agent. Should a compound concomitantly inhibit carcinogenesis and reduce the rate of animal body weight gain, the utility of the finding will be severely compromised. It is then unclear whether the inhibition was mediated via a true anti-carcinogenic activity of the agent, or was secondary to caloric restriction, reduced body weight and/or the induction of other toxicity in test animals.

Dose tolerance studies for the transgenic mice can be conducted using female non-transgenic litter mates (FVB) of the parent strain. Previous studies in our laboratory have shown that the parent non-transgenic female FVB mouse exhibits similar toxicity and/or dose tolerance profiles as exhibited by the C3(1)/Tag female transgenic mouse. Such studies for the rat can employ the female Sprague-Dawley rat. All animals begin treatment at the same age at which agent administration would begin in the anti-cancer study; in the mouse, seven weeks of age, and in the rat,

Table 14.1. Protocol for dose tolerance assay in female non-transgenic FVB mice or Sprague-Dawley rats.

Group	No. of mice or rats	Dose
1	10	Water
2	10	No dilution
3	10	1:1
4	10	1:2
5	10	1:4
6	10	1:8

approximately ten weeks of age. Prior to beginning treatment, animals should be randomized by body weight into treatment groups. Animals are observed twice daily and weighed twice weekly in order to assess any possible adverse effects. After six weeks of treatment, all animals are killed and necropsies are performed in order to detect possible gross toxicity of the herbal preparation. The highest dose of the herbal preparation selected for the anti-cancer studies should that dose which does not affect body weight gain or present any gross effect (maximum tolerated dose, MTD), compared with vehicle controls. The mice and rats selected for the MTD should continue on the dose until the end of the anti-carcinogenesis studies to determine whether or not there is any evidence of delayed toxicity. Sample protocols for dose tolerance studies in the transgenic mouse and Sprague-Dawley rat are given in Table 14.1.

14.4.2 *N-Methyl-N-nitrosourea rat mammary*

The rat mammary adenocarcinoma model system, which can employ as carcinogens polycyclic aromatic hydrocarbons such as DMBA, 3-methylcholanthrene or benzo(*a*)pyrene (BP), or *N*-nitroso compounds such as *N*-methyl-*N*-nitrosourea (MNU), has been widely used to screen for anti-carcinogenic activity of chemical agents. In our laboratory, this model has been used in studies of the anti-carcinogenic activity of retinoids, antioxidants, modifiers of arachidonic acid metabolism, anti-hormones, endocrine ablation, biological response modifiers, and natural products (Park and Pezzuto, 2002).

The MNU model, as originally described (Gullino *et al.*, 1975) and subsequently extensively modified in Moon's laboratory (McCormick *et al.*, 1981), provides a rapid and reliable assay for anti-carcinogenic activity, and the tumors induced in this experimental model have many similarities to the human disease in terms of histology, biology, and hormone dependence which make it useful for studies of modification of carcinogenesis and/or the effect of potential anti-cancer agents on established tumors. These unique features are:

- mammary cancers can be induced with a single dose of carcinogen;
- tumor induction is specific for the mammary gland;
- tumors are induced in a dose-related manner with little or no systemic toxicity, and the majority of MNU-induced mammary cancer is hormone dependent;
- our experience with this model over the past several years has shown it to be extremely reproducible in terms of both dose-response and time-response parameters;
- the latency period of induced tumors is such that, at the MNU dose to be used in this protocol, sufficient tumor numbers can be attained within 100 days, making this a relative short *in vivo* assay;
- tumors are locally invasive and metastasize to distant sites; and
- histopathologically, the tumors resemble human breast tumors more closely than those of other animal models.

The experimental model to be used in these studies is the rat mammary carcinoma induced by a single intravenous injection of *N*-methyl-*N*-nitrosourea (MNU) at 50 days of age. Our experience with this model has shown it to be extremely reproducible in terms of its dose-response and time-response parameters. The experimental animal to be used for the mammary study is the virgin, female Sprague-Dawley [Hsd:(SD)BR] rat. All animals are obtained at 42 days of age from Harlan/Sprague-Dawley, Indianapolis, IN. Sprague-Dawley animals were chosen because they are readily available, relatively healthy animals which are extremely susceptible to mammary cancer induction by MNU, and have been successfully used in anti-cancer studies.

The experimental approach follows. Virgin, female Sprague-Dawley rats are received at 42 days of age from the supplier, and maintained for

Table 14.2. Protocol for effects of various herbal preparations on growth of palpable mammary tumors.

Group	No. of animals	Tumors/Group	MNU	Agent
1	12	12–15	+	Basal diet
2	12	12–15	+	i.g. control
3	12	12–15	+	A
4	12	12–15	+	B
5	12	12–15	+	C
6	12	12–15	+	D
7	12	12–15	+	E
8	12	12–15	+	F
9	12	12–15	+	G
10	12	12–15	+	H

seven days in isolation. Animals are housed in polycarbonate cages (two to three per cage) in a windowless room that is illuminated for 12 hours each day and is maintained at 22 ± 1°C and at 50% relative humidity. At 49 days of age, animals are randomized by body weight into groups.

At age 50 days, rats receive a single intravenous injection of 50 mg MNU/kg b.w. dissolved in sterile saline (pH 5) via the jugular. Control animals receive sterile saline only. Beginning three weeks at MNU administration, animals are palpated weekly to monitor mammary tumor appearance. The date of appearance and location of all tumors are recorded. Growth of the tumors are monitored twice weekly and measurements taken with Vernier caliper. When an animal's first palpable tumor becomes ~6–8 mm in diameter, the animal is placed into one of the ten treatment groups. Animals are observed twice daily to assess their general health, and weighed weekly for the duration of the study. In the protocol (Table 14.2), the administration of the traditional medicine should begin when the first tumor to appear attains a size of ~6–8 mm in diameter and continue for six weeks at which time the animals are sacrificed. We have previously conducted such studies using similar protocols (Ratko *et al.*, 1989; Moon *et al.*, 1989; Dowlatshahi *et al.*, 1989).

14.4.3 *Transgenic mouse*

Several transgenic mouse models are available for studying the "spontaneous" development of cancer at several target sites. Most of these models involve the alteration for overexpression of one or more oncogenes. Frequently used oncogenes for such transgenic mice have been certain transforming antigens of the simian virus 40 (SV 40). Other models have used specific oncogenes (c-*ras*, c-*myc*, c-*neu*), particularly as related to mammary oncogenesis. Recent efforts by Green and associates (Maroulakou *et al.*, 1994) have resulted in the development of a transgenic mouse line in which the SV 40 large tumor antigen (Tag) was combined with a hormone responsive promoter. The specific regulatory control element was derived from the 5α flanking region of the rat prostatic steroid binding protein, C3(1) gene and this regulatory region directs expression of Tag to the prostate and mammary glands resulting in a sequence of histopathologic changes.

In the male, the prostatic epithelium exhibits atypical hyperplasia and dysplasia as early as three months of age and about a third of the animals possess prostatic adenomas at age six to eight months. Further, in those animals surviving for eight months or more, a majority exhibit prostatic adenocarcinomas. The mammary glands of the female mice exhibit a typical ductal and acinar hyperplasia in 75% of the mice within three months of age and virtually a 100% incidence of adenocarcinoma in animals surviving four months or more.

Although lesions of the mammary gland develop in these female transgenic mice, a disadvantage of the model is the relative short life-span of these animals. For example, females in which mammary adenocarcinomas appear at four months exhibit a survival rate of only about 40%. However, the model appears highly relevant for determining the chemopreventive efficacy of various agents against early lesions of the mammary gland which subsequently progress to carcinomas.

The experimental model to be used in these studies is the transgenic mouse model developed for mammary and prostatic adenocarcinomas by Green and colleagues (Maroulakou *et al.*, 1994). Transgenic female mice bearing a recombinant gene expressing the SV 40 early-region transforming sequence under the regulatory control of rat prostatic steroid binding

Table 14.3. Protocol for anti-cancer assay in mammary glands of female transgenic mice.

Group	No. of animals	Dose
1	20	Water
2	20	MTD
3	10	None

protein [C3(1)] gene can be obtained from the Biological Testing Branch/ NCI at six weeks of age.

The protocols for evaluating the anti-cancer potential of the various agents against tumorigenesis in the female transgenic mice are detailed in Table 14.3. Transgenic mice are received at six weeks of age and acclimated for at least one week. Animals will be housed in polycarbonate cages (four or five per cage) in a windowless room that is illuminated for 14 hours each day and is maintained at 22 ± 1°C and at 50% relative humidity. After one week of quarantine, animals are randomized by body weight into groups. Mice are sacrificed at the time indicated in the protocols. The herbal preparation is administered intragastrically three times per week at the maximum tolerated dose as determined by a dose tolerance study. Animals are observed twice daily to assess their general health, and weighed weekly for the duration of the study.

Moribund animals are killed by CO_2 asphyxiation. All moribund animals and any animals found dead during the course of the study are promptly necrospied. At the termination of the experiment, all remaining animals are killed by CO_2 asphyxiation.

Mice are palpated for mammary tumors on a weekly basis. The number and location of mammary tumors observed are recorded. At sacrifice, tumors are fixed in 10% buffered formalin, embedded in paraffin, sectioned at 5 μ, stained with hematoxylin eosin, and are evaluated histopathologically for tumor type.

14.5 Conclusions

The proposed evaluation procedure is designed to select the complex formulas of traditional Chinese medicine for prevention or therapeutic control of human breast cancer on the basis of *in vitro* and *in vivo* bioactivities pertinent to the modulation of growth and differentiation of cancer cells. Since the selected complex formulas are reputed to be of use in treating human breast cancer, data obtained with *in vitro* systems are not definitive, and further mechanistic studies are meaningless with test substances incapable of mediating *in vivo* anti-tumor responses. The most appropriate approach to assess their potential clinical efficacy is first to establish their efficacy in a clinically relevant animal model. The animal models were selected based on our experience, and their close relevance to the human cancer situation. Determining MDT is a necessary precursor for the performance of anti-tumor studies, but this work should also provide insight regarding the potential toxicity of the test substances. Studies with the transgenic mouse model should indicate potential to alter tumorigenesis, even though it would not be clear if a positive response is due to a cancer preventive effect or a cancer therapeutic effect. Nonetheless, in either case, a positive response would be of great interest, and future studies could readily be designed to differentiate these activities. In addition, of course, the MNU rat studies are explicitly designed to explore the therapeutic effects, and this response mimics current clinical use. In future studies, the MNU model, as well as the DMBA model, could be used to assess cancer chemopreventive activity.

Acknowledgments

Experimental work in this area is supported by program project P01 CA48112 awarded by the US National Cancer Institute.

References

Adler, S. (1999) Complimentary and alternative medicine use among women with breast cancer. *Med. Anthropol. Q.* **13**, 214–222.

Adwankar, M.K. and Chitnis, M.P. (1982) *In vivo* anti-cancer activity of RC-18: A plant isolate from *Rubia cordifolia*, Linn. Against a spectrum of experimental tumour models. *Chemotherapy* **28**, 291–293.

Aggarwal, B.B., Kumar, A. and Bharti, A.C. (2003) Anticancer potential of curcumin: Preclinical and clinical studies. *Anticancer Res.* **23**, 363–398.

Aliev, A.A., Dzhafarova, S.D., Rustamova, A.M. and Medzhidov, M.M. (2002) Protection of mammalian genome from the mutagenicity of styrene and aniline using the extract from unabi (*Zizyphus mil*) fruit and a composite preparation. *Tsitol. Genet.* **36**, 26–29.

Arun, B. and Hortobagyi, G.N. (2002) Progress in breast cancer prevention. *Endocr. Relat. Cancer* **9**, 15–32.

Bespalov, V.G., Alexandrov, V.A., Limarenko, A.Y., Voytenkov, B.O., Okulov, V.B., Kabulov, M.K., Peresunko, A.P., Slepyan, L.I. and Davydov, V.V. (2001) Chemoprevention of mammary, cervix and nervous system carcinogenesis in animals using cultured *Panax* ginseng drugs and preliminary clinical trials in patients with precancerous lesions of the esophagus and endometrium. *J. Korean Med. Sci.* **16**, S42–53.

Brignall, M.S. (2001) Prevention and treatment of cancer with indole-3-carbinol. *Altern. Med. Rev.* **6**, 580–589.

Chan, H.Y., Chen, Z.Y., Tsang, D.S.C. and Leung, L.K. (2002) Baicalein inhibits DMBA-DNA adduct formation by modulating CYP1A1 and CYP1B1 activities. *Biomed. Pharmacother.* **56**, 269–275.

Chan, K. and Morris, G.J. (2006) Chemoprevention of breast cancer for women at high risk. *Semin. Oncol.* **33**, 642–646.

Chang, Y.C., Tseng, T.H., Lee, M.J., Hsu, J.D. and Wang, C.J. (2002) Induction of apoptosis by penta-acetyl geniposide in rat C6 glioma cells. *Chem. Biol. Interact.* **141**, 243–257.

Chemoprevention Working Group (1999) Prevention of cancer in the next millenium: Report of the chemoprevention working group to the American Association for Cancer Research. *Cancer Res.* **59**, 4743–4758.

Chen, X.G., Li, Y., Yan, C.H., Li, L.N. and Han, R. (2001) Cancer chemopreventive activities of S-3-1, a synthetic derivative of danshinone. *J. Asian Nat. Prod. Res.* **3**, 63–75.

Cheung, C.S. (1999) *Breast Cancer Supportive Management: A Collective Works from Traditional Chinese Medicine Practitioners of China.* Harmonious Sunshine Press, San Francisco, CA.

Chin, Y.W., Lim, S.W., Kim, S.H., Shin, D.Y., Suh, Y.G., Kim, Y.B., Kim, Y.C. and Kim, J. (2003) Hepatoprotective pyrrole derivatives of *Lycium chinense* fruits. *Bioorg. Med. Chem. Lett.* **13**, 79–81.

Chung, H.S., Jeong, H.J., Hong, S.H., Kim, M.S., Kim, S.J., Song, B.K., Jeong, I.S., Lee, E.J., Ahn, J.W., Baek, S.H. and Kim, H.M. (2002) Induction of nitric oxide synthase by *Oldenlandia diffusa* in mouse peritoneal macrophages. *Biol. Pharm. Bull.* **25**, 1142–1146.

Cohen, I., Tagliferri, M. and Tripathy, D. (2002) Traditional Chinese medicine in the treatment of breast cancer. *Semin. Oncol.* **29**, 563–574.

Crowell, P.L., Ren, Z., Lin, S. and Vedejs, E.M.N. (1994) Structure-activity relationships among monoterpene inhibitors of protein isoprenylation and cell proliferation. *Biochem. Pharmacol.* **47**, 1405–1415.

Cuzick, J., Powles, T., Veronesi, U., Forbes, J., Edwards, R., Ashley, S. and Boyle, P. (2003) Overview of the main outcomes in breast cancer prevention trials. *Lancet* **361**, 296–300.

Day, S.H., Lin, Y.C., Tsai, M.L., Tsao, L.T., Ko, H.H., Chung, M.I., Lee, J.C., Wang, J.P., Won, S.J. and Lin, C.N. (2002) Potent cytotoxic lignans from *Justicia procumbens* and their effects on nitric oxide and tumor necrosis factor-alpha production in mouse macrophages. *J. Nat. Prod.* **65**, 379–381.

Dowlatshahi, K., Mehta, R.G., Thomas, C.F., Dinger, N.M. and Moon, R.C. (1989) Therapeutic effect of *N*-(4-hydroxyphenyl)retinamide on *N*-methyl-*N*-nitrosourea-induced rat mammary cancer. *Cancer Lett.* **47**, 187–192.

Duan, H., Takaishi, Y., Momota, H., Ohmoto, Y. and Taki, T. (2002) Immunosuppressive constituents from Saussurea medusa. *Phytochemistry* **59**, 85–90.

Forman, M.R., Ballard-Barbash, R. and Kipnis, V. (2003) Nutritional strategies for breast cancer prevention, What have we learned and where do we go from here? *Cancer* **98**, 1782–1785.

Fukuda, K., Hibiya, Y., Mutoh, M., Koshiji, M., Akao, S. and Fujiwara, H. (1999) Inhibition by berberine of cyclooxygenase-2 transcriptional activity in human colon cancer cells. *J. Ethnopharmacol.* **66**, 227–233.

Gali Muhtasib, H.U. and Affara, N.I. (2000) Chemopreventive effects of sage oil on skin papillomas in mice. *Phytomedicine* **7**, 129–136.

Gan, L., Wang, J. and Zhang, S. (2001) Inhibition the growth of human leukemia cells by *Lycium barbarum* polysaccharide. *Wei Sheng Yen Chiu/J. Hyg. Res.* **30**, 333–335.

Gordaliza, M., Garcia, P.A., Corral, M.D., Castro, M.A. and Gomez-Zurita, M.A. (2004) Podophyllotoxins: distribution, sources, applications and new cytotoxic derivatives. *Toxicon* **44**, 441–459.

Gray, A.I., Bhandari, P. and Waterman, P.G. (1988) New protolimonoids from the fruits of *Phellodendron chinense*. *Phytochemistry* **27**, 1805–1808.

Gullino, P.M., Pettigrew, H.M. and Grantham, F.H. (1975) *N*-nitrosomethylurea as mammary gland carcinogen in rats. *J. Natl. Cancer Inst.* **54**, 401–414.

Hanf, V. and Gonder, U. (2005) Nutrition and primary prevention of breast cancer: Foods, nutrients and breast cancer risk. *Eur. J. Obstet. Gynecol. Reprod. Biol.* **123**, 139–149.

Heo, M.Y., Kim, S.H., Yang, H.E., Lee, S.H., Jo, B.K. and Kim, H.P. (2001) Protection against ultraviolet B- and C-induced DNA damage and skin carcinogenesis by the flowers of *Prunus persica* extract. *Mutat. Res.* **496**, 47–59.

Hirose, M., Yamaguchi, T., Lin, C., Kimoto, N., Futakuchi, M., Kono, T., Nishibe, S. and Shirai, T. (2000) Effects of arctiin on PhIP-induced mammary, colon and pancreatic carcinogenesis in female Sprague-Dawley rats and MeIQx-induced hepatocarcinogenesis in male F344 rats. *Cancer Lett.* **155**, 79–88.

Hong, C.H., Hur, S.K., Oh, O.J., Kim, S.S., Nam, K.A. and Lee, S.K. (2002) Evaluation of natural products on inhibition of inducible cyclooxygenase (COX-2) and nitric oxide synthase (iNOS) in cultured mouse macrophage cells. *J. Ethnopharmacol.* **83**, 153–159.

Hsieh, T.C., Lu, X., Guo, J., Xiong, W., Kunicki, J., Darzynkiewicz, Z. and Wu, J.M. (2002) Effects of herbal preparation Equigard on hormone-responsive and hormone-refractory prostate carcinoma cells: Mechanistic studies. *Int. J. Oncol.* **20**, 681–689.

Hsu, H.Y. (1982) *Treating Cancer with Chinese Herbs*. Oriental Healing Art Institute, Los Angeles, CA.

International Breast Cancer Intervention Study Investigators (2002) First results from the International Breast Cancer Intervention Study: A randomized prevention trial. *Lancet* **360**, 817–824.

Itoh, H., Noda, H., Amano, H. and Ito, H. (1995) Immunological analysis of inhibition of lung metastases by fucoidan (GIV-A) prepared from brown seaweed *Sargassum thunbergii*. *Anticancer Res.* **15**, 1937–1947.

Jemal, A., Siegel, R., Ward, E., Murray, T., Xu, J. and Thun M.J. (2007) Cancer statistics, 2007. *CA Cancer J. Clin.* **57**, 43–66.

Jeong, S.J., Itokawa, T., Shibuya, M., Kuwano, M., Ono, M., Higuchi, R. and Miyamoto, T. (2002) Costunolide, a sesquiterpene lactone from *Saussurea lappa*, inhibits the VEGFR KDR/Flk-1 signaling pathway. *Cancer Lett.* **187**, 129–133.

Kamangar, F., Dores, G.M. and Anderson W.F. (2006) Patterns of cancer incidence, mortality, and prevalence across five continents: Defining priority to reduce cancer disparities in different geographic regions of the world. *J. Clin. Oncol.* **24**, 2137–2150.

Kapadia, G.J., Azuine, M.A., Tokuda, H., Hang, E., Mukainaka, T., Nishino, H. and Sridhar, R. (2002) Inhibitory effect of herbal remedies on 12-*O*-tetradecanoylphorbol-13-acetate-promoted Epstein-Barr virus early antigen activation. *Pharmacol. Res.* **45**, 213–220.

Kim, D.S.H.L., Ashendel, C.L., Zhou, Q., Chang, C.T., Lee, E.S. and Chang C.J. (1998) Novel protein kinase C inhibitors: α-Terthiophene derivatives. *Bioorg. Med. Chem. Lett.* **50**, 8661–8670.

Kim, H.M., An, C.S., Jung, K.Y., Choo, Y.K., Park, J.K. and Nam, S.Y. (1999) *Rehmannia glutinosa* inhibits tumour necrosis factor-α and interleukin-1 secretion from mouse astrocytes, *Pharmacol. Res.* **40**, 171–176.

Kim, S.H., Kang, I.C., Yoon, T.J., Park, Y.M., Kang, K.S., Song, G.Y. and Ahn, B.Z. (2002) Antitumor activities of a newly synthesized shikonin derivative, 2-hyim-DMNQ-S-33. *Cancer Lett.* **172**, 171–175.

Kishi, K., Yoshikawa, K. and Arihara, S. (1992) Limonoids and protolimonoids from the fruits of *Phellodendron amurense*. *Phytochemistry* **31**, 1335–1338.

Kris-Etherton, P.M., Hecker, K.D., Bonanome, A., Coval, S.M., Binkoski, A.E., Hilpert, K.F., Griel, A.E. and Etherton, T.D. (2002) Bioactive compounds in foods: Their role in the prevention of cardiovascular disease and cancer. *Am. J. Med.* **113**, 71S–88S.

Kong, M., Ke, Y.B., Zhou, M.Y., Ke, X.Y., Lu, B. and Nie, H.L. (1998) Study on Trichosanthin induced apoptosis of leukemia K562 cells. *Shih Yen Sheng Wu Hsueh Pao/J. Exp. Biol.* **31**, 233–243.

Koyama, J., Morita, I., Tagaharra, K., Nobukuni, Y., Mukainaka, T., Kuchide, M., Tokuda, H. and Nishino, H. (2002) Chemopreventive effects of emodin and cassiamin B in mouse skin carcinogenesis. *Cancer. Lett.* **182**, 135–139.

Kwak, D.H., Kim, J.K., Kim, J.Y., Jeong, H.Y., Keum, K.S., Han, S.H., Rho, Y.I., Woo, W.H., Jung, K.Y., Choi, B.K. and Choo, Y.K. (2002) Anti-angiogenic activities of *Cnidium officinale* Makino and *Tabanus bovinus*. *J. Ethnopharmacol.* **81**, 373–379.

Lam, J., Christensen, L.P. and Thomasen, T. (1991) Thiophene derivatives from *Echinops* species. *Phytochemistry* **30**, 1157–1159.

Lang, W.J. and Mung, L.C. (1992) *One Thousand Anticancer Chinese Herbal Formulas*. Chinese Medical Science Publisher.

Lau, K.M., He, Z.D., Dong, H., Fung, K.P. and But, P.P.H. (2002) Anti-oxidative, anti-inflammatory and hepto-protective effects of *Ligustrum robustum*. *J. Ethnopharmacol.* **83**, 63–71.

Lee, H. and Lin Y.Y. (1988) Antimutagenic activity of extracts from anticancer drugs in Chinese medicine. *Mutat. Res.* **204**, 229–234.

Lee, M.S., Oh, W.K., Kim, B.Y., Ahn, S.C., Kang, D.O., Sohn, C.B., Osada, H. and Ahn, J.S. (2002a) Inhibition of VHR dual-specificity protein tyrosine phosphatase activity by flavonoids isolated from *Scutellaria baicalensis*: Structure-activity relationships. *Planta Med.* **68**, 1063–1065.

Lee, S.M.Y., Li, M.L.Y., Tse, Y.C., Leung, S.C.L., Lee, M.M.S., Tsui, S.K.W., Fung, K.P., Lee, C.Y. and Waye, M.M.Y. (2002b) *Paeoniae radix*, a Chinese herbal extract, inhibit hepatoma cells growth by inducing apoptosis in a p53 independent pathway. *Life Sci.* **71**, 2267–2277.

Liang, A., Xue, B., Wang, J., Hao, J., Yang, H. and Yi, H. (1999) A study on hemostatic and immunological actions of fresh and dry dihuang. *Zhongguo Zhong Yao Za Zhi* **24**, 663–666, 702.

Mai, le P., Guenard, D., Franck, M., Van, T.M., Gaspard, C. and Sevenet, T. (2002) New cytotoxic cucurbitacins from the pericarps of *Trichosanthes tricuspidata* fruits. *Nat. Prod. Lett.* **16**, 15–19.

Manson, M.M. (2003) Cancer prevention — the potential for diet to modulate molecular signalling. *Trends Mol. Med.* **9**, 11–18.

Maroulakou, I.G., Anver, M., Garrett, L. and Green, J.E. (1994) Prostate and mammary adenocarcinoma in transgenic mice carrying a rat C3(1) simian virus 40 large tumor antigen fusion gene. *Proc. Natl. Acad. Sci. USA* **91**, 11236–11240.

Matsuda, H., Murakami, T., Ninomiya, K., Inadzuki, M. and Yoshikawa, M. (1997) New hepatoprotective saponins, bupleurosides III, VI, IX, and XIII, from Chinese Burpleuri Radix: Structure-requirements for the cytoprotective activity in primary cultured rat hepatocytes. *Bioorg. Med. Chem. Lett.* **7**, 2193–2198.

Matulka, L.A. and Wagner, K. (2005) Models of breast cancer. *Drug Discov. Today* **2**, 1–6.

McCormick, D.L., Adamowski, C.B., Fiks, A. and Moon, R.C. (1981) Lifetime dose-response relationships for mammary tumor induction by a single administration of *N*-methyl-*N*-nitrosourea. *Cancer Res.* **41**, 1690–1694.

Minakata, H., Komura, H., Tamura, S.Y., Ohfune, Y., Nakanishi, K. and Kada, T. (1985) Antimutagenic unusual amino acids from plants. *Experientia* **41**, 1622–1623.

Moon, R.C., Pritchard, J.F., Mehta, R.G., Nomides, C.T., Thomas, C.F. and Dinger, N.M. (1989) Suppression of rat mammary cancer development by *N*-(4-hydroxyphenyl)retinamide (4-HPR) following surgical removal of first palpable tumor. *Carcinogenesis* **10**, 1645–1649.

Morita, H., Yun, Y.S., Takeya, K., Itokawa, H., Yamada, K. and Shirota, O. (1997) Thionation of segetalins A and B, cyclic peptides with estrogen-like activity from seed of *Vaccaria segetalis*. *Bioorg. Med. Chem.* **5**, 631–636.

Morita, K., Kada, T. and Namiki, M. (1984) A desmutagenic factor isolated from burdock (*Arctium lappa* Linne). *Mutat. Res.* **129**, 25–31.

Muños, G.H. and Pluchino, S. (2003) *Cimicifuga racemosa* for the treatment of hot flushes in women surviving breast cancer. *Maturitas* **44**, S59–S65.

Murakami, A., Takahashi, D., Kinoshita, T., Koshimizu, K., Kim, H.W., Yoshihiro, A., Nakamura, Y., Kiwajinda, S., Terao, J. and Ohigashi, H. (2002) Zerumbone, a Southeast Asian ginger sesquiterpene, markedly suppresses free radical generation, proinflammatory protein production, and cancer cell proliferation accompanied by apoptosis: The α, β-unsaturated carbonyl group is a prerequisite. *Carcinogenesis* **23**, 795–802.

Nangia-Makker, P., Hogan, V., Honjo, Y., Baccarini, S., Tait, L., Bresalier, R. and Raz, A. (2002) Inhibition of human cancer cell growth and metastatis in nude mice by oral intake of modified citrus pectin. *J. Natl. Cancer Inst.* **94**, 1854–1862.

Navarro, E., Alonso, S.J., Trujillo, J., Jorge, E. and Perez, C. (2001) General behavior, toxicity, and cytotoxic activity of elenoside, a lignan from *Justicia hyssopifolia*. *J. Nat. Prod.* **64**, 134–135.

Niikawa, M., Hayashi, H., Sato, T., Nagase, H. and Kito, H. (1993) Isolation of substances from glossy privet (*Ligustrum lucidum* Ait.) inhibiting the mutagenicity of benzo[*a*]pyrene in bacteria. *Mutat. Res.* **319**, 1–9.

Oh, G.S., Pae, H.O., Oh, H., Hong, S.G., Kim, I.K., Chai, K.Y., Yun, Y.G., Kwon, T.O. and Chung, H.T. (2001) *In vitro* anti-proliferative effect of 1, 2, 3, 4, 6-penta-*O*-galloyl-β-D-glucose on human hepatocellular carcinoma cell line, SK-HEP-1 cells. *Cancer Lett.* **174**, 17–24.

Pae, O., Oh, H., Yun, Y.G., Oh, G.S., Jang, S.I., Hwang, K.M., Kwon, T.O., Lee, H.S. and Chung, H.T. (2002) Imperatorin, a furanocoumarin from *Angelica dahurica* (Umbelliferae), induces cytochrome c-dependent apoptosis in human promyelocytic leukaemia, HL-60 cells. *Pharmacol. Toxicol.* **91**, 40–48.

Park, E.J. and Pezzuto, J.M. (2002) Botanicals in cancer chemoprevention. *Cancer Metastasis Rev.* **21**, 231–255.

Park, S., Lee, D.K., Whang, Y.H. and Yang C.H. (2000) Momordin I, a compound of ampelopsis radix, inhibits AP-1 activation induced by phorbal ester. *Cancer Lett.* **152**, 1–8.

Peraza-Sanchez, S.R., Chai, H.B., Shin, Y.G., Santisuk, T., Reutrakul, V., Farnsworth, N.R., Cordell, G.A., Pezzuto, J.M. and Kinghorn, A.D. (2002) Constituents of the leaves and twigs of *Ficus hispida*. *Planta Med.* **68**, 186–188.

Popat, S. and Smith, I.E. (2006) Breast cancer. *Updated Cancer Ther.* **1**, 187–210.

Ratko, T.A., Detrisac, C.J., Dinger, N.M., Thomas, C.F., Kelloff. G.J. and Moon, R.C. (1989) Chemopreventive efficacy of combined retonoid and tamoxifen treatment following surgical excision of a primary mammary cancer in female rats. *Cancer Res.* **49**, 4472–4476.

Reddy, L., Odhav, B. and Bhooola, K.D. (2003) Natural products for cancer prevention: A global perspective. *Pharmacol. Ther.* **5544**, 1–13.

Ruso, J. and Ruso, I.H. (2004) *Molecular Basis of Breast Cancer — Prevention and Treatment.* Springer Verlag, New York.

Schinella, G.R., Tournier, H.A., Prieto, J.M., Mordujovich de Buschiazzo, P. and Rios, J.L. (2002) Antioxidant activity of anti-inflammatory plant extracts. *Life Sci.* **70**, 1023–1033.

Shi, J., Chen, X. and Wan, L. (1999) Hepatoprotective effect of several constituents of *Lonicera fulvotomentosa* Hsu et S.C. Cheng, and L. *macranthoide* Hand.-Mazz. on CC1(4) and D-galactosamine induced liver injuries in mice and rats. *Zhongguo Zhong Yao Za Zhi* **24**, 363–364.

Shi, Y.Q., Fukai, T., Sakagami, H., Kuroda, J., Miyaoka, R., Tamura, M., Yoshida, N. and Nomura, T. (2001) Cytotoxic and DNA damage-inducing activities of low molecular weight phenols from rhubarb. *Anticancer Res.* **21**, 2847–2853.

Simon, P.N., Chaboud, A., Darbour, N., Di Pietro, A., Dumontet, C., Lurel, F., Raynaud, J. and Barron, D. (2001) Modulation of cancer cell multidrug resistance by an extract of *Ficus citrifolia. Anticancer Res.* **21**, 1023–1027.

Stevan, F.R., Oliveira, M.B., Bucchi, D.F., Noseda Iacomini, M. and Duarte, M.E. (2001) Cytotoxic effects against HeLa cells of polysaccharides from seaweeds. *J. Cytol. Pathol.* **33**, 477–484.

Su, B.N., Cuendet, M., Farnsworth, N.R., Fong, H.H., Pezzuto, J.M. and Kinghorn, A.D. (2002) Activity-guided fractionation of the seeds of *Ziziphus jujuba* using a cyclooxygenase-2 inhibitory assay. *Planta Med.* **68**, 1125–1128.

Tang, W., Hemm, I. and Bertram, B. (2003a) Recent development of antitumor agents from Chinese herbal medicines: Part I. Low molecular compounds. *Planta Med.* **69**, 97–108.

Tang, W., Hemm, I. and Bertram, B. (2003b) Recent development of antitumor agents from Chinese herbal medicines, Part II. High molecular compounds. *Planta Med.* **69**, 193–201.

Teas, J. (1983) The dietary intake of *Laminaria*, a brown seaweed, and breast cancer prevention. *Nutr. Cancer* **4**, 217–222.

Tsai, I.L., Hung, C.H., Duh, C.Y. and Chen, I.S. (2002a) Cytotoxic butanolides and secobutanolides from the stem wood of Formosan *Lindera communis. Planta Med.* **68**, 142–145.

Tsai, T.H. (2001) Analytical approaches for traditional Chinese medicine exhibiting antineoplastic activity. *J. Chromatogr.* **764**, 27–48.

Tsai, Y.J., Chen, I.L., Horng, L.Y. and Wu, R.T. (2002b) Induction of differentiation in rat C6 glioma cells with Saikosaponins. *Phytother. Res.* **16**, 117–121.

Tuchinda, P., Pompimon, W., Reutrakul, V., Pohmakotr, M., Yoosook, C., Kongyai, N., Sophasan, S., Sujarit, K., Upathum, S.E. and Santisuk, T. (2002) Cytotoxic and anti-HIV-1 constituents of *Gardenia obtusifolia* and their modified compounds. *Tetrahedron* **58**, 8073–8086.

Ukiya, M., Akihisa, T., Tokuda, H., Hirano, M., Oshikubo, M., Nobukuni, Y., Kimura, Y., Tai, T., Kondo, S. and Nishino, H. (2002) Inhibition of tumor-promoting effects by poricoic acids G and H and other lanostane-type triterpenes and cytotoxic activity of poricoic acids A and G from *Poria cocos. J. Nat. Prod.* **65**, 462–465.

van Poppel, G., Verhoeven, D.T., Verhagen, H. and Goldbohm, R.A. (1999) Brassica vegetables and cancer prevention: Epidemiology and mechanisms. *Adv. Exp. Med. Biol.* **472**, 159–168.

Veronesi, U. and Bonanni, B. (2005) Chemoprevention from research to clinical oncology. *Eur. J. Cancer* **41**, 1833–1841.

Villasenor, I.M., Echegoyen, D.E. and Angelada, J.S. (2002) A new antimutagen from *Mentha cordifolia Opiz. Mutat. Res.* **515**, 141–146.

Vimala, S., Norhanom, A.W. and Yadav, M. (1999) Anti-tumor promoter activity in Malaysian ginger rhizobia used in traditional medicine. *Br. J. Cancer* **80**, 110–116.

Wakita, K., Minami, M., Venkateswarlu, A., Sharma, V.M., Ramesh, M. and Akahane, K. (2001) Antitumor bicyclic hexapeptide RA-VII modulates cyclin D1 protein level. *Anti-Cancer Drugs* **12**, 433–439.

Wang, C.C., Huang, Y.J., Chen, L.G., Lee, L.T. and Yang, L.L. (2002) Inducible nitric oxide synthase inhibitors of Chinese herbs III. *Rheum palmatum. Planta Med.* **68**, 869–874.

Wang, C.N., Shiao, Y.J., Kuo, Y.H., Chen, C.C. and Lin, Y.L. (2000) Inducible nitric oxide synthase inhibitors from *Saposhnikovia divaricata and Panax quinquefolium. Planta Med.* **66**, 644–647.

Wang, Z.Y. and Nixon, D.W. (2001) Licorice and cancer. *Nutr. Cancer* **39**, 1–11.

Watanabe, M., Hayakawa, S., Isemura, M., Kumazawa, S., Nakayama, T., Mori, C. and Kawakami, T. (2002) Identification of licocoumarone as an apoptosis-inducing component in licorice. *Biol. Pharm. Bull.* **25**, 1388–1390.

Winchester, D.J., Winchester, D.P., Hudis, C.A. and Norton, L. (2006) *Breast Cancer.* B.C. Decker, Hamilton, ON, Canada.

Wong, B.Y., Lau, B.H., Tadi, P.P. and Teel, R.W. (1992) Chinese medicinal herbs modulate mutagenesis, DNA binding and metabolism of aflatoxin B1. *Mutat. Res.* **279**, 209–216.

Wong, C.K., Leung, K.N., Fung, K.P. and Choy, Y.M. (1994) The immuno-stimulating activities of anti-tumor polysaccharides from *Pseudostellaria heterophylla. Immunopharmacology* **28**, 47–54.

Xie, W. (1997) *Cancer and Death: Treatment of Cancer the Chinese Way*. New World Press, Beijing, China 1997.

Yang, S.-E., Hsieh, M.-T., Tsai, T.-H. and Hsu, S.-L. (2002) Down-modulation of Bcl-X_L, release of cytochrome c and sequential activation of caspases during honokiol-induced apoptosis in human squamous lung cancer CH27 cells. *Biochem. Pharmacol.* **63**, 1641–1651.

Ye, Q., Qin, G. and Zhao, W. (2002) Immunomodulatory sesquiterpene glycosides from *Dendrobium nobile*. *Phytochemistry* **61**, 885–890.

Yin, M.L. and Chen, Z.L. (1989) Chemical constituents of *Dysosma aurantiocaulis* (H.-M.) Hu and *Dysosma pleianthum* Woods. *Zhongguo Zhong Yao Za Zhi* **14**, 420–421.

Yoshida, Y., Wang, M.Q., Liu, J.N., Shan, B.E. and Yamashita, U. (1997) Immunomodulating activity of Chinese medicinal herb and *Oldenlandia diffusa in particular*. *Int. J. Immunopharmacol.* **19**, 359–270.

Yu, K.W., Kiyohara, H., Matsumoto, T., Yang, H.C. and Yamada, H. (2001) Characterization of pectic polysaccharides having intestinal immune system modulating activity from rhizomes of *Atractylodes lancea* DC. *Carbohyd. Polym.* **46**, 125–134.

Yun, T.K. (2003) Experimental and epidemiological evidence on non-organ specific cancer preventive effect of Korean ginseng and identification of active compounds. *Mutat. Res.* **523–524**, 63–74.

Zheng, G.Q., Kenney, P.M., Zhang, J. and Lam, L.K. (1993) Chemoprevention of benzo[a]pyrene-induced forestomach cancer in mice by natural phthalides from celery seed oil. *Nutr. Cancer* **19**, 77–86.

Zhu, L. and Xu, X. (2003) Selective separation of active inhibitors of epidermal growth factor receptor from *Caragana jubata* by molecularly imprinted solid-phase extraction. *J. Chromatogr.* **991**, 151–158.

Chapter 15

Functional Magnetic Resonance Imaging Studies of Acupuncture

Gary Deng & Barrie Cassileth

Abstract

Background: Acupuncture has been evaluated in functional magnetic resonance imaging (fMRI) studies to determine its modulating effect on neuronal activity in the central nervous system. However, the methodology and results vary across reported studies. A review of this research helps illuminate the possible mechanisms of action of acupuncture. *Methods*: Clinical studies of acupuncture with fMRI technology, published in English language, are reviewed. The data are summarized and discussed. *Results*: No two studies showed identical results, even when the same acupuncture points were used. One common finding is that acupuncture is associated with functional signal changes in somatosensory areas and the limbic system. How the needle is stimulated also appears important, as it causes varying patterns of activation and deactivation. Direct comparison across studies is difficult due to absence of stable methodology across studies. *Conclusion*: fMRI technology opens a new field of acupuncture research. Studies conducted to date provide insight into how acupuncture renders its physiologic effects. Better and less variable study design, plus additional data from several study groups, are needed to realize the full potential of this powerful neuroscience research tool in understanding the mechanisms behind acupuncture activity.

Keywords: Acupuncture; Neuroimaging; fMRI; Functional Magnetic Resonance Imaging; Complementary Therapies.

15.1 Introduction

Acupuncture is an ancient component of traditional Chinese medicine (TCM). Historically, it has been used to treat a variety of clinical conditions. For some indications, its clinical efficacy is demonstrated in randomized controlled trials; effectiveness for other indications remains to be studied. The exact mechanisms of action of acupuncture are an area of active research. Many clinical responses observed during acupuncture can be explained by the effect of acupuncture on the nervous system. Most mechanistic research used neurophysiologic techniques, focusing on acupuncture's ability to regulate neurotransmitter activity. Such research shows that acupuncture regulates the expression and activity of a variety of neurotransmitters, most notably endogenous opioids, although most of this research was conducted in analgesia animal models (Han, 2004; Kaptchuk, 2002).

However neurologic reactions are seldom the result of a linear pathway. Rather, they tend to be products of multidimensional interaction among many parts of the central nervous system (CNS). Neurophysiologic approaches are suboptimal for identification of complex neuronal networks involved in acupuncture. Non-invasive neuroimaging technology, developed and refined in recent years, offers a powerful, superior research tool for this purpose. It enables measuring the activation and deactivation of specific areas of the brain in real time in human subjects, thus providing deeper and broader understanding of how acupuncture may induce clinical responses.

One of the most common non-invasive neuroimaging techniques is functional magnetic resonance imaging (fMRI). A full review of fMRI can be found in Matthews *et al.* (2006). In brief, fMRI measures the hemodynamic response related to neural activity in the brain or spinal cord of humans or other animals. The magnetic resonance signal of blood is slightly different depending on the level of oxygenation. Changes in the concentration of deoxygenated hemoglobin can be detected using a special MR pulse sequence known as blood-oxygen-level dependent (BOLD) contrast. In general, changes in BOLD signal are well correlated with changes in blood flow, which is an indicator of neuronal activity. By comparing the BOLD signals in the presence versus absence of acupuncture stimulation, areas of the brain that are activated or deactivated

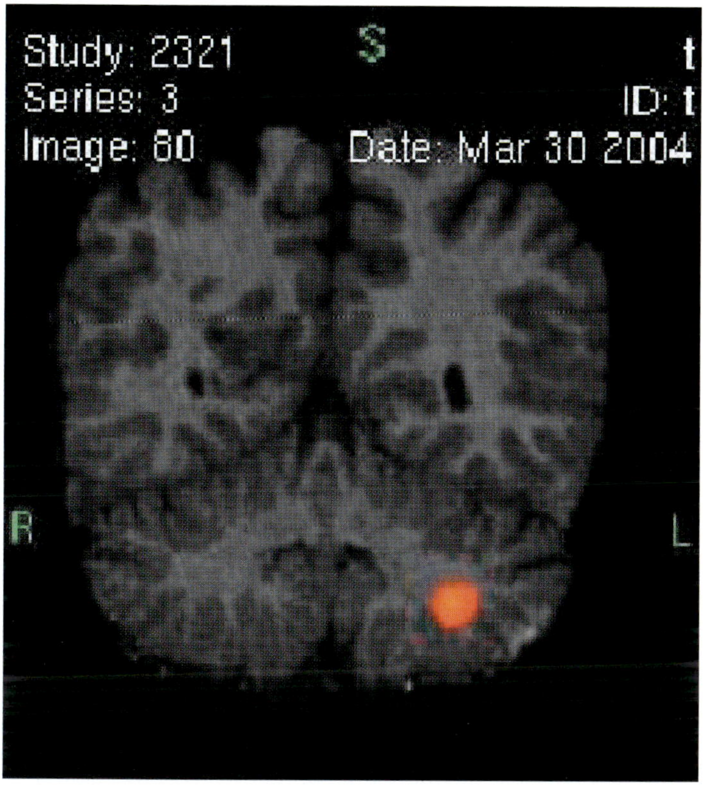

Figure 15.1. An example of fMRI images during acupuncture.

by acupuncture can be identified. These areas can be illustrated in a pseudocolor image, usually with warm colors (red or yellow) indicating activation and cool colors (blue or green) deactivation. A typical fMRI image is shown in Fig. 15.1.

To interpret fMRI acupuncture data, it is necessary to know the study population (healthy volunteers or people with specified disorders), the specific acupuncture points used, and whether different acupoints were compared in the same study, how results compare to previous data using those acupoints, the nature of any control intervention (pharmacologic, behavioral intervention, sham acupuncture) and any sham acupuncture must be detailed. It is necessary also to describe any measures of physiologic response and their correlation with neuroimaging change.

The many fMRI acupuncture studies published in the last decade were conducted using different methodologies, and therefore producing different results. Here we review those studies, summarize their data and discuss the significance of results.

15.2 Methods

Medline was searched in February 2007 using "acupuncture" and "resonance" as keywords, with limits to English language and Clinical Trials. The search results in 22 publications. Additional search efforts using "acupuncture" and "resonance" in the titles and abstracts, or "acupuncture," "resonance" or "MRI" as medline subject heading, yielded no additional publications. Those not published in medical journals, unrelated to fMRI or describing non-needling technique (e.g. laser acupuncture) were then excluded, resulting in the nine publications that were extracted and analyzed for this review.

15.3 Results

The target studies were categorized by year of publication, study population, sample size, acupuncture points tested, key neural areas of activation or deactivation, and whether clinical responses were measured. The results are summarized in Table 15.1. The five representative papers are described below.

In an early study by Wu *et al.* reported in 1999, two groups of nine healthy volunteers were subjected to four stimulation paradigms: Real acupuncture at acupoints ST 36 and LI 4 and control stimulations (minimal acupuncture and superficial pricking on the leg). Stimulations were performed in semi-randomized, balanced order nested within two experiments. Imaging data were averaged for a group analysis. Acupuncture at LI 4 and ST 36 resulted in activation of the hypothalamus and nucleus accumbens and deactivation of the rostral part of the anterior cingulate cortex, amygdala formation, and hippocampal complex. Control stimulations, such as simple skin stimulation by needle pricking, failed to elicit such activations and deactivations. Instead, activation of the sensory cortices was observed. This study demonstrated for the first time specific

Table 15.1. Summary of fMRI studies of acupuncture.

First author	Sample size	Acupuncture point	Activated area	Deactivated area
Li *et al.* (2006a)	n = 24	LI 4, LI 11	Somatosensory cortex (greater activation in stroke patients)	
Li *et al.* (2006b)	n = 9	LI 4	Bilateral middle frontal gyri, secondary somatosensory cortex, middle temporal gyri, occipital lobe, anterior cingulate cortex, insula, and cerebellum (posterior lobe); right superior parietal lobule	Bilateral medial frontal gyri and occipital lobe, right precentral gyrus, precuneus, and pons; left superior frontal gyrus, temporal pole, parahippocampus, ACC, and midbrain
Hui *et al.* (2005)	n = 15	ST 36	Mixed in limbic and paralimbic structures in telencphalon, diencephalon, brainstem and cerebellum. During tactile stimulation	Limbic and paralimbic structures in telencephalon, diencephalon, brainstem and cerebellum
Jeun *et al.* (2005)	n = 10	GB 34	Bilateral sensorimotor areas	

Table 15.1. (*Continued*)

First author	Sample size	Acupuncture point	Activated area	Deactivated area
Fang *et al.* (2004)	n = 15	Liv 3, G40, sham point (rotating versus non-rotating needle stimulation)	Secondary somatosensory cortical areas, secondary frontal areas, thalamus (right side), cerebellum (right side)	
Zhang *et al.* (2003)	n = 48	ST 36, SP 6 (2 versus 100 Hz electrical stimulation)	Secondary somatosensory area and insula, contralateral anterior cingulate cortex and thalamus	Hippocampus, contralateral amygdala
Li *et al.* (2003)	n = 18	BL60, BL65, BL66, BL67 (electroacupuncture versus traditional acupuncture versus visual stimulation)	Visual cortex	Bilateral occipital lobes, temporal gyri, frontal gyri
Kong *et al.* (2002)	n = 11	LI 4 (electroacupuncture versus manual acupuncture)	Electroacupuncture: precentral gyrus, postcentral gyrus/inferior perital lobule and putamen/insula	Manual acupuncture: posterior cingulate, superior central gyrus putamen/ insula
Wu *et al.* (1999)	n = 9	ST36, LI 4 (traditional acupuncture versus needle prick and "minimal acupuncture")	Hypothalamus, nucleus accumbens	Rostral anterior cingulate cortx, amygdala, hippocampus

neuronal substrates that are activated and deactivated with acupuncture. Acupuncture at ST 36 and LI 4 was found to activate structures of the descending antinociceptive pathway and deactivate pain-related areas of the limbic system. Such changes appeared specific to the unique way acupuncture needles were manipulated, as simple stimulation of the skin by needle pricking was not associated with these changes Wu *et al.*, 1999).

Kong *et al.* compared manual and electroacupuncture stimulation of LI4 in an fMRI study of 11 healthy volunteers. The needle was inserted to a depth of 1 cm. Either low frequency (3 Hz) electrical pulses was delivered or the needle was rotated manually back and forth at about 3 Hz (180 times/minute). The order of the stimulations was randomized. Electroacupuncture mainly produced fMRI signal increases in precentral gyrus, postcentral gyrus/inferior parietal lobule, and putamen/insula; in contrast, manual needle manipulation produced prominent decreases of fMRI signals in posterior cingulate, superior temporal gyrus, and putamen/insula. This study shows that manual versus electrical stimulation of the same acupuncture point produces different neuroimaging changes (Kong *et al.*, 2002).

In a largest study reported to date (N = 48), Zhang *et al.* compared low frequency (2 Hz) versus high frequency (100 Hz) electrical acupuncture at ST 36 and SP 6 on the left leg of healthy volunteers. Both induced activation at bilateral secondary somatosensory area and insula, contralateral anterior cingulate cortex and thalamus. In the low frequency group, activation in contralateral primary motor area, supplementary motor area, and ipsilateral superior temporal gyrus were also observed, along with suppression in bilateral hippocampus. In the high frequency group, activation was observed in contralateral inferior parietal lobule, ipsilateral anterior cingulate cortex, nucleus accumbens, and pons, while suppression was detected in contralateral amygdala. Four subjects receiving "minimal electrical acupuncture" were included as controls. In these subjects, contralateral primary somatosensory area and bilateral secondary somatosensory area were activated. What is notable in this study is that the investigators measured the analgesic effect of acupuncture during the sessions and correlated clinical response to neuroimaging changes. They found that, in subjects demonstrating greater neuroimaging changes, acupuncture tended to produce a greater analgesic effect as well. The report suggests that electroacupuncture-induced analgesia with low and high frequencies seems to be mediated by different, though overlapped, brain networks (Zhang *et al.*, 2003).

Fang *et al.* tested different needle manipulation techniques — rotating stimulation versus non-rotating stimulation. Two real acupoints (LV3 and G40) and a sham point were stimulated in 15 healthy volunteers who were blinded to group assignment. When compared to the non-rotating stimulation method, rotating stimulation resulted in activation in both secondary somatosensory cortical areas, frontal areas, the right side of the thalamus and the left side of the cerebellum. Such differential effects were not seen when the sham point was needled (Fang *et al.*, 2004).

In clinical practice, the therapeutic effect of acupuncture is thought to be related to "deqi" (literally getting the "chi" — energy), a constellation of sensation such as pressure, fullness, soreness and/or heaviness experienced by the recipient. Hui *et al.* compared fMRI changes in healthy volunteers who experience deqi or simply sharp pain from needle manipulations. They found deactivation in the limbic and paralimbic structures of cortical and subcortical regions in the telencephalon, diencephalon, brainstem and cerebellum associated with deqi. In individual experiencing deqi mixed with sharp pain, signal in the cerebro-cerebellar and limbic systems exhibited a predominantly activation pattern. Simple tactile stimulation as control also induced mainly signal increases. The report is notable for its data on the correlation of deqi and functional neuroimaging changes (Hui *et al.*, 2005).

The above studies were done in healthy volunteers. Li *et al.* evaluated neuroimaging differences between stroke patients and healthy volunteer controls during acupuncture. Tactile stimuli (brushing the subject's palm and fingers with a rough sponge) and electroacupuncture LI 4 and LI 11 acupoint on the affected side of the body were performed in 12 clinically stable strok patients with left side somatosensory deficits and 12 control subjects. Both tactile stimuli and electroacupuncture induced greater activation in the somatosensory cortex. Activation appeared greater during the tactile stimulation in both patients and normal controls (Li *et al.*, 2006a).

15.4 Discussion

Acupuncture has been shown to elicit physiologic response in many clinical studies. However, the underlying mechanisms are not clearly understood. Non-invasive functional neuroimaging offers a powerful technique to evaluate the involvement of the central nervous system in acupuncture in humans. This field of research is still in its developmental stage with a limited number of published studies. Although many limitations and unanswered questions remain, some common themes emerge from existing data reviewed here.

Variability of data: No two studies found identical neural response patterns, even when the same acupuncture points were used. This inconsistency is likely attributable to even minor differences in acupuncture needle placement, variability in the way the needle is stimulated/manipulated, the exact fMRI paradigm used, the software used to process voxel data, and individualized subject response to needling. The fMRI technology itself is still evolving. Despite hundreds of publication and its great potential in neuroscience research, there are still disagreements concerning how fMRI data should be interpreted and the level of clinical significance of fMRI results (Matthews *et al.*, 2006).

The second common scheme is the involvement of somatosensory areas and the limbic system in acupuncture activation. Although the areas of activation and deactivation differ across studies, there is considerable overlap in areas involved in the detection and processing of sensory signals (Wu *et al.*, 1999; Kong *et al.*, 2002; Zhang *et al.*, 2003; Fang *et al.*, 2004; Hui *et al.*, 2005; Li *et al.*, 2006a; Jeun *et al.*, 2005). This is not surprising considering that acupuncture starts as a somatosensory stimulation by skin penetration. The limbic system is involved in secondary and tertiary processing of somatosensory signal. It may serve a bridge to link sensory stimuli to other parts of the CNS that leads to downstream responses in the afferent arm of the nervous system such as reduction of distress and avoidance, or reactions in the autonomic nervous system.

The third common theme is that how the needle is manipulated appears to induce different patterns of functional neuroimaging changes. Electroacupuncture versus manual stimulation, low frequency versus high frequency electrical stimulation, or rotating versus non-rotating manual stimulation of the needles are associated with both common and specific areas of activities (Kong *et al.*, 2002; Zhang *et al.*, 2003; Fang *et al.*, 2004). Studies attempting to distinguish true acupuncture stimulation with its "deqi" sensation from simple needle pricking showed that true acupuncture is associated with both deactivation of the limbic system and activation of the somatosensory area, whereas needle pricking is associated with only the later (Wu *et al.*, 1999; Hui *et al.*, 2005). This may explain the pleiotropic clinical reactions frequently observed in patients receiving acupuncture treatment.

One of the major hurdles of acupuncture is how to standardize the intervention to ensure valid comparison from one study to another. Acupuncture is a procedural intervention, akin more to a surgical intervention than a pharmacologic intervention. The human factor makes it difficult to completely eliminate variability among those who deliver the intervention and in recipients of the intervention. This is reflected in the fMRI studies that show non-identical areas of activation or deactivation, despite sharing common patterns of signal change. It is therefore important to have a critical mass of acupuncture fMRI data to enable emergence of a stronger consensus.

Another major limitation of fMRI acupuncture research is the interpretation of imaging data. Prior to functional imaging research, understanding of the neural substrates involved in acupuncture was limited at the molecular and cellular level, with imprecise and non-real-time anatomical localization. fMRI studies take us one step closer to identifying components modulated by acupuncture at the neuronal network level. They put changes induced by acupuncture in the larger perspective of how the nervous system functions. They show reactions more complex than simple reflex. This may be explained by concerted involvement of various parts of the CNS. On the other hand, pictures painted by fMRI studies are incomplete and may also be misleading. The organization of the CNS is such that many functional centers co-inhabit the same anatomic location. Most areas of activation and deactivation are not uniquely associated with a single neurological response. Data from fMRI studies reveal which parts of the brain are activated or deactivated by acupuncture, but there is no direct evidence that such activation or deactivation is responsible for the clinical response observed. Functional imaging research to date can establish only an association, but not a causal relationship. More sophisticated tasks and paradigms for fMRI will help move the field forward in that direction (Buracas and Boynton, 2002; Liu, 2004; Amaro and Barker, 2006).

In summary, fMRI technology opens a new field of acupuncture research. Studies conducted to date provide insight into how acupuncture render its physiologic effects, but considerable variability across studies makes interpretation unclear. Better study design and more data from many study groups will help realize the full potential of this powerful neuroscience research tool in the acupuncture treatment setting.

Acknowledgments

The authors wish to thank Carrie Trevisan for her assistance in the preparation of this manuscript.

References

Amaro, E., Jr. and Barker, G.J. (2006) Study design in fMRI: Basic principles. *Brain Cogn.* **60**(3), 220–232.

Buracas, G.T. and Boynton, G.M. (2002) Efficient design of event-related fMRI experiments using M-sequences. *Neuroimage* **16**(3 Pt. 1), 801–813.

Fang, J.L., Krings, T., Weidemann, J., Meister, I.G. and Thron, A. (2004) Functional MRI in healthy subjects during acupuncture: Different effects of needle rotation in real and false acupoints. *Neuroradiology* **46**(5), 359–362.

Han, J.S. (2004) Acupuncture and endorphins. *Neurosci. Lett.* **361**(1–3), 258–261.

Hui, K.K., Liu, J., Marina, O., *et al.* (2005) The integrated response of the human cerebro-cerebellar and limbic systems to acupuncture stimulation at ST 36 as evidenced by fMRI. *Neuroimage* **27**(3), 479–496.

Jeun, S.S., Kim, J.S., Kim, B.S., *et al.* (2005) Acupuncture stimulation for motor cortex activities: A 3T fMRI study. *Am. J. Chin. Med.* **33**(4), 573–578.

Kaptchuk, T.J. (2002) Acupuncture: Theory, efficacy, and practice. *Ann. Intern. Med.* **136**(5), 374–383.

Kong, J., Ma, L., Gollub, R.L., *et al.* (2002) A pilot study of functional magnetic resonance imaging of the brain during manual and electroacupuncture stimulation of acupuncture point (LI-4 Hegu) in normal subjects reveals differential brain activation between methods. *J. Altern. Complement. Med.* **8**(4), 411–419.

Li, G., Cheung, R.T., Ma, Q.Y. and Yang, E.S. (2003) Visual cortical activations on fMRI upon stimulation of the vision-implicated acupoints. *Neuroreport* **14**(5), 669–673.

Li, G., Jack, C.R., Jr. and Yang, E.S. (2006) An fMRI study of somatosensory-implicated acupuncture points in stable somatosensory stroke patients. *J. Magn. Reson. Imaging* **24**(5), 1018–1024.

Li, K., Shan, B., Xu, J., *et al.* (2006) Changes in FMRI in the human brain related to different durations of manual acupuncture needling. *J. Altern. Complement. Med.* **12**(7), 615–623.

Liu, T.T. (2004) Efficiency, power, and entropy in event-related fMRI with multiple trial types. Part II: Design of experiments. *Neuroimage* **21**(1), 401–413.

Matthews, P.M., Honey, G.D. and Bullmore, E.T. (2006) Applications of fMRI in translational medicine and clinical practice. *Nat. Rev. Neurosci.* **7**(9), 732–744.

Wu, M.T., Hsieh, J.C., Xiong, J., *et al.* (1999) Central nervous pathway for acupuncture stimulation: Localization of processing with functional MR imaging of the brain — preliminary experience. *Radiology* **212**(1), 133–141.

Zhang, W.T., Jin, Z., Cui, G.H., *et al.* (2003) Relations between brain network activation and analgesic effect induced by low versus high frequency electrical acupoint stimulation in different subjects: A functional magnetic resonance imaging study. *Brain Res.* **982**(2), 168–178.

Index

acupuncture 1–4, 9, 10, 14, 19, 20, 22, 23, 25–30, 166, 168–170, 348
adaptogen 260
adjuvant therapy 257
adriamycin 108
Aegle marmelos 96
alchemy rejuvenation 86
alcoholic liver disease 83
alpha-fetoprotein 93
alternative therapy 164
Amura rohitaka 94
amygdala 350, 353
Anacartin forte 93
Andrographis paniculata 88, 96
andrographolide 88
angiogenesis 11, 20, 21
Annona atemoya 88
anterior cingulate cortex 350, 353
anthracycline 108
anti-angiogenic 8, 13
anti-cancer herb 77
anticoagulant 24
anti-inflammatory 11, 15
antioxidant 129–131, 134–136
anti-tumor 7, 11, 16–20, 24, 273
apoptosis 4, 7, 8, 12, 18, 20, 21, 132, 134, 135, 236, 237, 242, 243
arbuda 78–80
Aristolochia 167
Arogyavardhini 95
Asparagus racemosus 259
autonomic nervous system 3, 4, 9, 25
autopoietic process 4
ayurveda 77, 87, 256
  anti-cancer drug 87
  drug 87, 94
  hepatoprotective formulation 94
  practitioner 97

Bacopa monnieir 96
beta-glucan 17, 18
biological response 1, 10
blood flow 12–14, 25, 26, 28
blood-oxygen-level dependent (BOLD) 348
body-mind 2, 3, 5, 9, 14, 20, 22, 23, 30
Boerhavia diffusa 89
Bonucci, Massimo 113, 114
breast cancer 321–324, 330, 331, 337
bullatacin 88

cancer 1–29, 31, 32, 65–67, 69–75, 77, 129–135, 141, 142, 145–147, 149, 150, 179–193, 201, 203, 204, 206, 233–235, 238, 239, 242–244, 247, 285–292
  definition 78
  prevention 20
  symptom relief 96
  treatment 55–57, 61
case study 97

causative factor 81
cell cycle 236, 238, 242, 243
cell proliferation 133, 134, 136
cerebellum 354
Charaka 78
chemoprevention 118
chemoprotection 264
chemotherapy 5, 7, 10–15, 21, 23–27, 94, 121, 122, 130, 136, 141, 145, 150, 164
cirrhosis 83
Citrullus lanthus 96
clinical trial 1, 5, 7–9, 14, 17, 18, 30, 32
Codetron™ 27, 29
colon cancer 111, 112
comfrey 167
complementary and alternative medicine (CAM) 129, 130, 233
complementary therapy 97, 164, 165, 167, 173
copper powder 94
curcumin 239–241, 244
cyclooxygenase-2 (COX-2) 240
cytochrome 129, 131, 140
cytochrome P450 (CYP) isoenzymes 245, 246
cytokine 9, 12, 14–16, 18, 25, 27
cytotoxic 6–8, 15, 16, 19

deqi 354
destagnation 13
Di Bella, Luigi 107, 109, 110
diagnosis 84
dosha 79
Draksnadi arkom 94
drug formulation 87
dynamical system 4

Eclipta alba 89, 96
efficacy assessment 302
emotion 2, 5, 21
energy 1, 4, 5, 12, 14, 30, 31
epidemiology 83
epigallocatechin gallate (EGCg) 236, 241, 242
Essiac 166
ethnopharmacology 258
evaluation 55, 57, 58, 63
extract 133, 135, 146

fatigue 23, 25, 27, 28, 31
Fu Zheng 14, 15
functional magnetic resonance imaging (fMRI) 29, 348, 357

G40 354
gene expression profiling 7
genistein 238, 239, 241, 245, 246
glucan 286, 287, 289
Glycyrrhiza glabra 94
Granthi 78, 80
Gudapippali 94

HBSAg 89
hepatitis 83
hepatocellular carcinoma (HCC) 77, 83, 87
  marker 89
hepatoprotective herb 78
Hepax 95
herb 1, 2, 5–8, 11–17, 19, 23–25, 30, 86, 179–183, 185, 190, 193–206
herbal formula decoction 301, 302, 305, 315–317
herbal supplement 166, 167
hippocampal complex 350
hippocampus 353
hormonal effect 19
hypnotherapy 168
hypoglycemia 93

immune homeostasis 276
immune stimulant 93

immune suppression 16, 18
immune system 5, 11, 15–18, 22, 129, 130, 132, 133, 140
immunity 2, 4, 14–18, 21–23, 31
immunosensitizer 18
immunotherapy 107, 111–113, 256, 287
inferior parietal lobule 353
integrative care 1
integrative medicine 173
interaction 129–132, 134, 140, 145, 147, 148, 150, 151
interferon-alpha 112
interleukin-2 112
intracellular signaling 20
irradiation 123
Italy 107–110, 112–115
    Bologna 107, 108, 112
    Modena 107, 109
    Monza 107, 110

Kamalahar forte 95
Kampo medicine 117, 118, 124, 125
kapha 80
Kava kava 167

LI 4 350
LI 11 354
limbic system 9, 354, 355
liposarcoma 107, 113
Lissoni, Paolo 107, 110, 111
Liv 52 96
liver
    description 82
    disorder 87
    fibrosis 92
    primary cancer 78
LSA-CM 113, 114
LV3 354
lymphocyte-activated killer (LAK) cell 112

Ma huang 167
mammary tumor 321, 322, 331, 334, 336
Mancini, Aldo 107, 113, 114
manganese super oxide dismutase (Mn-SOD-2) 107, 114
massage 171
    therapy 170
medicinal plant preparation 86
meditation 168
Mediterranean diet 115
melanoma 111
melatonin 107, 109, 111, 112
meridian 9, 10
metastasis 118, 124
microsome 93
mind-body technique 167
mood disorder 22
multi-drug resistance 12, 129–131, 135, 140, 141, 149
multitarget approach 257
music therapy 172
myofascial 9

National Institutes of Health (NIH) 97
natural killer (NK) cell 15, 17, 19
natural product 179–183, 193, 203–206
nausea 23–26
necrosis 91
neoplasm pathology 84
neuropeptide 3, 9, 21, 25
neurotransmitter 9
N-methyl-*N*-nitrosourea (MNU) 322, 323, 332–334, 337
non-small cell lung cancer 111, 301–303, 317
normal tissue 12, 14, 15
nucleus accumbens 353

oestrogen receptor 133, 134, 136

Office of Alternative Medicine (OAM) 97
ov valiliv 95

pain 22–24, 26, 27, 31
palliative care 124
pancha karma 86
pathogenesis 84
peptide 3, 12
P-glycoprotein (Pgp) 91, 243–245
phase I and phase II biotransformation enzyme 93
Phyllanthus amarus 89
Phyllanthus asperulatus 96
Phyllanthus niruri 89, 96
phytochemical 87, 233–235, 240, 241, 244–247
  profiling 5
Picroliv 90, 91
Picrorrhiza kurroa 90, 96
Piper longum 96
Pitta 80
Pizza, Giancarlo 107, 112
placebo 10, 21, 22, 27, 29
Plumbago zeylanica 96
podophyllotoxin 91
Podophyllum hexandrum 91
polysaccharide 285–292
pons 353
postcentral gyrus/inferior parietal lobule 353
posterior cingulate 353
precentral gyrus 353
primary motor area 353
psychoneuroimmunology (PNI) 2, 21
psycho-spiritual 1, 29, 30, 32
putamen/insula 353

qi 5, 12, 13, 23, 31
Qi Gong 166
quality of life 10, 21–23, 28, 29, 31, 32, 301, 302, 305–307, 315–317

radioprotection 271
radiotherapy 10, 13–15, 19, 23–25, 27, 28, 31, 94, 129–131, 136, 147, 149, 150
Rasayana 256, 259
rating scale 301, 302
receptor tyrosine kinase (RTK) 241
recommended research design 97
recurrence 118, 124
reflexology 171
Reiki 166
renal-cell carcinoma 112
research 97

Semecarpus anacardium 92–94
shark cartilage 166
Shiatsu 171
side effect 5, 12, 22–26, 28, 31, 130, 131, 133
somatosensory area 353–355
somatostatin 107, 109
SP 6 353
Sphaeramthus indicus 96
ST 36 350
St. John's Wort 167
stagnation 12
stroke 354
superior temporal gyrus 353
supplementary motor area 353
supportive care 1, 10, 23, 32
Sushruta Samhita 78
Swedish massage 171
symptom control 1, 10, 22, 25, 164

Tai Chi 171, 172
Tephrosia purpurea 96
Th1-Th2 balance 276
thalamus 353
therapeutic
  gain 10, 12, 14
  touch 171

Tibetan yoga 168
Tinospora cordifolia 92, 259
toll-like receptor (TLR) 17, 18, 287, 288
toxicity 146
traditional Chinese medicine (TCM) 1, 2, 3, 5, 10–14, 20–24, 29, 32, 55–64, 65, 71, 166, 285, 286, 288, 290–292, 321–324, 336
traditional medical system 163
transgenic mice 321, 322, 331, 335, 336
treatment modality 85
Tui Na 166, 171
tumor response 11

vaccine 15–19
Vasagulu chyadi arkom 94
vasomotor symptom 29
Vata 80
viral hepatitis 90
viral hepatitis B 89
vomiting 23, 25, 26
VP-16 91

Withania somnifera 259

xerostomia 23, 28, 29

Yakrit 82
Yakrut 82